PEDIATRIC DERMOSCOPY, TRICHOSCOPY AND ONYCHOSCOPY

PEDIATRIC DERMOSCOPY, TRICHOSCOPY AND ONYCHOSCOPY

Editor-in-Chief

Subrata Malakar
MD (Dermatology) DCH
Director
Rita Skin Foundation
Kolkata, West Bengal, India

Associate Editors

Surit Malakar
MD
Consultant Dermatologist
Rita Skin Foundation
Kolkata, West Bengal, India

Harshal Ranglani
MD DNB MRCP SCE
Consultant Dermatologist
Rita Skin Foundation
Kolkata, West Bengal, India

Assistant Editors

Seujee Das
MD
Resident Physician
Department of Dermatology
Gauhati Medical College and Hospital
Guwahati, Assam, India

Rashmi Agarwal
MD FRGUHS (Pediatric Dermatology)
Junior Pediatric Consultant
Cutis Academy of Cutaneous Sciences
Bengaluru, Karnataka, India

Foreword

Antonella Tosti

JAYPEE

JAYPEE BROTHERS MEDICAL PUBLISHERS

The Health Sciences Publisher

New Delhi | London

Jaypee Brothers Medical Publishers (P) Ltd.

Headquarters
Jaypee Brothers Medical Publishers (P) Ltd
EMCA House, 23/23-B, Ansari Road, Daryaganj
New Delhi 110 002, India
Landline: +91-11-23272143, +91-11-23272703
+91-11-23282021, +91-11-23245672
Email: jaypee@jaypeebrothers.com

Corporate Office
Jaypee Brothers Medical Publishers (P) Ltd
4838/24, Ansari Road, Daryaganj
New Delhi 110 002, India
Phone: +91-11-43574357
Fax: +91-11-43574314
Email: jaypee@jaypeebrothers.com

Overseas Office
J.P. Medical Ltd
83 Victoria Street, London
SW1H 0HW (UK)
Phone: +44 20 3170 8910
Fax: +44 (0)20 3008 6180
Email: info@jpmedpub.com

Website: www.jaypeebrothers.com
Website: www.jaypeedigital.com

Pediatric Dermoscopy, Trichoscopy and Onychoscopy

First Edition: **2022**

ISBN: 978-93-89188-28-8

Printed at Replika Press Pvt. Ltd.

Dedicated to

My late wife Dr Rita Shah Malakar

Contributors

Antonella Tosti MD
Fredric Brandt Endowed Professor of Dermatology
Dr Phillip Frost Department of Dermatology
and Cutaneous Surgery
University of Miami Miller School of Medicine
Miami, Florida, USA

Bikash Ranjan Kar MD
Professor and Head
Department of Dermatology
Institute of Medical Sciences and
SUM Hospital
Bhubaneswar, Odisha, India

Chander Grover MD DNB MNAMS
Professor
Department of Dermatology and STD
University College of Medical Sciences and
Guru Teg Bahadur Hospital
New Delhi, India

Deepak Jakhar MD
Department of Dermatology
NDMC Medical College and Hindu Rao Hospital
New Delhi, India

Gabriella Fabbrocini MD
Section of Dermatology
Department of Clinical Medicine and Surgery
University of Naples Federico II
Naples, Italy

Harshal Ranglani MD DNB MRCP SCE
Consultant Dermatologist
Rita Skin Foundation
Kolkata, West Bengal, India

Liane Zwetzich BS
Affiliated with Herbert Wertheim
Medical School Florida
International University
Section of Dermatology
Department of Clinical Medicine and Surgery
University of Naples Federico II
Naples, Italy

Madhuchhanda Mohapatra MD
Senior Resident
Department of Dermatology
Institute of Medical Sciences and
SUM Hospital
Bhubaneswar, Odisha, India

Maria Carmela Annunziata MD
Section of Dermatology
Department of Clinical Medicine and Surgery
University of Naples Federico II
Naples, Italy

Mariateresa Cantelli MD
Section of Dermatology
Department of Clinical Medicine and Surgery
University of Naples Federico II
Naples, Italy

Purva Mehta DNB
Consultant Dermatologist
Nucleus Eye and Skin Clinic
Mumbai, Maharashtra, India

Rashmi Agarwal MD FRGUHS (Pediatric Dermatology)
Junior Pediatric Consultant
Cutis Academy of Cutaneous Sciences
Bengaluru, Karnataka, India

Seujee Das MD
Resident Physician
Department of Dermatology
Gauhati Medical College and Hospital
Guwahati, Assam, India

Subrata Malakar MD (Dermatology) DCH
Director
Rita Skin Foundation
Kolkata, West Bengal, India

Surit Malakar MD
Consultant Dermatologist
Rita Skin Foundation
Kolkata, West Bengal, India

Foreword

It is a real pleasure to present this new book from a very special doctor!

I had the honor to receive the Trichology book as a present from Professor Subrata Malakar, 3 years ago and I was really impressed: a very beautiful book, everything more than perfect, with pictures of the best possible quality. I know how much work is necessary to write a good book and I admire his capacity of pursuing in this task. His dermoscopy book was another example of perfection and now this book on *Pediatric Dermoscopy, Trichoscopy and Onychoscopy* completes the series. I am honored to have contributed with a chapter to this book specifically dedicated to all aspect of dermoscopy in children, the first ever published book of this kind.

No doubts, it will be a bestseller and I am sure that most dermatologists and pediatricians will have it on their desk.

Antonella Tosti MD
Fredric Brandt Endowed Professor of Dermatology
Dr Phillip Frost Department of Dermatology
and Cutaneous Surgery
University of Miami Miller School of Medicine
Miami, Florida, USA

Preface

When my book "*Trichoscopy: A Text and Atlas*" was published in 2017, a very few dermatologists in India were trained to utilize dermoscope for the diagnosis and evaluation of trichological and dermatological disorders. In 2018, when I published my next book "*Dermoscopy: Text and Atlas*", things were changing because of more and more published articles in the major journals and the subject was gaining importance in most of the conferences; conferences dedicated only to dermoscopy and trichoscopy were also successful to attract dermatologists in India and some other countries. As this novel technique is becoming popular in India and across the world and it became a passion for me, I wrote this book "*Pediatric Dermoscopy, Trichoscopy and Onychoscopy*" entirely devoted to pediatric population. As dermoscopy is noninvasive and the findings are almost instant, it is very suitable for use in pediatric patients in whom invasive diagnostic procedures are truly difficult to carry out.

I spent more than 5 hours a day for last 3 to 4 years working on dermoscopy and trichoscopy. Thanks to my son, Dr Surit Malakar and some dedicated and talented junior colleagues such as Dr Purva Mehta, Dr Sushrut Save, Dr Samipa Mukherjee, Dr Harshal Ranglani, Dr Seujee Das, and Dr Rashmi Agarwal for constantly supporting me.

I am sure readers of this book will get their own findings and discoveries. I encourage all the dermatologists to share their findings and experiences with others in this developing field of diagnosis.

Keeping in mind that *we find only what we look for*, I wish all of you the very best to discover more and more in dermoscopy, trichoscopy, and onychoscopy in pediatric populations.

Subrata Malakar

Acknowledgments

We would like to acknowledge our patients who have inspired us to work on this project.

We acknowledge the support of Dr Uday Khopkar, Dr Uttam Banerjee, Dr Pratibha Pradhan, Dr Subal Chandra Mondal, Dr Vaswatee Madhab, Dr Sarina Jain, Dr Milan Kumar Ghosh who have been instrumental in the formation of the book.

We appreciate the efforts of Mr Suman Das for his technical assistance.

We are especially thankful to Shri Jitendar P Vij (Group Chairman), Mr Ankit Vij (Managing Director), Mr MS Mani (Group President), Ms Chetna Malhotra Vohra (Associate Director—Content Strategy), Ms Pooja Bhandari (Production Head), Dr Rajul Jain (Development Editor) and Mr Sabyasachi Hazra (Commissioning Editor, Kolkata Branch) of M/s Jaypee Brothers Medical Publishers (P) Ltd, New Delhi, India, for giving the go-ahead at the very beginning and helping us in every way possible to bring out this book.

Contents

SECTION 3: TRICHOSCOPY

SECTION 4: ONYCHOSCOPY

SECTION 5: INTERESTING CASES AND DIFFERENTIALS

SECTION 1

Pediatric Dermoscopy

CHAPTERS

CHAPTER 1

Pediatric Dermoscopy: Introduction

Seujee Das, Rashmi Agarwal

Dermoscopy, considered as the dermatologist's stethoscope in recent times, is an ex vivo noninvasive method which enables us to look beyond what our naked eyes cannot perceive. It helps in examining the subsurface features of the skin and in appreciating the epidermal and superficial dermal features of a lesion at a greater magnitude by decreasing the scattering of light and increasing transillumination, either through polarized light or through usage of a linkage fluid. Therefore, it serves as an important diagnostic aid in the practice of dermatology.

There are three ways to perform dermoscopy:

1. Nonpolarized dermoscopy—requires direct contact with the skin surface in addition to a liquid interface (mineral oil or alcohol) placed between the dermoscope and the skin.
2. Polarized contact dermoscopy.
3. Polarized noncontact dermoscopy.

Polarized dermoscopy has the advantage of eliminating the reflected light from the skin surface by using cross-polarized filters, thus allowing the reflected light from deeper layers to reach the observer's retina, making visualization of structures below the stratum corneum possible.

A few extra minutes is what the dermoscope demands and henceforth the clinical examination stands complete. Apart from enhancing the subtle clinical features, the dermoscope gives an insight into the pigment network as well as the vascular pattern of the skin. Any alteration in them can be very well-detected through a dermoscope, thereby, contributing to the diagnosis. Dermoscopy improves the clinician's diagnostic accuracy and can help correctly classify numerous skin lesions based on the presence or absence of specific dermoscopic structures. Dermoscopy also helps in monitoring the response to treatment and in predicting the prognosis of a disease.

The wide array of colors that we see through a dermoscope actually corroborates to the histology of the normal or diseased skin. Pin-point white dots represent eccrine gland/hair follicles openings while white patches, white shiny structures denote fibrosis. Red color denotes cutaneous vessels and extravasated blood. Superficial cutaneous vessels that form hair pin loops and are perpendicular to the skin appear as dots and globules while the subpapillary plexus which is parallel to the skin appear as red linear structures. Black, light to dark brown, grey, and blue relate to melanin at different depths in the skin. Therefore, the color concept, the different size and shapes in which the colors are configured give rise to various patterns. A constellation of these features contribute to the dermoscopic diagnosis of various skin diseases. For example, the arrangement of red dots in a lesion can differentiate psoriasis from lichen planus and eczema, which actually corresponds to the morphology of different vascular arrangement histologically.

Even the inflammatory infiltrate gives rise to different colors. Orange-yellow background or structures on dermoscopy points toward a granulomatous infiltrate while a violaceous hue usually corresponds to a lichenoid infiltrate.

The pediatric population constitutes a special population in our society with very specific needs. The practice of pediatric dermatology differs greatly from general dermatology since the challenges faced are diverse ranging from inability of the child to correctly specify their problems to handling them in a hospital setup. Handling parental queries and anxieties also form one of the corner stones of pediatric practice. As dermoscopy is a noninvasive and painless tool, it is very well accepted by children and their parents. The ease with which it can be handled and the minimum time required for examination of lesions under a dermoscope, makes it an ideal tool for examining pediatric skin lesions in day-to-day practice. Dermoscopy definitely contributes to the overall satisfaction of the parents as it imparts the idea in their mind that a proper thorough examination of their child has been carried out and this in turn improves the doctor-patient relationship as well as compliance.

It is very difficult to perform biopsies in a child because of their low-pain threshold and is often very restless. Moreover, even the parents are hesitant to let their child undergo such invasive procedures. Therefore, it is always better to avoid such procedures in a child and this is where dermoscopy come into play.

Hair disorder in children is very common and raises substantial amount of concern in the parents as well as children. The most common sign is alopecia and can be either due to congenital or acquired causes and the pathology can involve either the hair itself or the scalp skin. Trichoscopy is considered to be as reliable as microscopy in the detection of most hair shaft diseases and thus assist in the diagnosis of multiple genetic disorders, such as trichorrhexis invaginata, trichorrhexis nodosa, monilethrix, pili torti, and pili annulati. Prompt diagnosis of these features with the help of dermoscopy can give the clinician an insight into a broader syndrome, for example, the presence of trichorrhexis invaginata points toward the diagnosis of Netherton syndrome. Presence of corkscrew and comma hair, exclamation mark hair, flame hairs, and carpet of vellus hair can point toward the diagnosis of tinea capitis, alopecia areata, trichotillomania, and congenital triangular alopecia, respectively, in cases of patchy hair loss. Trichoscopy is a practical, painless, and tolerable method for examining various hair disorders, obviating the need for plucking or cutting the hair for microscopic examination.

Many dermatological diseases involve the nails in children. Dermoscopy of the nail, i.e., onychoscopy, helps in differentiating onychomycosis from nail psoriasis and nail lichen planus. Visualization of the nail fold capillaries helps in the diagnosis and prognostication of various connective tissue diseases in children.

Dermoscopy is indeed a revelation in the practice of pediatric dermatology. With the ever increasing horizons of dermoscopy literature we are soon progressing to a stage where many skin conditions can be diagnosed with a dermoscope, thus obviating the need for histopathological examination and making it an indispensable tool in our daily practice.

CHAPTER 2

Instrument

Bikash Ranjan Kar, Madhuchhanda Mohapatra

DERMOSCOPE

INTRODUCTION

Rightly called as a dermatologist's stethoscope, a dermatoscope (a.k.a. dermoscope, skin surface microscope, epiluminescence microscope, episcope) is a noninvasive device which helps in visualization of the minute clinical details of not only the lesions on surface of the skin but also of the subsurface structures up to the superficial dermis. Basically dermoscope is a handheld microscope along with a magnification lens and an inbuilt illumination system.

ADVANTAGES OF DERMOSCOPE OVER A SIMPLE MAGNIFICATION LENS

Now, it is essential that a dermoscope should not be viewed as any other magnification device. Although the fundamental function of a dermoscope is magnification, it has several additional features:

- Self-built illumination system
- Image capturing and recording ability
- Allowing visualization of deeper dermal structures
- Analytical capacity (for follow-up of melanoma especially in western countries, e.g., DermoGenius MoleMap and FotoFinder dermoscope).

BASIC MODEL OF A DERMOSCOPE

The following integral components are assembled into a dermoscope:[1]

- *Achromatic lens*: The basic purpose of a lens is magnification. Majority of the dermoscope models provide magnification in the range of 10–20×. But higher magnification up to 1000× for better results can be attained with special lenses in modern videodermoscopes.
- *Inbuilt illuminating system*: Currently, light-emitting diodes (LEDs) are the standard sources of light providing high-intensity white light with less power consumption than the traditionally used halogen lamps. The illumination and the color (hence the wavelength) of light can be controlled which in turn determines the depth of penetration into the skin by the incident light. Structures under the surface of skin are made visible by the use of polarized light sources.
- *Power source*: Batteries like rechargeable battery (DermLite MSO), AA battery (mini 2000 dermoscope), lithium ion battery (DermLite DL1000), and rechargeable handles (DELTA 200) power the device.
- *Display system*: This can be the dermoscope itself (handheld dermoscopes) having a see-through viewing window, or having the ability to be connected to mobiles and using mobile screen as display, or the videodermoscopes that can be connected to the computer or other devices with their own display screen.
- *Inbuilt image capturing system*: Dermoscopes can be grouped on the basis of this feature as:[2]
  - Instruments without image capturing facility, e.g., dermatoscope

- Instruments with image capturing facility, e.g., Dermaphot
- Instruments with image capturing facility and analytical capability, e.g., DermoGenius Molemap.

Devices without image capturing facility: In these models, an adapter can be used for attaching cameras to some of these devices. Some examples of this type of dermoscope are DermoGenius Basic, DermaliteMSO, DELTA 10, and Mini 2000 Dermatoscope.

Devices with image capturing facility: Dermoscopes under this category have either an inbuilt image recording system or an attached camera. An apparatus like Mole Max I is also capable of whole body photography (body mapping). Video dermatoscopes (Video dermoscope, Videocap100) come under this category that can record small videos in addition to high resolution pictures, which can be seen on the computer screen. Delta20, Dermaphot, DermLite Foto, etc., are some of the models of this type.

Dermoscopes with image capturing facility and analytical capability: These devices have the additional feature of interpreting the images taken and are mostly used for follow-up of melanoma in western countries. New images of the patient are compared with the recorded ones and different color signals are generated in case of any significant change. Similarly, the benignness of a melanocytic nevus is decided by an artificial neural network mechanism. Some examples of this type are DermoGenius MoleMap, Fotofinder dermoscope, etc.

OPTICS IN DERMOSCOPY[3,4]

Optical Properties of Light without the Use of Dermoscopy

Any light ray incident on the skin undergoes reflection, refraction, diffraction, and absorption governed by the optical properties of two different media—skin and air. Refractive index of skin is 1.55 which is higher than that of air 1.00. Whenever light travels from skin to air, it follows Snell's law of refraction which states that when light travels from a denser medium (higher refractive index) to a lighter medium (lower refractive index) it speeds up and bends away from the normal **(Fig. 1)**.

Hence, most of the incident light reflected back from the stratum corneum known as *Surface glare* blinds the retina and prevents the observer from visualizing the light reflected from the deeper layers of skin.

Optical Properties of Light with Dermoscopy

There are two types of dermoscopy:[5]

1. Nonpolarized
2. Polarized.

Nonpolarized Dermoscopy

These dermoscopes require a liquid interface with refractive index equal to or closely matching that of the skin. The use of a liquid interface converts the skin-air interface to skin-liquid-glass (of the dermoscope) interface. Since the refractive indices of glass (1.52) and the liquid medium are almost similar to that of skin (1.55), the incident light reflected back from the surface of the skin undergoes minimal reflection and the observer is able to visualize the epidermis. Nonpolarized dermoscopy (NPD) can visualize

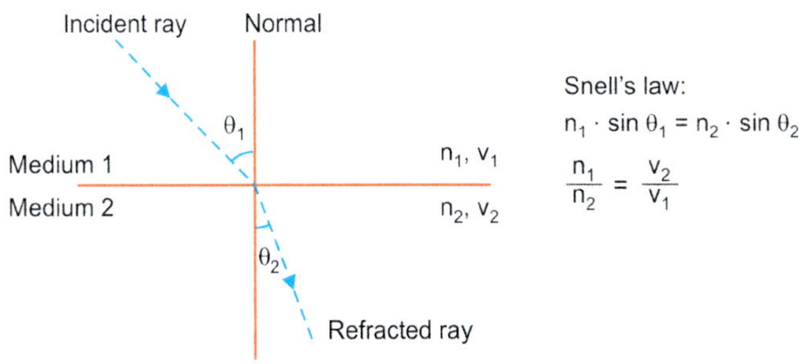

Fig. 1: Snell's law.

structures up to the dermoepidermal junction. This is because incident light ray penetrating the superficial layers of skin [up to the dermal-epidermal junction (DEJ)] undergoes minimal scattering but there occur multiple scattering events, decay of light and decrease in reflected back light with increase in depth of penetrating light.

Various immersion liquids that can be used are 70% alcohol, ultrasound gel, water, liquid paraffin, or mineral oil. One should be particular to avoid formation of air bubbles in between the skin-liquid-glass interface as this would create a skin-air interface which causes back-scatter of light and the visualization of structures below the stratum corneum is prevented. 70% alcohol and water cause fewer air bubbles but come with the drawback of rapid evaporation. Ultrasound gels are best suited for onychoscopy and periorbital areas. Mineral oils are better avoided because they are fetotoxic, carcinogenic, and teratogenic.[6] Multicoated silicone glass is used to manufacture the glass plates of dermoscope. Graduated scales are inscribed into the glass plates for measuring the lesion.

Polarized Dermoscopy

This type of dermoscopes uses two polarizers in orthogonal axes to achieve cross polarization. Light emitted from the polarized dermoscopy (PD) passes through the polarizer and becomes unidirectional (polarized) light. The reflected light must first pass through the second polarizer that is orthogonal (perpendicular) to the first. For this to happen, the original polarized light must undergo sufficient scattering events in the skin (randomization of polarization) that changes its direction by 90°.

Light reflected from the stratum corneum maintains its original polarization, cannot pass through the cross-polarized filter, hence PD is "blind" to surface glare.

Incident light penetrating the superficial layers of skin is not subjected to enough scattering events resulting in its direction change by 90° and pass through the cross-polarizer. Therefore, epidermal structures cannot be visualized with a PD.

Whereas the light penetrating deeply down the DEJ, through the superficial dermis encounters multiple scattering events leading to "randomization of polarization". Thus, reflected light from the deeper layers passes through the cross-polarized filter and enters observer's eyes permitting the visualization of structures below the DEJ up to the superficial dermis.

PDs do not need contact with skin or any immersion medium. This noncontact technique prevents nosocomial infections. Some PDs have the option of both noncontact and contact dermoscopy.

Difference between PD and NPD

Superficial structures (epidermis up to DEJ) are better seen in NPD whereas PD is better for visualizing deeper structures (DEJ to superficial dermis). Blood vessels and vascular blush are better seen with PD as blood vessels are located in deeper dermis, also due to the lack of pressure effect since PD uses noncontact technique.

Nonpolarized dermoscopy can specifically diagnose seborrheic keratosis by identifying milia-like cysts and comedo openings which are epidermal structures.[7]

Hybrid Demoscopes

Dermoscopes like DermLite DL 3N have PD and NPD modes which can be toggled by a switch. These devices improve dermoscopic diagnosis because one mode complements the other. These devices use contact technique with a liquid interface, or else dermoscopic features will be seen only in PD mode.

TYPES OF DERMOSCOPE[5]

There are two main types of dermatoscopes:

1. Handheld dermoscope
2. Video dermoscope.

Handheld Dermoscopes

These are portable, cheaper and easier to maintain but the major limitation that comes with these kinds of devices are their limited magnification, limited area of visualization at a time, and difficulty screening larger areas in a limited span of time.

The various handheld dermoscopes are:
- DermLite (3 gen)
- Delta 20 (Heine)
- Veos (Canfield).

DermLite Dermoscopes

DermLite line of dermoscopes are the often the first choice among dermatologists because of their portability, bright light source, good optics, and facility for being connected with mobile phones and tablets (iPhone, iPad, Samsung Galaxy). The latest DermLite dermoscope is DermLite DL4 among the many varieties of this line of dermoscopes. DL4 dermoscopes come with many advantages over the previous models like larger field of view, improved imaging of the deeper pigmentation, two levels of color spectrum control (PigmentBoost Plus), and all this in a smaller size. Along with this, they (DL4 dermoscopes) come with a unique facility for infection control with their Ice Cap (Infection Control and Epidemiology system) technology. These disposable caps can be attached with the spacer and greatly reduce the risk of contamination. Most of the dermoscopes of this series are hybrid with few only PD (DL 100, DL 200HR) models also available.

Heine Dermoscopes

Durability and high-resolution dermoscopic image capturing ability are the essential features of this series of devices. These sturdy dermoscopes are good option for academic institutions with multiple users. The dermoscopic images achieved with these devices are of high quality suitable for publication purpose. These devices are also hybrid and can be toggled between polarized and nonpolarized. But Heine dermoscopes need to be connected with a DSLR camera and adapter for DSLR for image capturing. Thus, even though the device is portable, it is impractical to carry the entire image capturing facility from one place to another.

Veos Dermoscopes

Veos dermoscopes are smart, flexible, and versatile. Veos HD1 is polarized and Veos HD2 is hybrid model. Both the devices come with an optional sleeve attachment for Iphone-enabling high-quality dermoscopic image capture and storage facility. Canfield has come up with whole body imaging systems like VECTRA WB 180 and VECTRA WB 360 which instantaneously capture the patient's skin surface and body shape of entire body in a single high-resolution 3D image. The Veos dermoscopes can be integrated with the DermaGraphix software, so that the dermoscopic images captured can be linked with their corresponding tagged lesions in the 3D body map. This has additional applications like the accurate body area assessment in case of psoriasis (PASI calculation), vitiligo, etc.

Video Dermoscopes

Video dermoscopes require a computer or any other screen for output of images and thus they provide options for recording of small videos. Video dermoscopes range from simple models with only NPD mode to complex models (marketed by DermaIndia TLS Ultracam) having multiple light sources (visible light, polarized light, and ultraviolet light). Ultraviolet light can be used as a Wood's lamp to differentiate pigmented lesions (e.g., vitiligo from other depigmented lesions). Video dermoscopes are very good for teaching purpose where exact structure can be shown to students.

Handheld Video Dermoscopes

These are small pocket-sized instruments having a screen like mobile to enable viewing of the dermoscopic images. These devices are inexpensive, high magnification, portable, do not need to be attached to a computer but have lower resolution. They also have an inbuilt camera for image capturing and storage **(Figs. 2 to 6)**.

CONCLUSION

In the current scenario, dermoscopes are like the bridge between clinical dermatology and dermatopathology. With increasing awareness about dermoscopy and development of specific dermoscopic signs, this noninvasive device has become an integral addition to the existing diagnostic armamentarium for dermatologists.

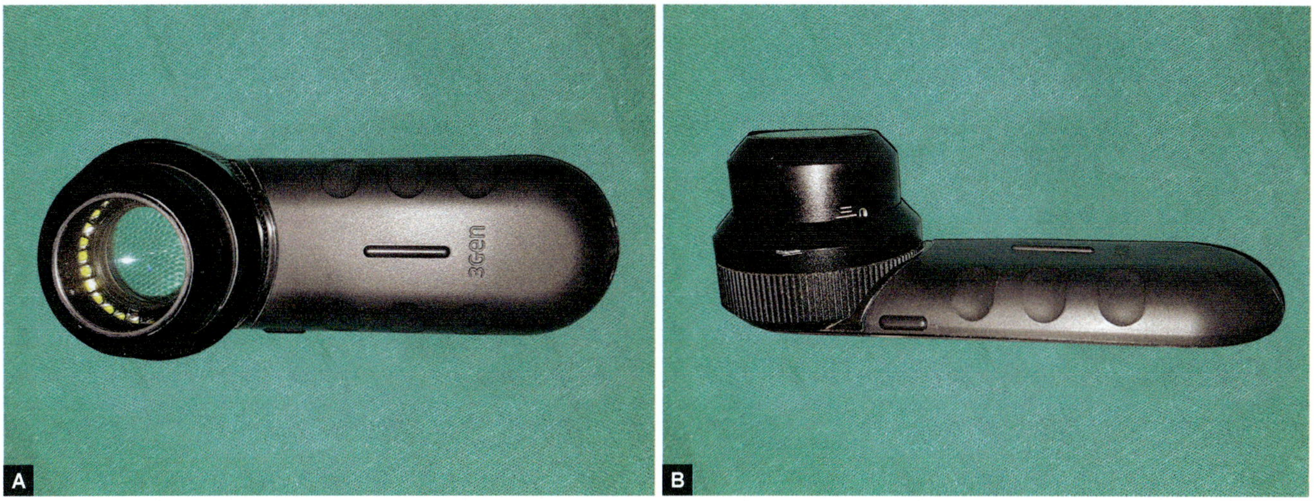

Figs. 2A and B: DermLite DL3.

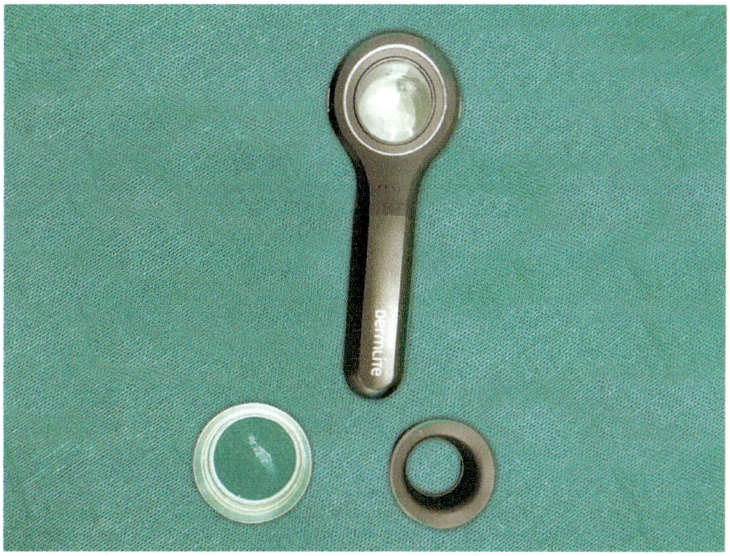

Fig. 3: DermLite DL4.

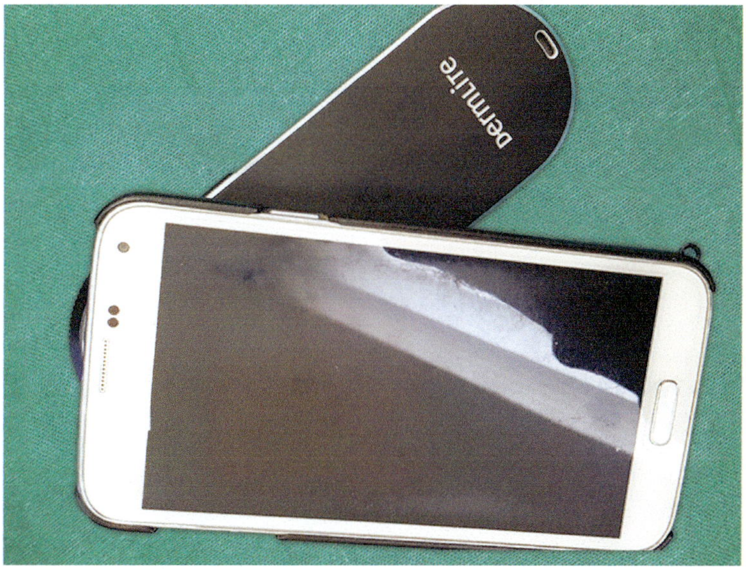

Fig. 4: DermLite with smart phone attachment.

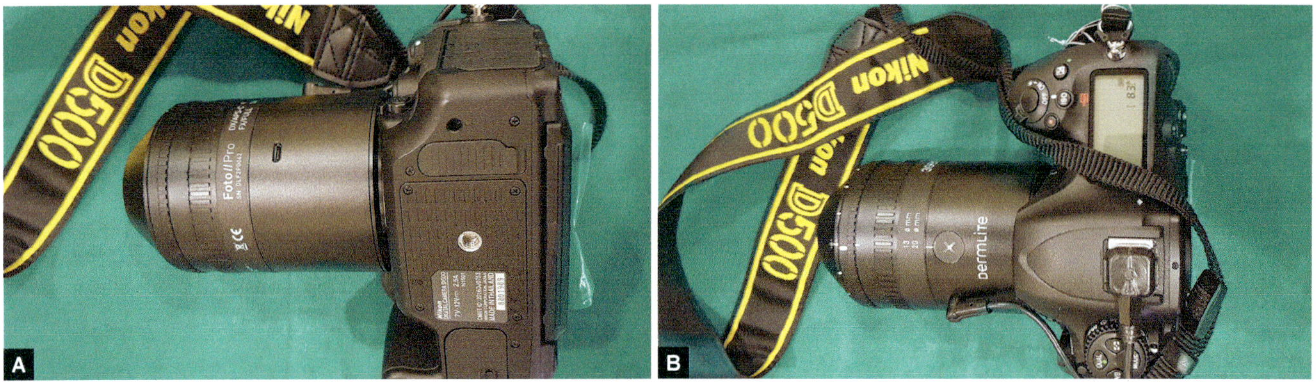

Figs. 5A and B: DermLite Photo II Pro.

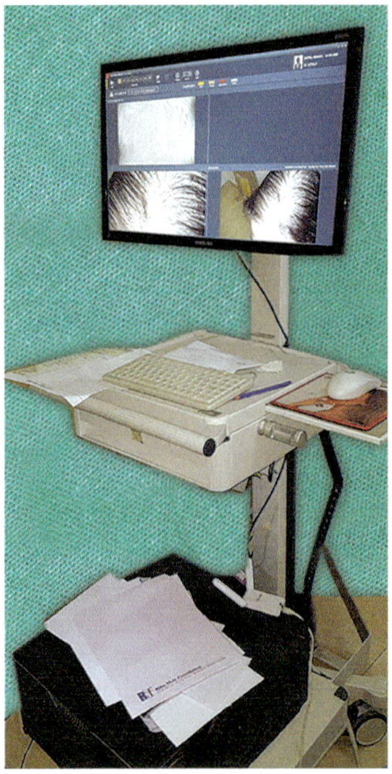

Fig. 6: Fotofinder.

REFERENCES

1. Nischal KC, Khopkar U. Principles and technique of dermoscopy and videodermoscopy. In: Khopkar U (Ed). Dermoscopy and Trichoscopy in Diseases of the Brown Skin: Atlas and Short Text, 1st edition. New Delhi: Jaypee Brothers Medical Publishers (P) Ltd; 2012. pp. 5-6.
2. Nischal KC, Khopkar U. Dermoscope. Indian J Dermatol Venereol Leprol. 2005;71:300-3.
3. Florentia D, Alon S. Principles of dermoscopy. [online] Available from: Dermoscopedia.org/Main_Page [Last accessed October, 2019].
4. Braun Ralph P. Dermoscopic equipment. [online] Available from: Dermoscopedia.org/Main_Page [Last accessed October, 2019].
5. Neema S, Chatterjee M. Types of dermoscope. In: Chatterjee M, Neema S, Malakar S (Eds). Dermoscopy in Darker Skin, 1st edition. New Delhi: Jaypee Brothers Medical Publishers (P) Ltd; 2017. pp. 7-11.
6. Vasudevan B, Neema S. Introduction to dermoscopy. In: Chatterjee M, Neema S, Malakar S (Eds). Dermoscopy in Darker Skin, 1st edition. New Delhi: Jaypee Brothers Medical Publishers (P) Ltd; 2017. pp. 3-6.
7. Benvenuto-Andrade C, Dsuza SW, Agero AL, et al. Differences between polarized light dermoscopy and immersion contact dermoscopy for the evaluation of skin lesions. Arch Dermatol. 2007;143:329-38.

SECTION 2

Dermoscopy

CHAPTERS

- Melanocytic Lesions
- Eczematous Eruptions in Childhood
- Papulosquamous
- Hereditary Disorders of Cornification
- Infections and Infestations
- Developmental Anomalies of the Newborn
- Genodermatoses
- Tumors
- Hypopigmented Lesions
- Vascular Lesions
- Connective Tissue Disorders
- Miscellaneous

CHAPTER 3

Melanocytic Lesions

Subrata Malakar

PEDIATRIC MELANOCYTIC LESIONS

INTRODUCTION

- Majority of pediatric melanocytic nevi (PMN) appear benign clinically but some of them may be confused with melanoma which may lead to unnecessary biopsies.
- Dermoscopic knowledge has been shown to increase the diagnostic accuracy and differentiation of PMN and melanoma.
- Dermoscopy is the ideal instrument to use during the evaluation of PMN/melanoma in children as it is painless and provides proper information for the clinician.
- Nevogenesis is a dynamic process in children and PMNs change with time where dermoscopy is a perfect instrument for evaluating these changing lesions.
- It is wise to note that melanomas in pediatric age commonly do not show the ABCD features [**A**symmetry, irregular **B**orders, uneven distribution of **C**olor, **D**iameter (greater than 6 mm)].
- Sometimes clinical appearance may not be alarming but dermoscopy may show some structures specific for melanoma such as atypical vascular structures and crystalline structures.

Congenital Melanocytic Nevi (CMN)

- They have a smooth surface, light to dark brown to black color, and their borders are well demarcated. They may darken or become lighter in color with time.
- Dermoscopic evaluation of CMN requires the knowledge of melanocytic network, and dots and globules. Presence of any one of them confirm that the lesion is melanocytic. The melanocytic or pigment network has two components, brown pigmented lines and the grids or holes among them. The brown pigmented lines correspond to rete ridge melanocytes and the holes can be correlated histologically with the suprapapillary basal epidermis.
- Dots and globules **(Fig. 1)** are well-circumscribed, round to oval aggregates which are nothing but nests of melanin-containing nevus cells. They reflect junctional nests of melanocytes and when seen at the periphery of a lesion they are considered as dynamic process of nevus evolution. Cobblestone **(Fig. 2)** is another type of globules with angulated borders and it reflects large dermal nests of melanocytes on histology.
- Dermoscopy of CMN not uncommonly may show other structures such as hypertrichosis **(Fig. 3)**, perifollicular pigment changes, milia-like cysts and comma vessels; serpentine and dotted vessels may also be seen rarely.
- Once the first step of the dermoscopic examination, i.e. categorization of the lesion is a melanocytic, is over, the next step is to determine the lesion has any of the benign dermoscopic patterns such as:
  1. Diffuse reticular **(Fig. 4)**—reticular network is present all throught the lesion. Observed in both congenital and acquired nevi.
  2. Patchy reticular—reticular network is patchy with homogeneous areas in between. Observed in both congenital and acquired nevi.

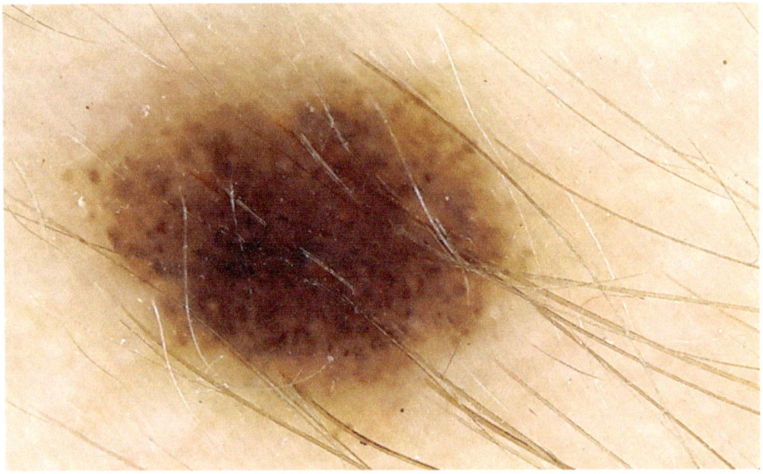

Fig. 1: Dots and globules.

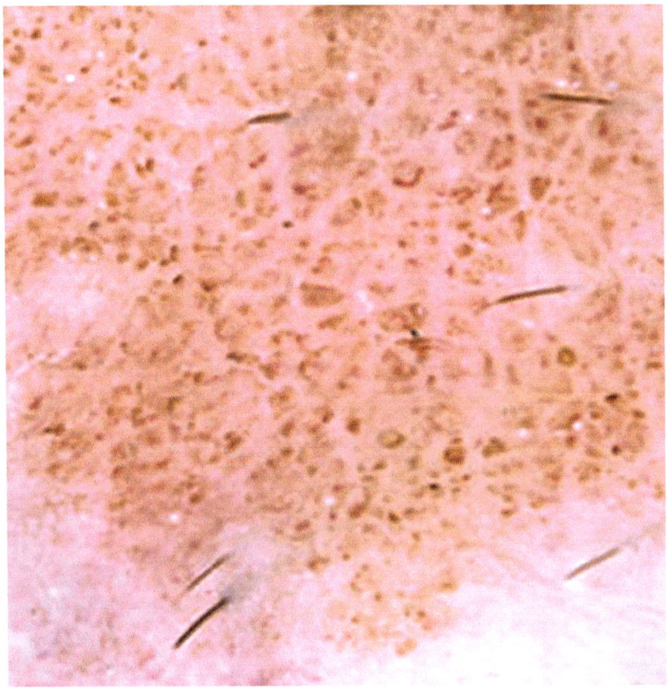

Fig. 2: Cobblestone.

3. Peripheral reticular with central hyperpigmentation **(Figs. 5 and 6)**—reticular network at the periphery with central homogeneous hyperpigmented area.
4. Peripheral reticular with central hypopigmentation—this is seen in acquired nevi mostly in darker skin.
5. Globular **(Fig. 7)**—found commonly in congenital nevi where dermoscopy shows brown to black globules of similar size, shape and color dispersed symmetrically throughout the lesion.
6. Central globular with peripheral reticular—seen commonly in congenital nevi.
7. Peripheral globular with central reticular—a ring of peripheral globules surrounds the entire reticular network which represents an acquired growing nevus.
8. Homogeneous brown **(Fig. 8)** or blue pigmentation **(Fig. 9)**—the entire nevus is totally structureless. Structureless brown is seen in congenital nevi whereas its blue component represent blue nevi.
9. Multicomponent—dermoscopy may show symmetrically distributed reticulation, dots and globules, blotches, veil, structureless areas and regression structures. At least three of them should be present to call it multicomponent.

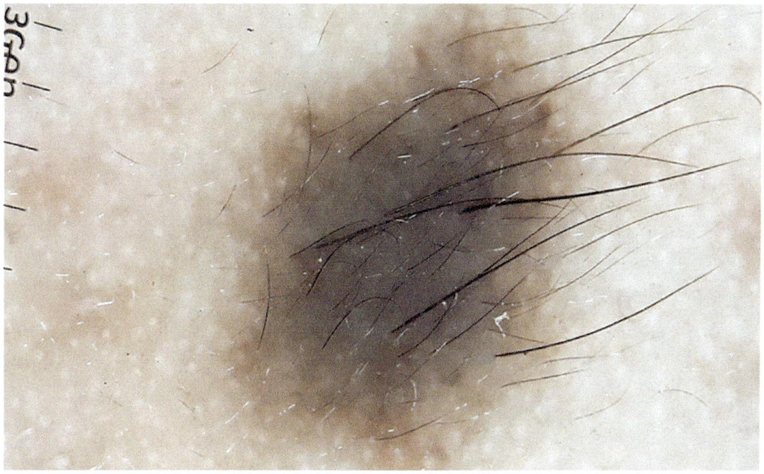

Fig. 3: Hypertrichosis associated with CMN.

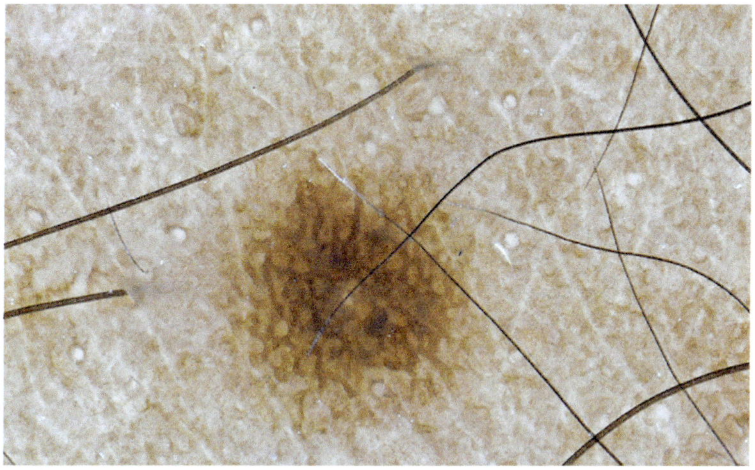

Fig. 4: Diffuse reticular.

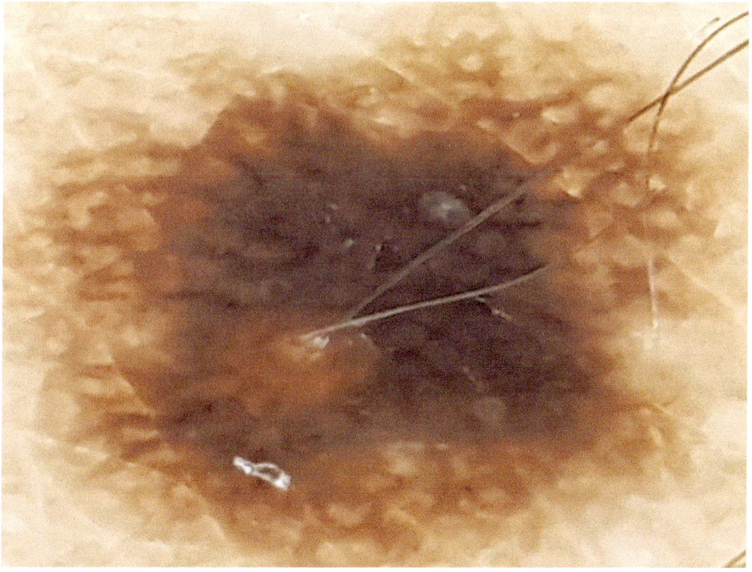

Fig. 5: Peripheral reticular with central hyperpigmentation.

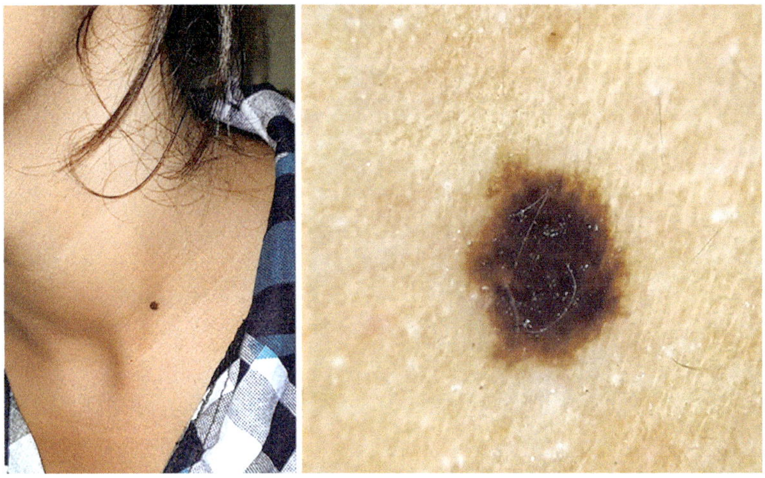

Fig. 6: Peripheral reticular with central hyperpigmentation.

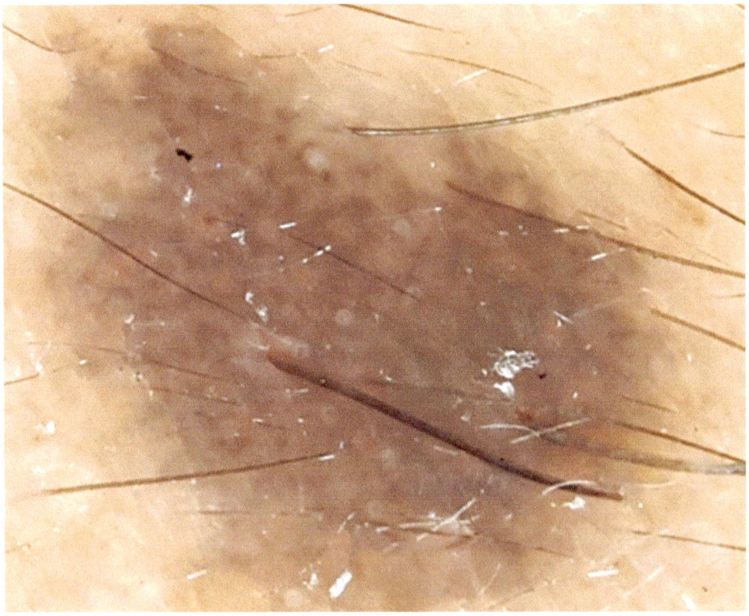

Fig. 7: Globular.

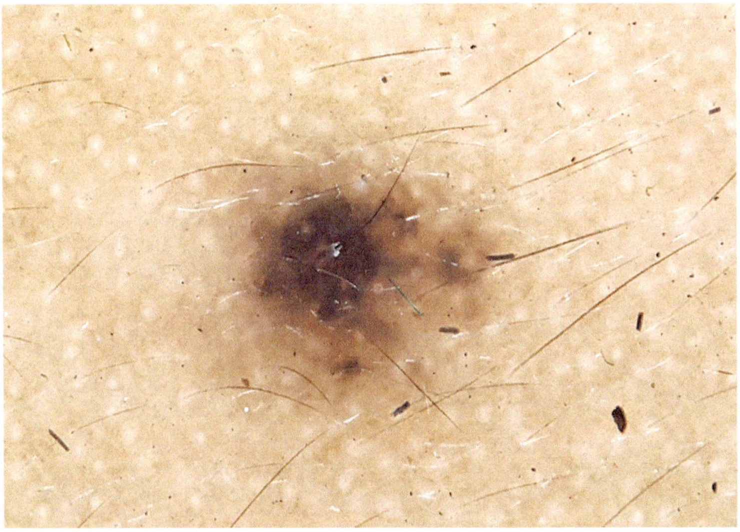

Fig. 8: Homogeneous brown.

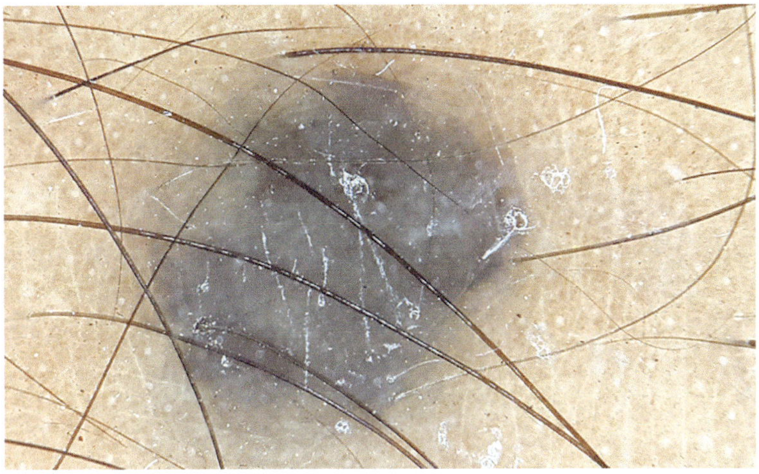

Fig. 9: Homogeneous blue pigmentation.

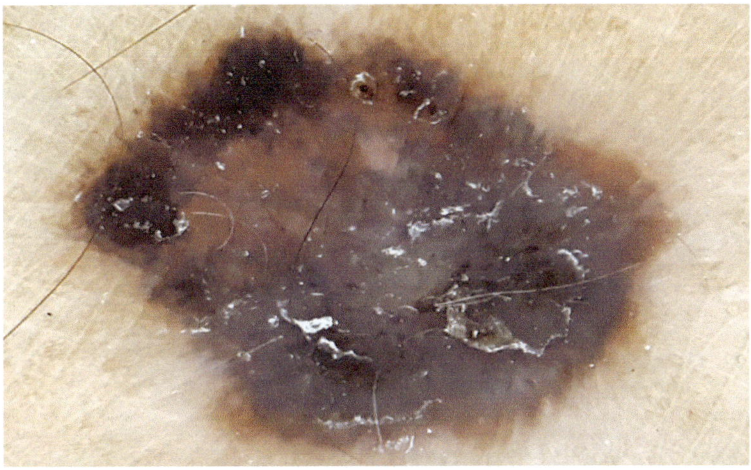

Fig. 10: Starburst pigmentation.

10. Two component—dermoscopy reveals two patterns in either half such as reticular-globular, globular-homogeneous, etc.
11. Starburst **(Fig. 10)**—it is a metaphor which reminds us of an exploding star which shows radial streaming or streaks surrounding the entire lesion.
12. Parallel **(Fig. 11)**—this pattern is often found in congenital nevi of pals and soles.

- Third step—if the dermoscopy shows none of the above benign patterns try to find out melanoma-specific dermoscopic structures such as:
  1. Atypical pigment network **(Fig. 12)**—dermoscopy reveals broadened, thickened and darkened lines of reticular network. Histological corroborates—proliferation of atypical nests of melanocytes.
  2. Atypical dots and globules **(Fig. 13)**—globules of varying size, shape and color which are not distributed symmetrically. Histological corroborates—junctional or dermal nests of melanocytes.
  3. Crystalline structures **(Fig. 14)**—polarized dermoscopy reveals shiny white lines oriented in an orthogonal manner. Histological corroborates—altered dermal collagen.
  4. Eccentric blotch—patch of diffuse pigmentation with sharp margins, irregular shapes or eccentric locations. Histological corroborates—melanin is present throught the epidermis and dermis.
  5. Eccentric streaks **(Fig. 15)**—pigmented projections located eccentrically. Histological corroborates: confluent junctional nests of melanoma cells at the periphery.
  6. Blue-white veil **(Fig. 16)**—bluish-white areas over a elevated portion of a lesion. Histological corroborates—compact orthokeratosis over melanophages in the papillary dermis.

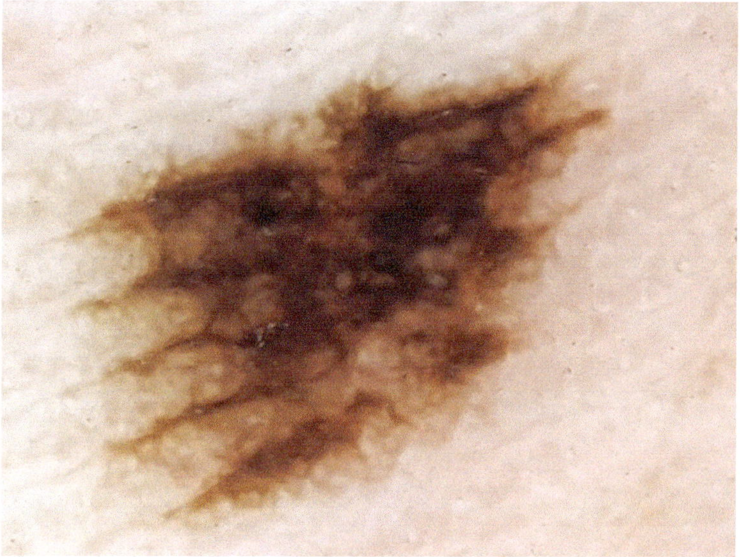

Fig. 11: Parallel pigmentation.

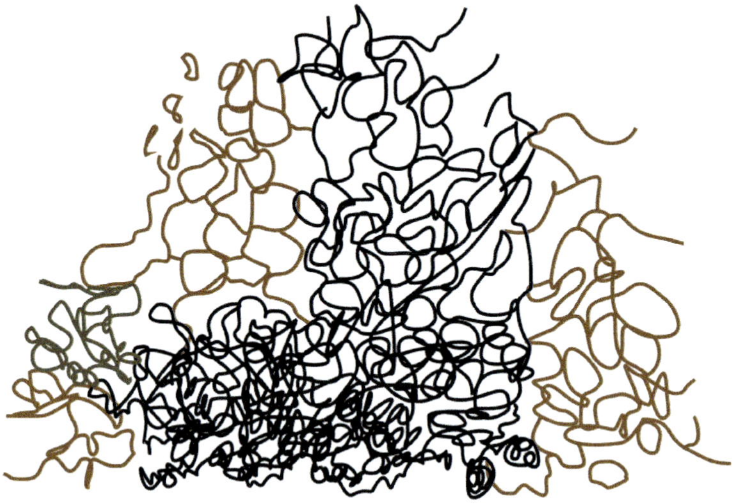

Fig. 12: Atypical pigment network.

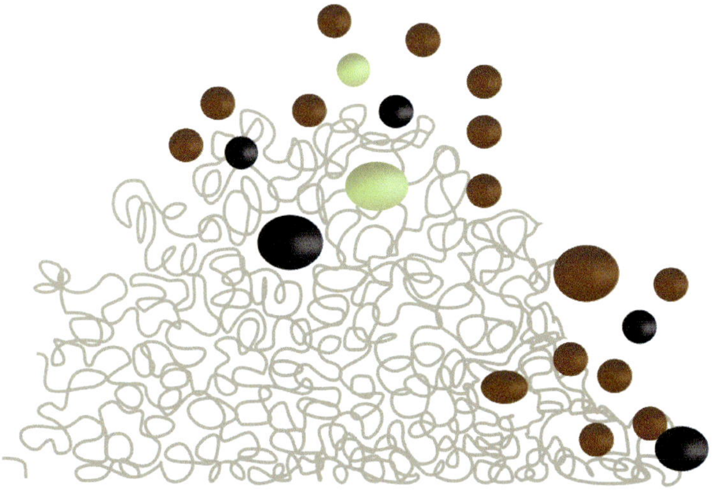

Fig. 13: Atypical dots and globules.

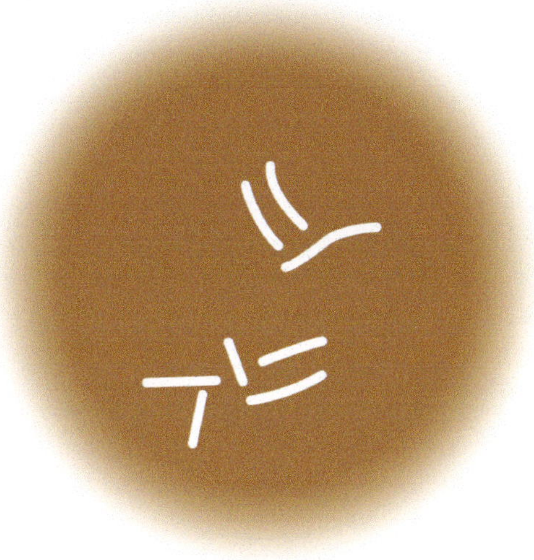

Fig. 14: Crystalline structures.

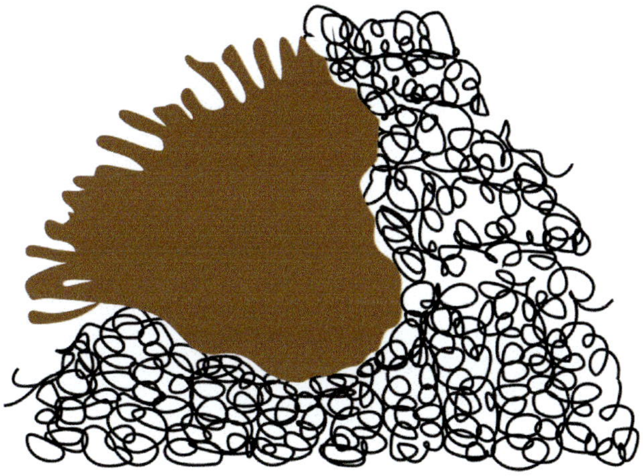

Fig. 15: Eccentric streaks.

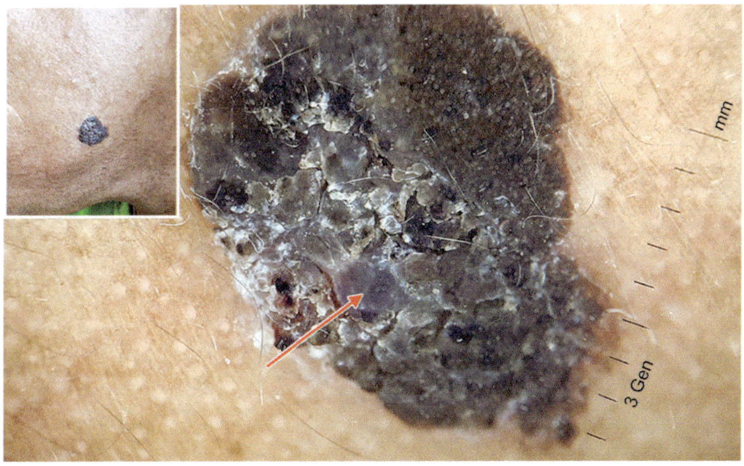

Fig. 16: Blue-white veil (red arrow).

7. Regression structures—white scar-like structures and or peppering over a flat portion of a lesion which appear as blue-white veil. Histological corroborates—melanosis and fibrosis in the papillary dermis.
8. Atypical vascular structures—dotted, linear irregular and twisted red vessels; sometimes milky red areas. Histological corroborates—neoangiogenesis induced by tumor.
9. Negative pigment network **(Fig. 17)**—dermoscopy shows the reverse of melanocytic network, i.e., the grid or holes are formed of dark areas and hypopigmented lines replace the brown lines. Histological corroborates—rete ridges are thin and elongated whereas papillary dermis is widened and contain tubular melanocytic nests.

- If dermoscopy shows any of the structures specific to melanoma then biopsy should be warranted. Lesions showing benign dermoscopic patterns do not need to be excised and can be monitored without risk. Hence, dermoscopy is a reliable tool to help differentiate smaller nevi from melanoma.

Acquired Melanocytic Nevi (AMN)

- They start appearing in early childhood and may gradually increase in numbers throughout adolescence.
- Dermoscopy shows reticular, globular and homogeneous patterns; of them globular pattern is the most common in childhood.
- *One should familiarize himself with the peripheral globular pattern* ***(Fig. 18)***: This pattern consists of peripherally placed globules surrounding the entire lesion. Over time these globules gradually become lesser in number and ultimately disappear, but preserve/manifest other melanocytic patterns such as melanocytic network. From the evaluation point of view, it is important to know that these changing nevi in pediatric age group are benign.

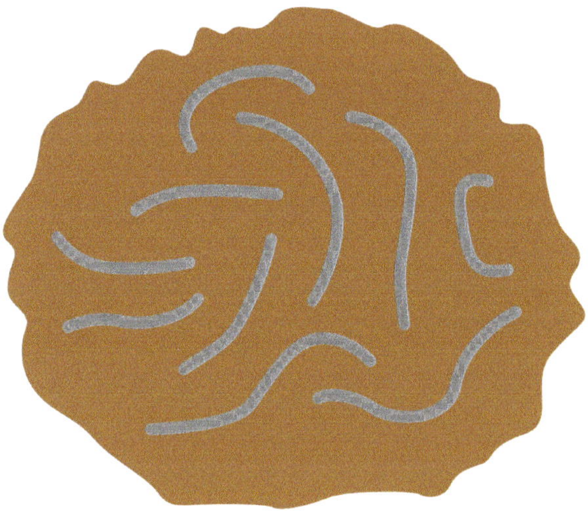

Fig. 17: Negative pigment network.

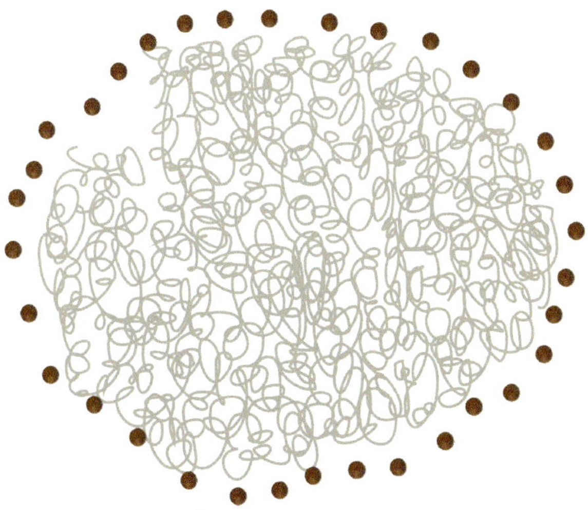

Fig. 18: Peripheral globular pattern.

Blue Nevi (Fig. 19)

- Blue nevi are benign in nature and composed of heavily pigmented dermal melanocytic nests. The classical dermoscopic pattern is homogeneous slate blue pigmentation. Any other melanocytic patterns such as network, dots and globules, and vascular structures are absent.
- Usually they appear during childhood or adolescence and present as solitary blue-black macule or papule and are located anywhere in the body including face.
- These dermal melanocytes became arrested below the dermoepidermal junction during development of the fetus.

Halo Nevi (Figs. 20A and B)

- Halo nevi are benign nevi that have a halo of hypopigmentation surrounding a central melanocytic nevus. They occur when the immune system attacks the melanocytes within a nevus and adjacent skin resulting in depigmentation of the surrounding skin. This phenomenon may be followed by depigmentation of the central nevus.

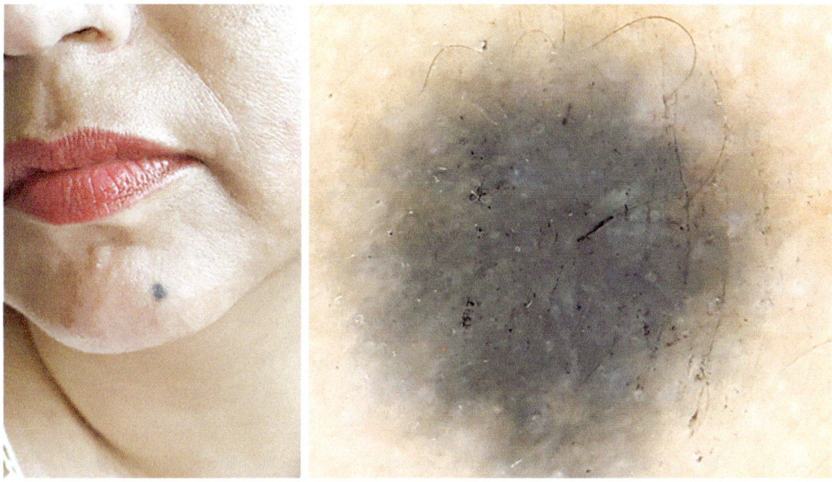

Fig. 19: Blue nevi.

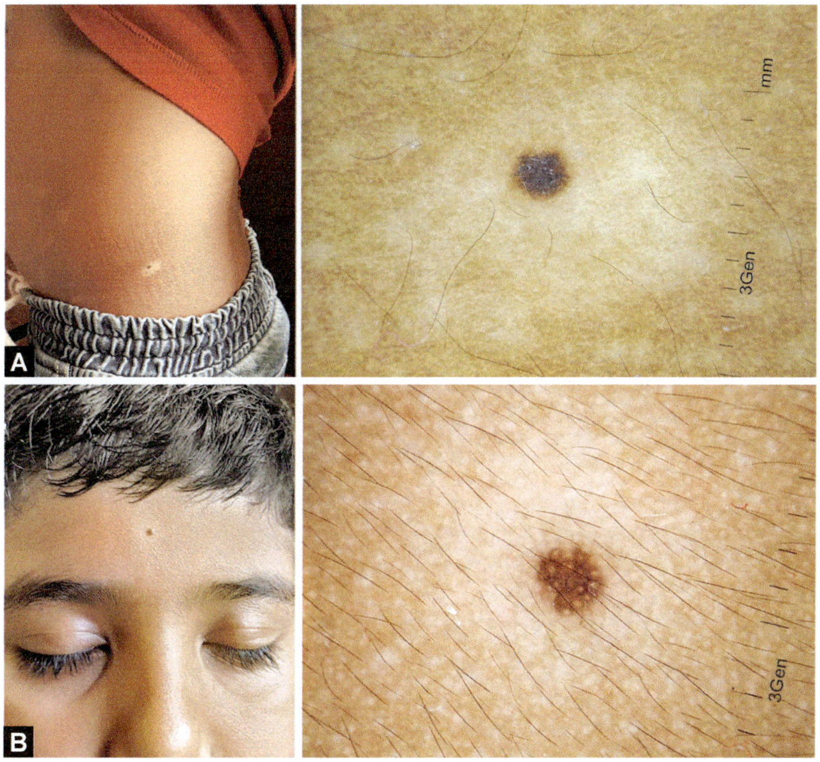

Figs. 20A and B: Halo nevus.

- Most halo nevi are inconsequential except for a very few, isolated lesions, where sudden appearance of multiple halo nevi can transform to melanoma.
- Dermoscopy of the central nevus exhibits reticular network, dots and globules, cobblestoning or homogeneous pattern; the zone of halo shows halo of depigmentation. In regressed nevi, dotted vessels and a light brown or pink central area may be noted.

Nevus Spilus (NS)

- It is a hyperpigmented patch which contains a variable number of darkly pigmented macules and papules. Also named speckled lentiginous nevus, it is considered a variant of CMN.
- Nevus spilus lesions are of two types, macular and papular. Histologically macular variety have nests of melanocytes at the tips of rete ridges whereas papular variety consists of dermal melanocytes.
- Multiple melanocytic lesions can develop within speckled lentiginous nevus such as intradermal, junctional, compound, blue, and spitz nevi; melanoma also has been reported to develop within it.
- Dermoscopy is highly helpful to evaluate the changes indicative of one of the above conditions. Biopsy is necessary when subtle changes suspective of melanoma is seen. Background of nevus spilus shows faint homogeneous color or faint melanocytic network on dermoscopy. Macular NS reveals reticular pattern whereas papular variety reveal reticular/globular/homogeneous or a combination of these features.

Melanoma

- The most common melanoma in pediatric age group are superficial spreading and nodular. Nodular melanomas grow rapidly and mostly they are amelanotic whereas superficial spreading melanomas are slowly growing.
- Dermoscopic diagnosis of amelanotic melanoma depends on its vascular features due to the lack of melanocytic structures.
- It is to be noted that pediatric melanomas usually do not manifest the ABCD features. in contrast, they are commonly symmetric, amelanotic and nodular. Sometimes the clinical appearance of pediatric melanomas are not alarming but under dermoscopy they will manifest at least one specific structures of melanoma, most often being crystalline structures and atypical vascular structures.

SUGGESTED READING

1. Berk DR, LaBuz E, Dadras SS, et al. Melanoma and melanocytic tumors of uncertain malignant potential in children, adolescents and young adults: the Stanford experience, 1995-2008. Pediatr Dermatol. 2010;27:244-54.
2. Changchien L, Dusza SW, Agero AL, et al. Age- and site-specific variation in the dermoscopic patterns of congenital melanocytic nevi: an aid to accurate classification and assessment of melanocytic nevi. Arch Dermatol. 2007;143:1007-14.
3. Ferrara G, Soyer HP, Malvehy J, et al. The many faces of blue nevus: a clinicopathologic study. J Cutan Pathol. 2007;34: 543-51.
4. Kittler H, Pehamberger H, Wolff K, et al. Diagnostic accuracy of dermoscopy. Lancet Oncol. 2002;3:159-65.
5. Kolm I, Di Stefani A, Hofmann-Wellenhof R, et al. Dermoscopy patterns of halo nevi. Arch Dermatol. 2006;142:1627-32.
6. Kovalyshyn I, Braun R, Marghoob A. Congenital melanocytic naevi. Australas J Dermatol. 2009;50:231-40; quiz 241-232.
7. Rhodes AR, Albert LS, Weinstock MA. Congenital nevomelanocytic nevi: proportionate area expansion during infancy and early childhood. J Am Acad Dermatol. 1996;34:51-62.
8. Schaffer JV. Pigmented lesions in children: when to worry. Curr Opin Pediatr. 2007;19:430-440. 292 Pediatric Dermatology Vol. 30 No. 3 May/June 2013.
9. Zalaudek I, Grinschgl S, Argenziano G, et al. Age related prevalence of dermoscopy patterns in acquired melanocytic naevi. Br J Dermatol. 2006;154:299-304.

CHAPTER 4

Eczematous Eruptions in Childhood

Subrata Malakar, Surit Malakar, Harshal Ranglani

ATOPIC DERMATITIS

INTRODUCTION

Atopic dermatitis (AD) is chronic, pruritic inflammatory dermatoses of unknown origin which usually starts in early infancy. It is common in children but can occur at any age. The eczematous lesion can occur at any part of the body but it is predominant over flexures.

KEY DERMOSCOPIC FEATURES

- Background erythema may be subtle or prominent, according to stage of the disease.
- A characteristic feature is seen at the flexural areas such as the antecubital fossa and the popliteal fossa, where the erythema and the pinpoint vessels are mostly evident along the creases.
- Patchy pinpoint vessels are characteristically seen in the early stage of the disease.
- Scales are haphazardly arranged.
- Resolving lesions are characterized by disappearance of the red dots; this serves as a marker for monitoring disease activity.

DISCUSSION

The histology in AD is a dynamic process and changes according to the stages of the disease. Similarly, erythema and scales change from prominent to subtle depending on whether the disease is acute, subacute, and chronic. Skin from atopic patients has been shown to contain thickened, flexuous blood vessels in the papillary dermis, which is responsible for the patchy pinpoint vessels, seen on dermoscopy.

The skin is relatively thinner in the flexural areas, more so in the skin creases, which explains the prominence of erythema and pinpoint vessels in this area. In the late stage of the disease, these morphological changes of the blood vessels are not seen, which correlates well with the disappearance of the red dots. This is extremely useful while monitoring the response to treatment.

KEYNOTE

Regularly distributed dotted vessels seen in psoriasis correspond histopathologically to dilated, elongated, and spiraled capillaries in the dermal papillae. In contrast, dermoscopy of AD shows dotted vessels arranged in a patchy distribution, with variable erythema **(Figs. 1 to 5)**.

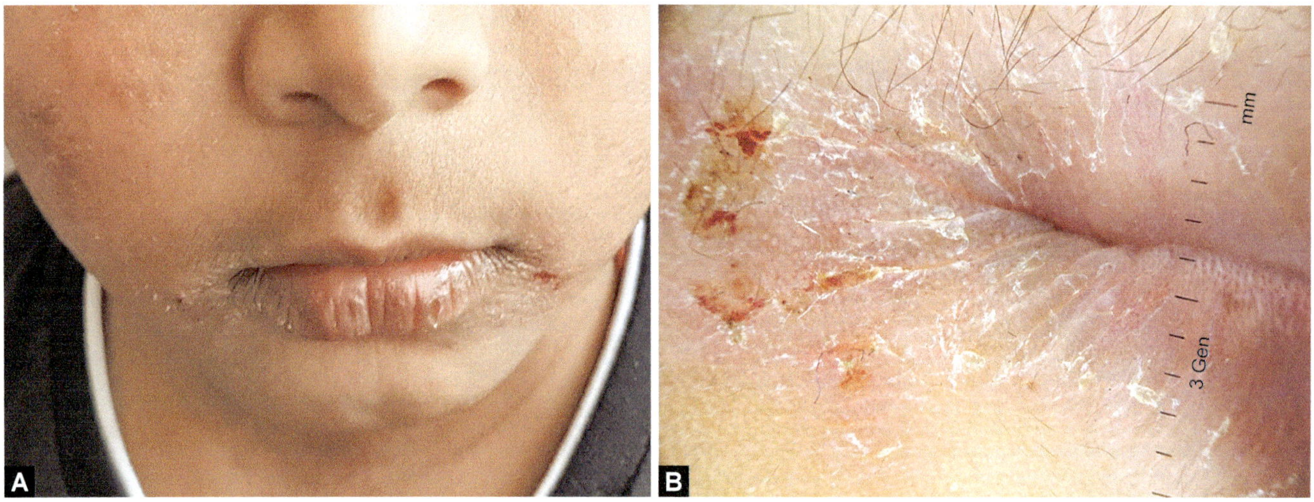

Figs. 1A and B: (A) Cheilitis in an 8-year old with atopy; (B) Dermoscopy shows haphazard arrangement of scales and patchy areas of pinpoint, dotted vessels along with some excoriations.

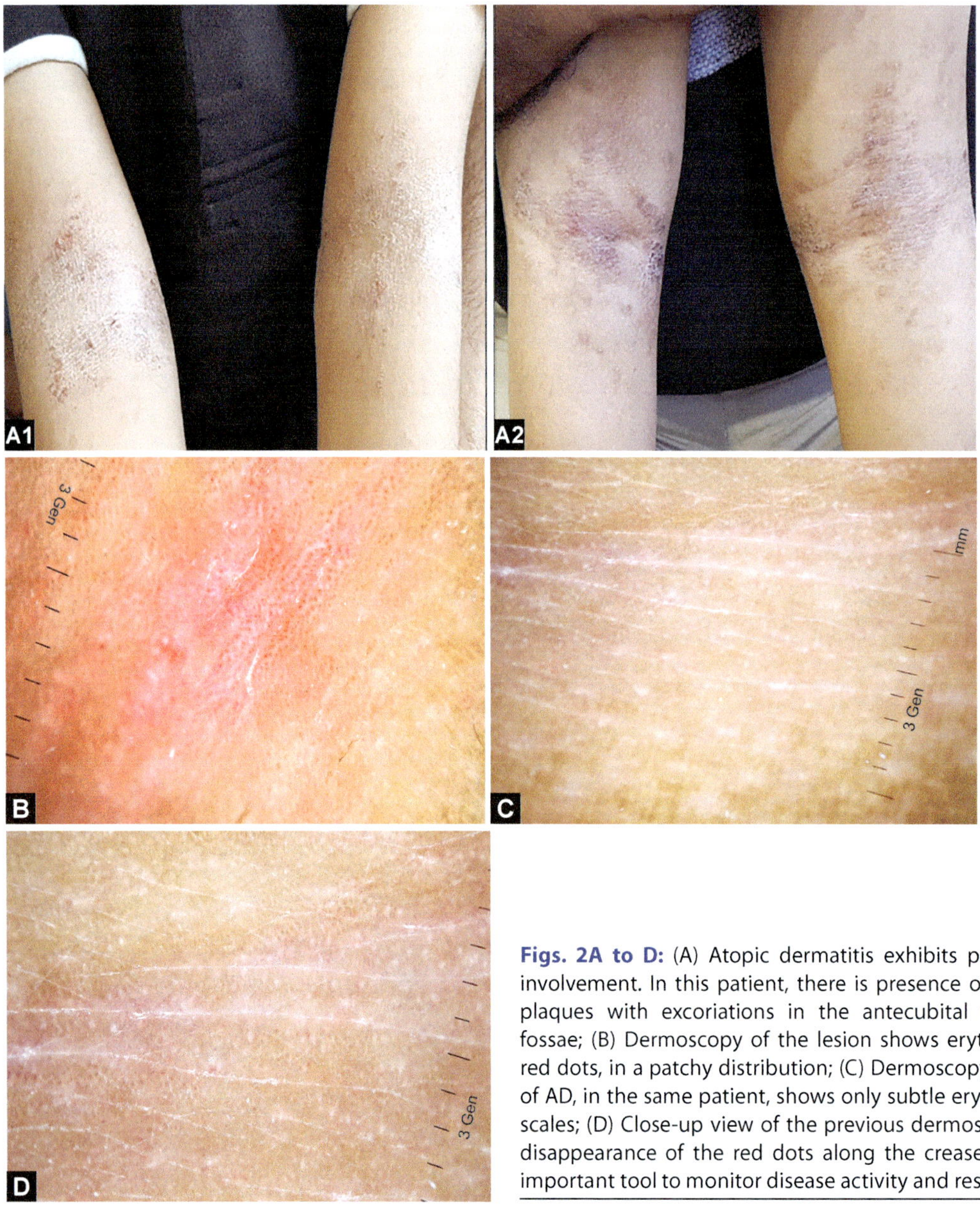

Figs. 2A to D: (A) Atopic dermatitis exhibits predominantly flexural involvement. In this patient, there is presence of erythematous, scaly plaques with excoriations in the antecubital fossae and popliteal fossae; (B) Dermoscopy of the lesion shows erythema and numerous red dots, in a patchy distribution; (C) Dermoscopy of the healing stage of AD, in the same patient, shows only subtle erythema and a few, tiny scales; (D) Close-up view of the previous dermoscopic image showing disappearance of the red dots along the creases, thus serving as an important tool to monitor disease activity and response to treatment.

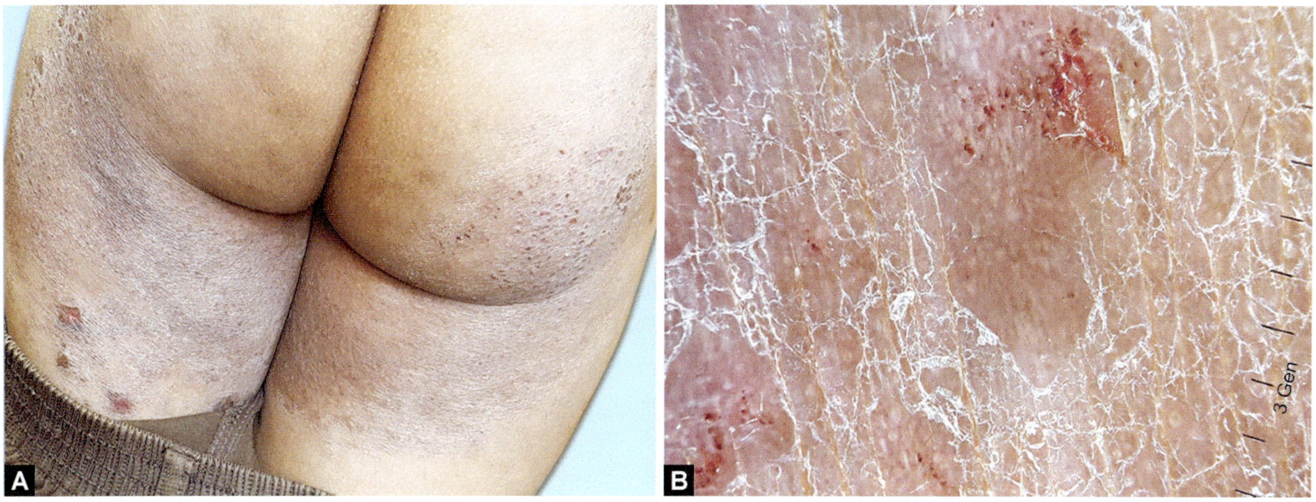

Figs. 3A and B: (A) Atopic dermatitis can affect many part of the body especially the intertriginous areas; (B) Dermoscopy of this patient shows haphazard scales, some excoriated areas with pinpoint bleeding spots. Subtle erythema is evident.

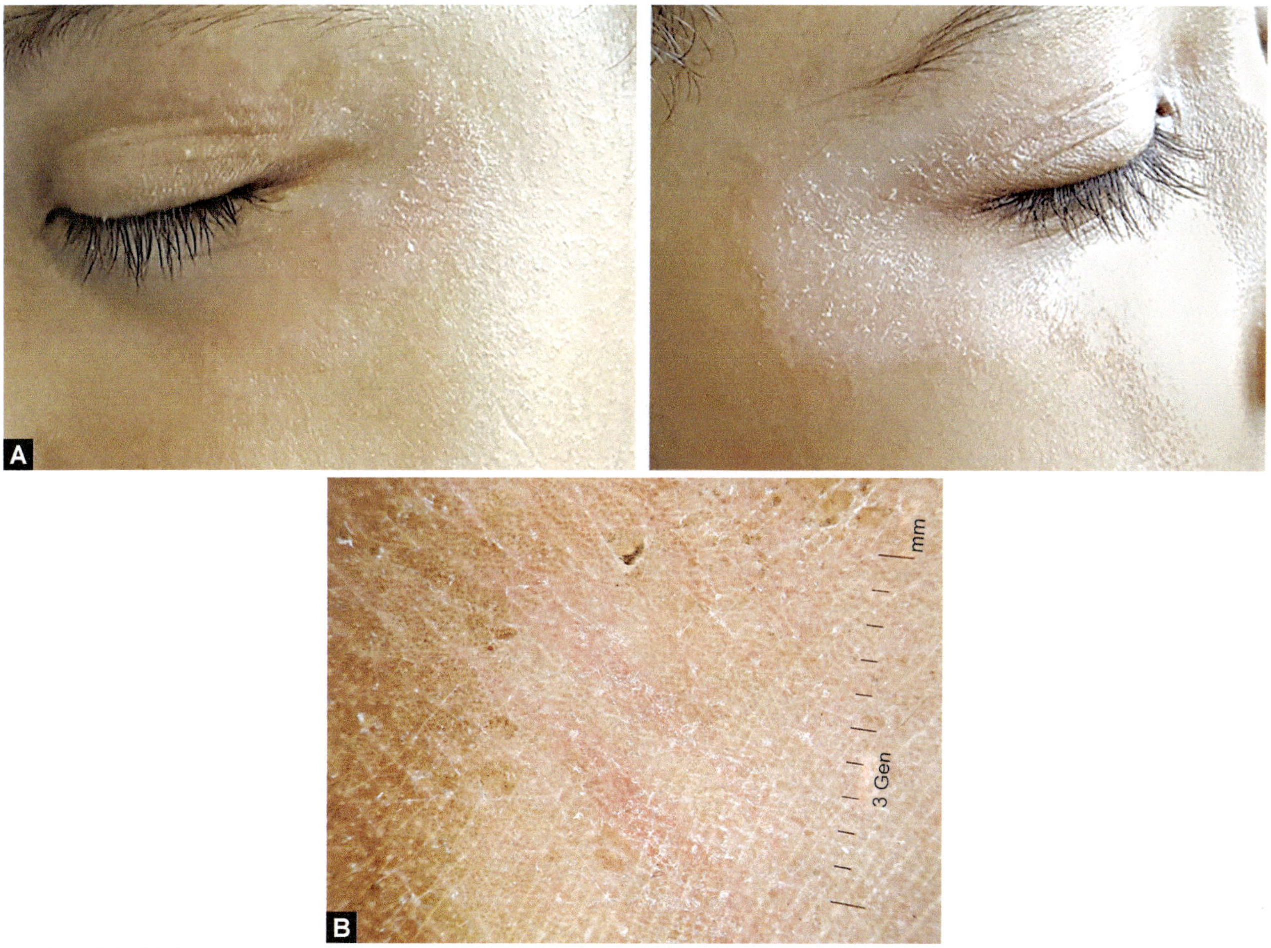

Figs. 4A and B: (A) Atopic dermatitis around the eyelids with scales and erythema; (B) Fine scales with subtle erythema, more prominent along the creases.

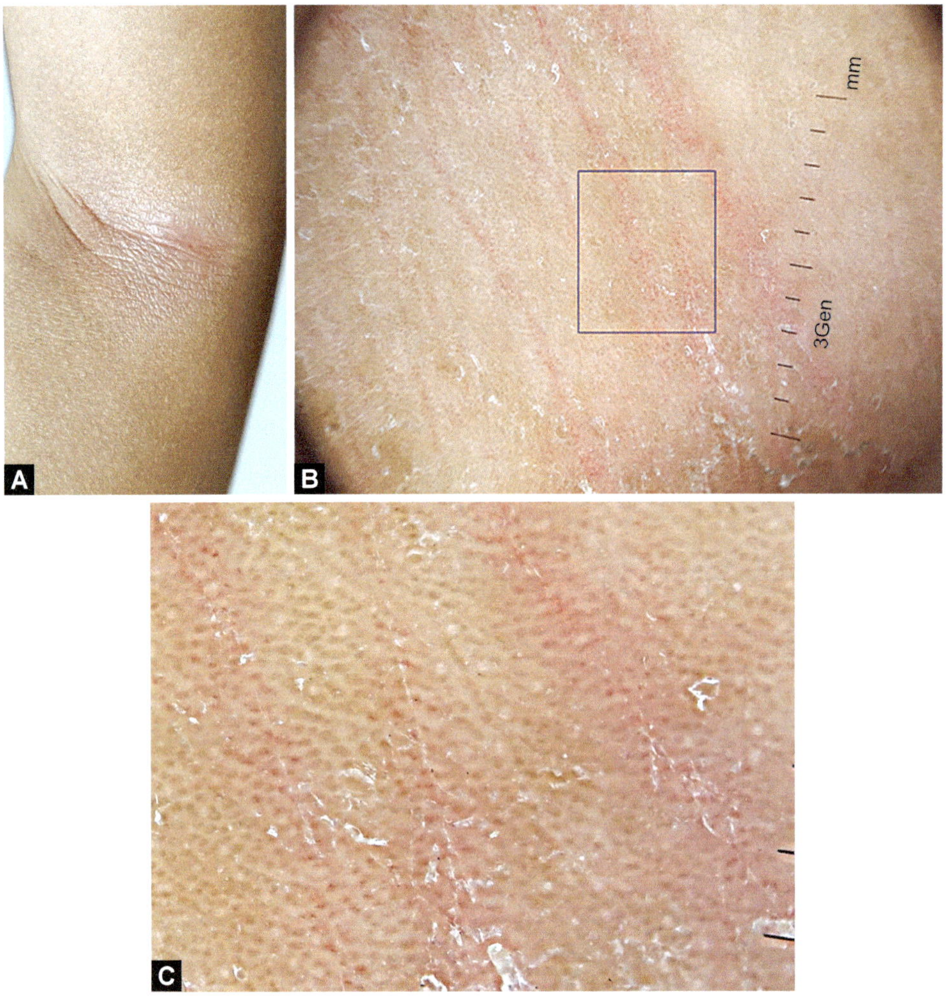

Figs. 5A to C: (A) Involvement of the antecubital fossa in the form of erythema and mild scaling in a case of AD; (B) The skin creases show prominent, pinpoint vessels with a background erythema and mild to moderate scaling; (C) Zoomed in view of the marked area of the previous dermoscopic image clearly showing the presence of erythema and red dots along the creases.

SUGGESTED READING

1. Abuabara K, Margolis D, Langan S. The long-term course of atopic dermatitis. Dermatologic Clinics. 2017;35(3);291-7.
2. Hale G, Davies E, Grindlay DJ, et al. What's new in atopic eczema? An analysis of systematic reviews published in 2017. Part 2: Epidemiology, aetiology and risk factors. Clin Exp Dermatol. 2019.
3. Tsutsumi M, Fukuda M, Kumamoto J, et al. Abnormal morphology of blood vessels in erythematous skin from atopic dermatitis patients. Am J Dermatopathol. 2016;38(5):363-4.

LICHEN SPINULOSUS

INTRODUCTION

Lichen spinulosus presents as solitary or multiple circumscribed patches, composed of tiny follicular papules studded with horny spines. It is believed to be a clinically distinct variant of keratosis pilaris and is also called "keratosis spinulosa".

It is commonly seen in children with dry skin and sometimes with atopic dermatitis. Usually, there are no other symptoms and signs. However, occasionally, itching may be present. They develop over extensor surfaces of arms, abdomen, buttocks, knees, etc.

At present, there are no specific laboratories or diagnostic tests that can confirm the diagnosis of lichen spinulosus. Keratosis pilaris and lichen spinulosus cannot be distinguished by histopathology.

KEY DERMOSCOPIC FEATURES

- Multiple round whitish structures surrounding the gray-black shadows at the centers
- Mild scaling
- Hairs embedded in the subcorneal layer along with deformed hair as well.

DISCUSSION

Round whitish structures correspond histologically to acanthosis. The gray-black shadows at the center of the whitish structures correlate to keratotic plugs on histopathological examination.

Embedded hair and deformed hair result from defective keratinization of the follicular epithelium **(Figs. 6 to 9)**.

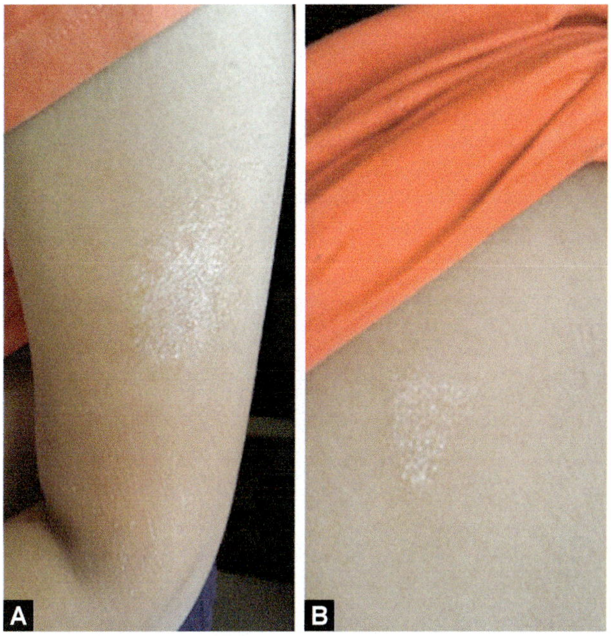

Figs. 6A and B: Well-circumscribed tiny pin-point flat topped grouped papules of lichen spinulosus.

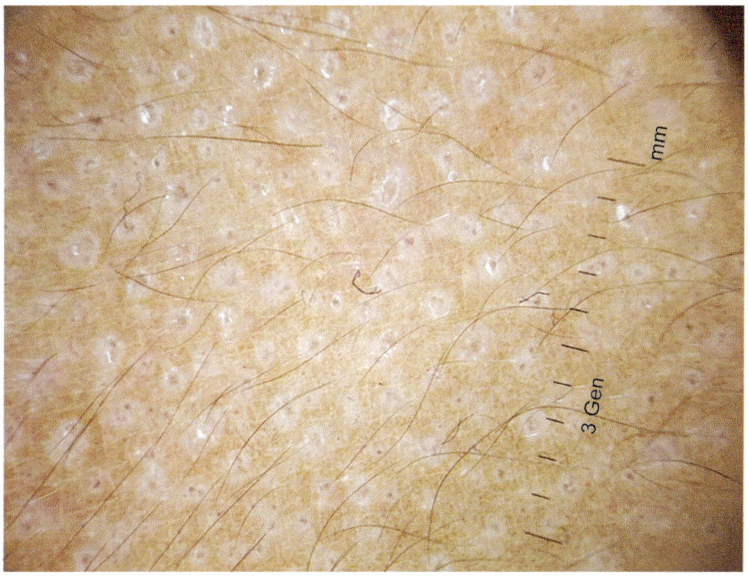

Fig. 7: Dermoscopy shows round whitish structures surrounding gray-black shadows at the centers, along with mild scaling.

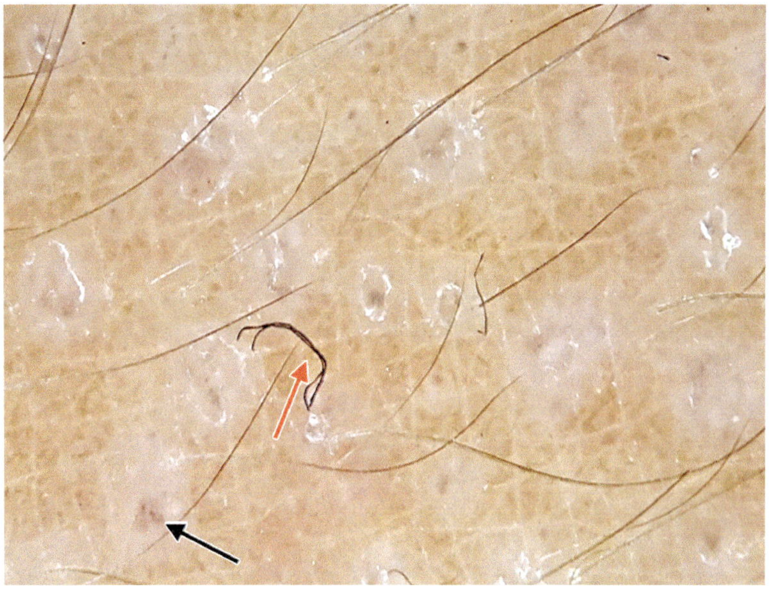

Fig. 8: Many hairs are embedded in the subcorneal layer (black arrow). Some hairs are deformed (red arrow).

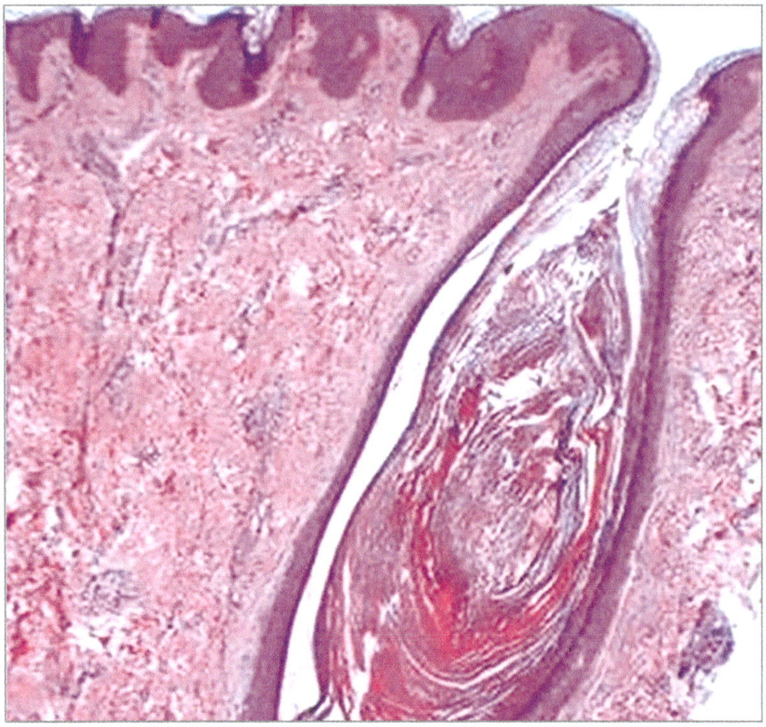

Fig. 9: Histopathology of lichen spinulosus shows dilated hair follicles are filled with keratotic plugs. These correspond to the gray-black shadows on dermoscopy.

SUGGESTED READING

1. Amy PS, Mancini AJ. Eczematous Eruption in Childhood. Hurwitz Clinical Pediatric Dermatology: A Textbook of Skin Disorders of Childhood and Adolescence, 5th edition. Edinburgh: Elsevier; 2016. pp. 43
2. Malakar S Body Hair. Trichoscopy: A Text and Atlas, 1st edition. New Delhi: Jaypee Brothers Medical Publishers; 2017. pp. 325-51.

LICHEN STRIATUS

INTRODUCTION

Lichen striatus is a self-limiting inflammatory dermatosis usually unilateral, linear, or curvilinear collection of flat-topped, hypopigmented to erythematous papules. It follows Blaschko lines.

The common differentials of lichen striatus include inflammatory linear verrucous epidermal nevus (ILVEN) and blaschkitis. Whether lichen striatus and blaschkitis are separate entities or are variations of the same disease remain controversial. ILVEN is psoriasiform whereas blaschkitis is eczematous.

KEY DERMOSCOPIC FEATURES

- Gray granular pigmentation
- White scar-like line
- Mild scaling.

DISCUSSION

Gray granular pigmentation corresponds histologically to pigment-laden melanophages in the superficial dermis. White scar-like line may be correlated to the acanthosis, which is a common histologic finding of lichen striatus.

KEYNOTE

Clinically, lichen striatus may be commonly confused with ILVEN. This confusion can be instantly resolved by examining the lesion with a dermoscope. ILVEN shows cerebriform pattern corresponding to papillated epidermal hyperplasia whereas lichen striatus will show gray granular pigment and white scar-like line **(Figs. 10 and 11)**.

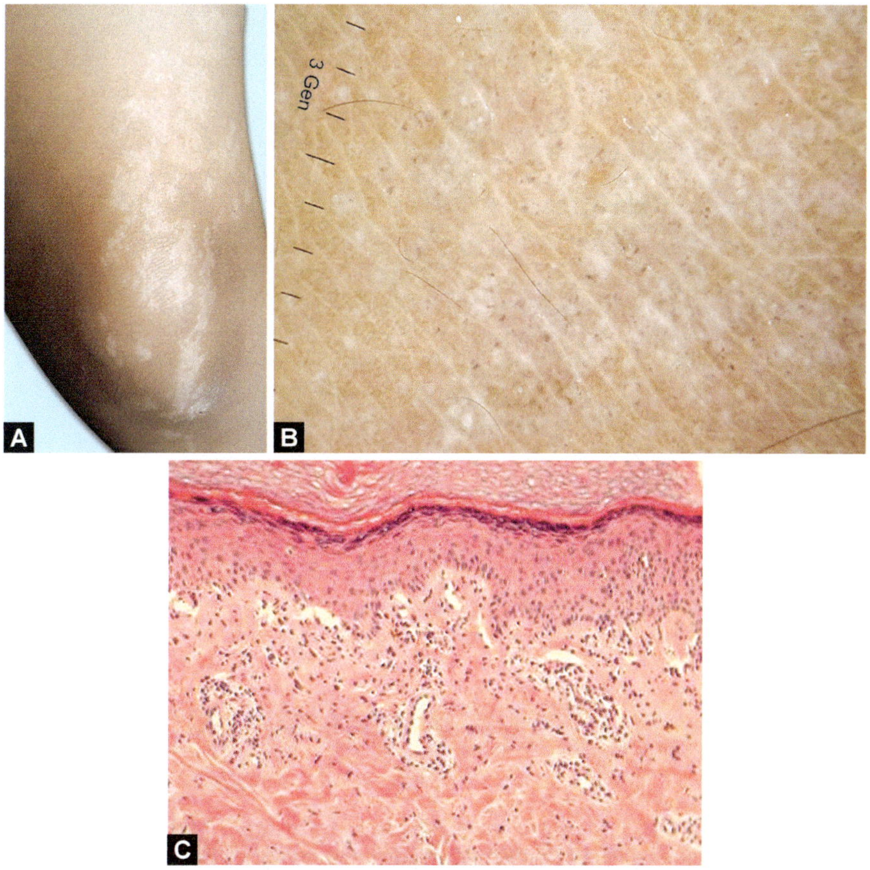

Figs. 10A to C: (A) Lichen striatus following Blaschko's lines in a 10-year-old boy; (B) The dermoscopy field is scattered with gray granular pigmentation which corresponds to melanophages histologically. Also, note the subtle background erythema and whitish structures; (C) Histopathology shows interface dermatitis, lymphohistiocytic infiltrate, and melanophages.

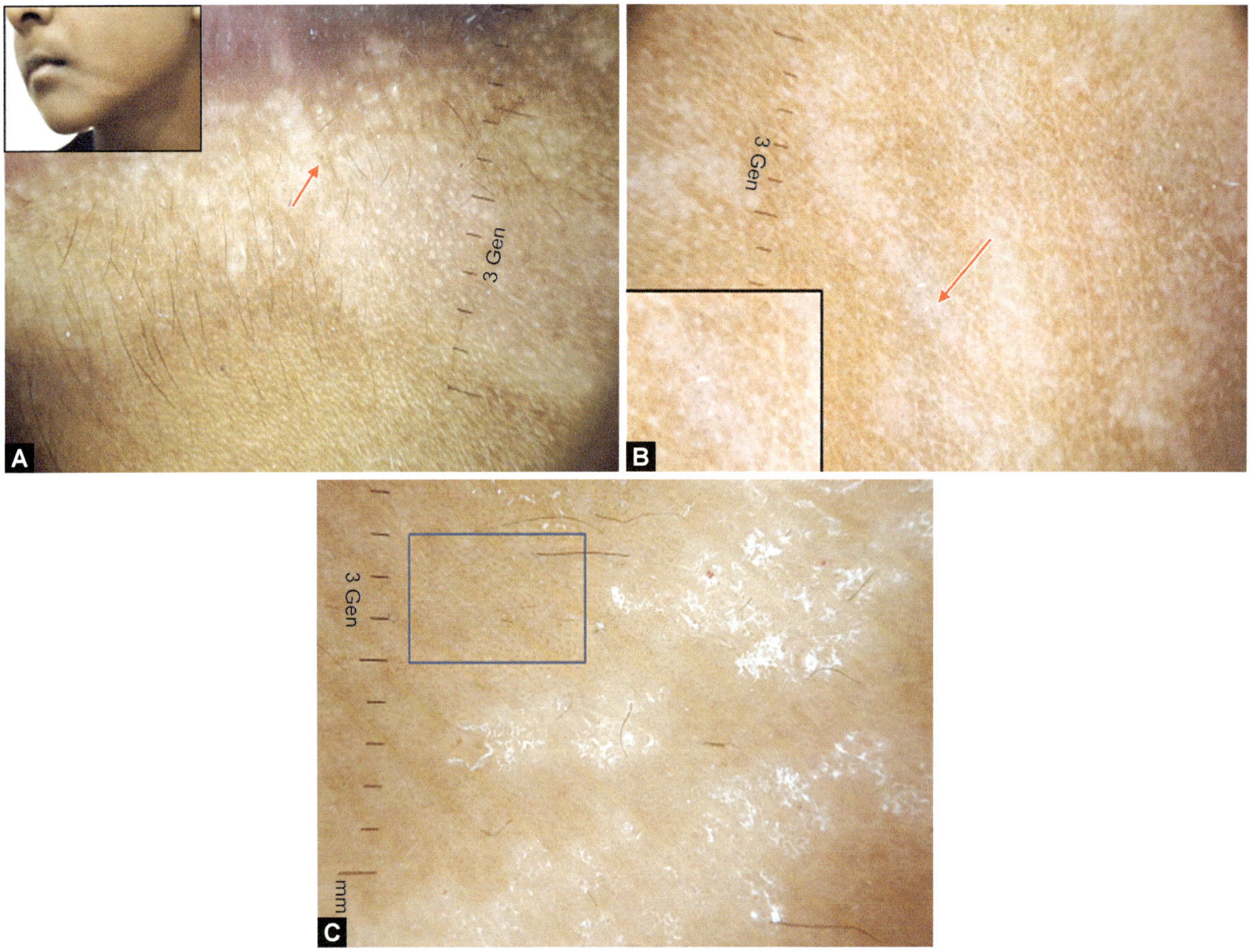

Figs. 11A to C: (A) Dermoscopy showing white scar-like line at the angle of the mouth and very few gray granular structure (red arrow). Inset: Clinical image of lichen striatus following Blaschko's lines; (B) Dermoscopy showing speckling of gray granular pigmentation (highlighted in inset) along white scar-like line (red arrow); (C) Dermoscopy showing moderate scaling with grey granular dots (blue box).

SUGGESTED READING

1. Amy PS, Mancini AJ, Hurwitz S. Eczematous eruption in childhood. Hurwitz Clinical Pediatric Dermatology: A Textbook of Skin Disorders of Childhood and Adolescence, 5th edition. Edinburgh: Elsevier; 2016. pp. 60-1.
2. Azizpour A, Nasimi M, Safaie-Naraghi Z, et al. A case of blaschkitis with features of both lichenoid and spongiotic dermatitis. Indian J Dermatol. 2016;61:348.
3. Carbotti M, Coppola R, Graziano A, et al. Dermoscopy of verrucous epidermal nevus: Large brown circles as a novel feature for diagnosis. Int J Dermatol. 2016;55:653-6.
4. Kim DW, Kwak HB, Yun SK, et al. Dermoscopy of linear dermatosis along Blaschko's line in childhood: Lichen striatus versus inflammatory linear verrucous epidermal nevus. J Dermatol. 2017;44(12):e355-6.

NUMMULAR ECZEMA

INTRODUCTION

Usually nummular eczema presents as distinct coin-shaped (nummular) patches or plaques over the skin. It often appears after a skin injury such as burn, abrasion, or insect bite. There may be single or multiple patches and lasts for weeks to months.

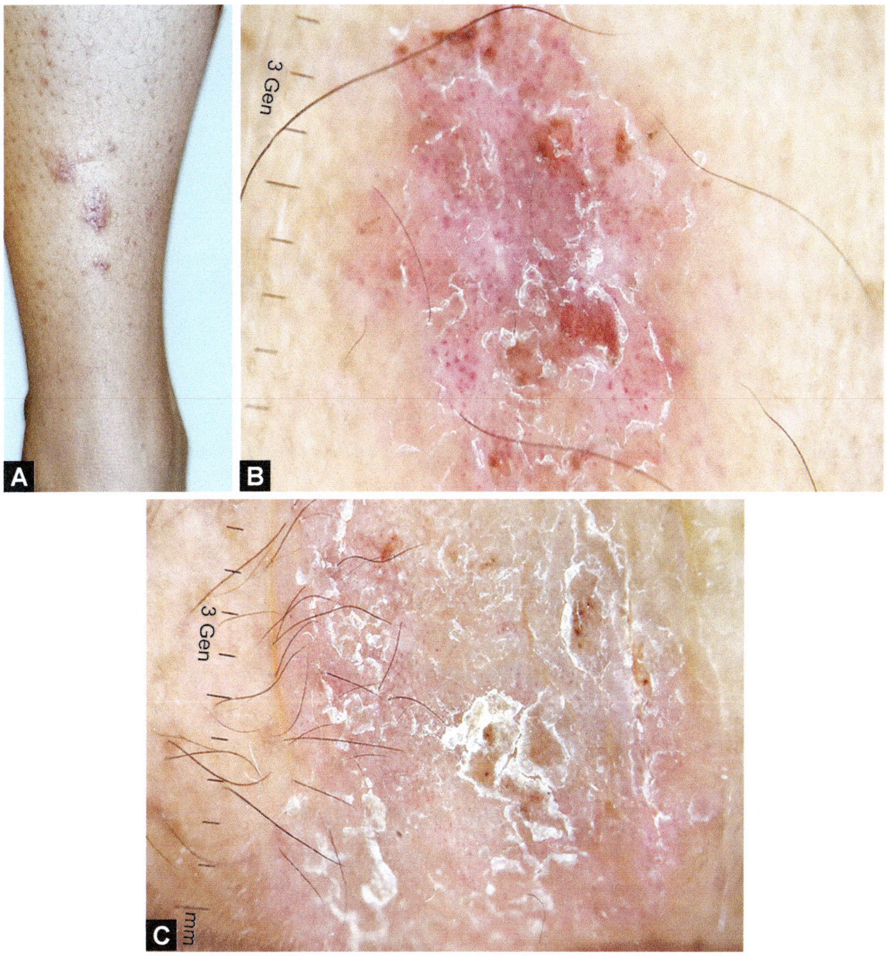

Figs. 12A to C: (A) Discoid plaques seen over the lower limb in a 15-year-old boy; (B) Arrangement of dotted vessels in a patchy distribution can be noted on dermoscopic examination of the above lesion; (C) Yellow clods, which represent serocrusts forming on the surface of lesions in dermatitis, are noted here. These are seen mainly in acute, exudative lesions.

KEY DERMOSCOPIC FEATURES

- Dotted vessels in a patchy distribution
- Yellow clods (representing serocrusts).

DISCUSSION

The dermoscopic findings in dermatitis are dotted vessels arranged in a patchy distribution and yellow serocrust ("yellow clod" sign). Depending on disease duration, eczematous dermatitis displays a spectrum of scaling and vascular changes. Acute exudative lesions exhibit yellow serocrusts. Chronic and lichenified lesions demonstrate dotted vessels arranged in a patchy fashion, along with scaling.

KEYNOTE

The pointers toward dermatitis include yellow-clods and the patchy distribution of dotted vessels **(Figs. 12A to C)**.

SUGGESTED READING

1. Lallas A, Argenziano G, Apalla Z, et al. Dermoscopic patterns of common facial inflammatory skin diseases. J Eur Acad Dermatol Venereol. 2013;28(5):609-14.
2. Lallas A, Kyrgidis A, Tzellos TG, et al. Accuracy of dermoscopic criteria for the diagnosis of psoriasis, dermatitis, lichen planus and pityriasis rosea. Br J Dermatol. 2012;166:1198-205.
3. Navarini AA, Feldmeyer L, Tondury B, et al. The yellow clod sign. Arch Dermatol. 2011;147:1350.

CHAPTER 5

Papulosquamous

Surit Malakar, Subrata Malakar

PSORIASIS

INTRODUCTION

Psoriasis is, more often than not, diagnosed clinically. However, atypical presentations such as a solitary plaque or guttate lesions may prove challenging to diagnose clinically, and histopathology may be needed in these cases. Dermoscopy can prove to be a valuable aid in the diagnosis of such cases, avoiding the need for a biopsy in pediatric patients.

Psoriasis is rarely present at birth. Approximately, one-third of adults with psoriasis noted the onset during the first two decades of life. Variants such as guttate psoriasis, napkin psoriasis, and facial psoriasis are more common in children than in adults.

KEY DERMOSCOPIC FEATURES[1-4]

- Regularly distributed dotted vessels on a diffuse pink background
- White scales
- Dermoscopic "Auspitz sign".

DISCUSSION

Dermoscopy of chronic plaque psoriasis is characterized by regularly arranged, red, dotted vessels against a pink background. "Red globular rings" and convoluted loops are other patterns, which may be seen. The "red globular ring" pattern is highly specific for psoriasis but rare. Convoluted loops correspond histopathologically to dilated, elongated, tortuous, and spiraled capillaries in the dermal papillae. They are visible only under higher magnification (100–400×).

Diffuse white scales are also seen in chronic plaque psoriasis, simply highlighting the clinical picture.

Dermoscopic auspitz sign: In case of lesions with marked hyperkeratosis, removal of the scales reveals an underlying vascular pattern with blood droplets under dermoscopy.

KEYNOTE

Several erythematosquamous conditions share similar clinical features, making their differentiation difficult. Regularly distributed dotted vessels over a dull red background along with white scales are the dermoscopic hallmark of psoriasis. Consequently, a dermoscope is a useful aid for rapid diagnosis of psoriasis in case of a diagnostic dilemma, obviating the need for biopsy in many cases. This is especially useful in pediatric patients **(Figs. 1 to 7)**.

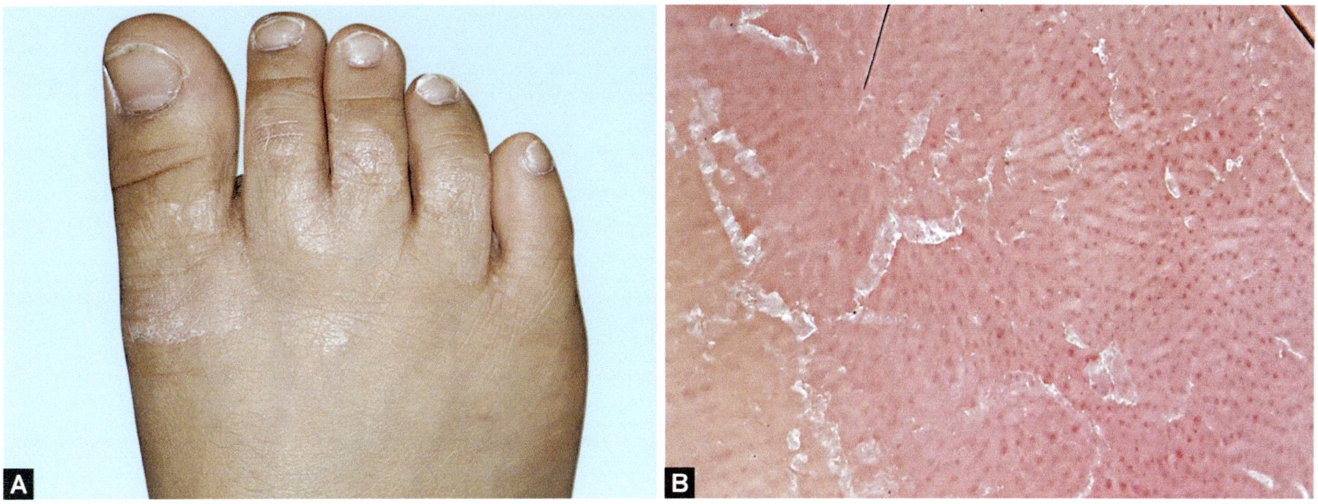

Figs. 1A and B: (A) Thin plaques with minimal erythema and scales over the dorsum of toes and foot pose a diagnostic challenge. The differentials considered could be forefoot eczema, tinea pedis, and psoriasis; (B) Dermoscopy of plaque over foot reveals regularly distributed red dots and diffuse silvery white scales. This characteristic pattern is due to dermal microvascular alterations, with presence of larger and spiraled capillaries within dermal papillae in association with psoriasiform epidermal hyperplasia.

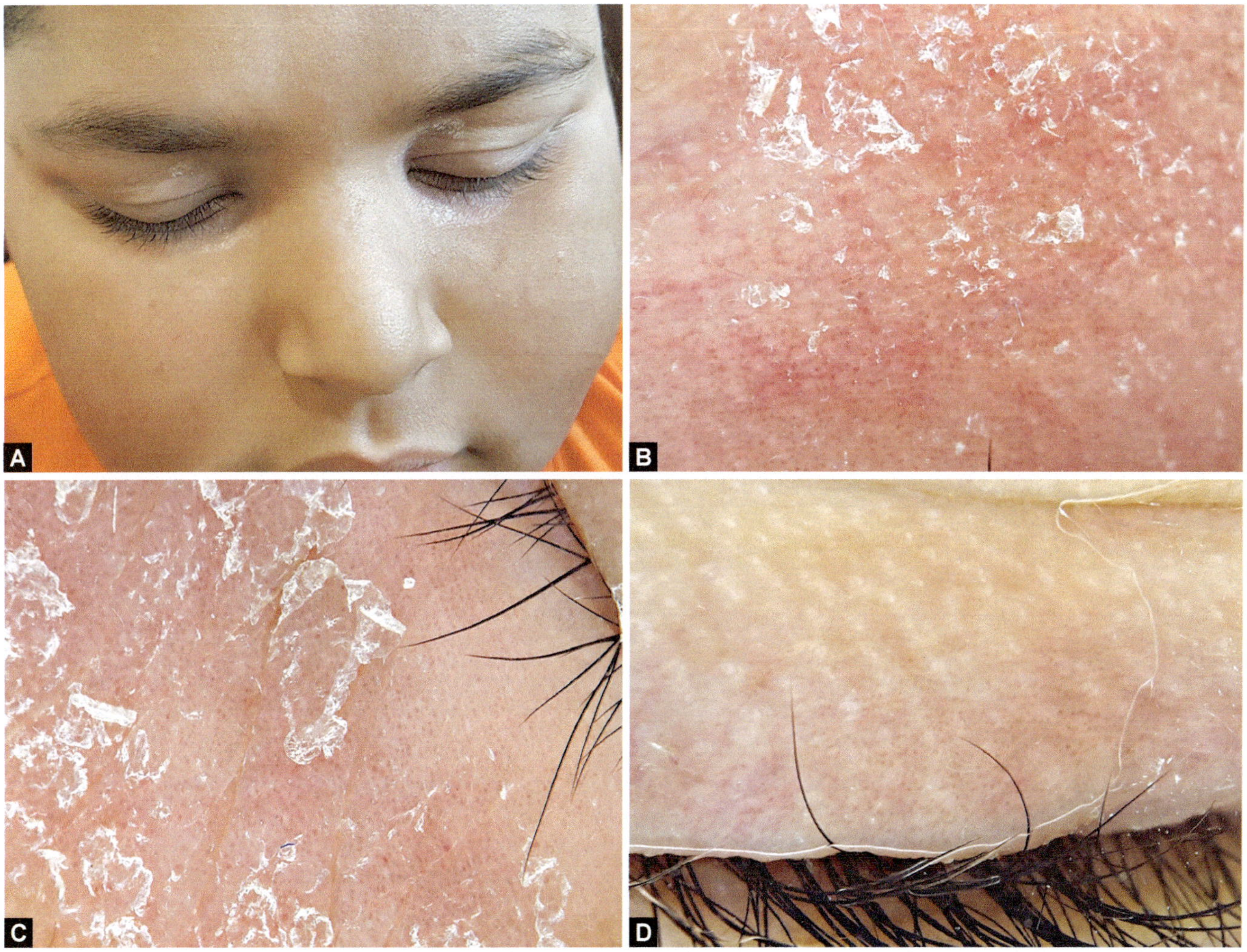

Figs. 2A to D: (A) A 10-year-old boy presented with erythematous, scaly plaques in bilateral periocular regions. Clinically, a diagnosis of eyelid dermatitis due to atopic dermatitis was made; (B) Dermoscopy of the infraorbital plaque revealed regular red dots on a pink background with white scales. Thus, a diagnosis of psoriasis could be based, with the help of dermoscopy; (C) Dermoscopy reveals whitish scales, on an underlying background of red dots and a few globules on the lower eyelid; (D) Regularly arranged red dots on a diffuse dull red background, seen on the upper eyelid.

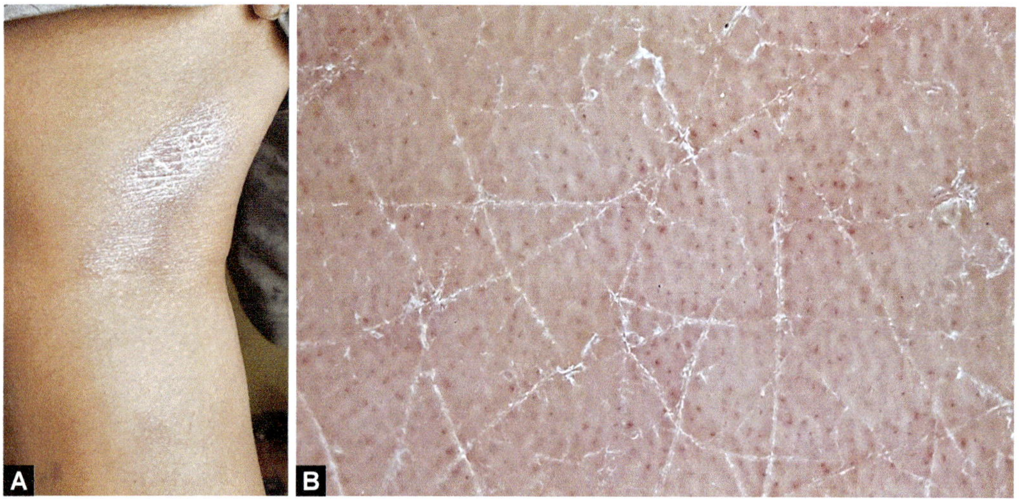

Figs. 3A and B: (A) Psoriasis may present as a single localized plaque where it becomes difficult to differentiate it from eczema; (B) Dermoscopy reveals red dots distributed regularly and symmetrically on a dull red background; white scales are present.

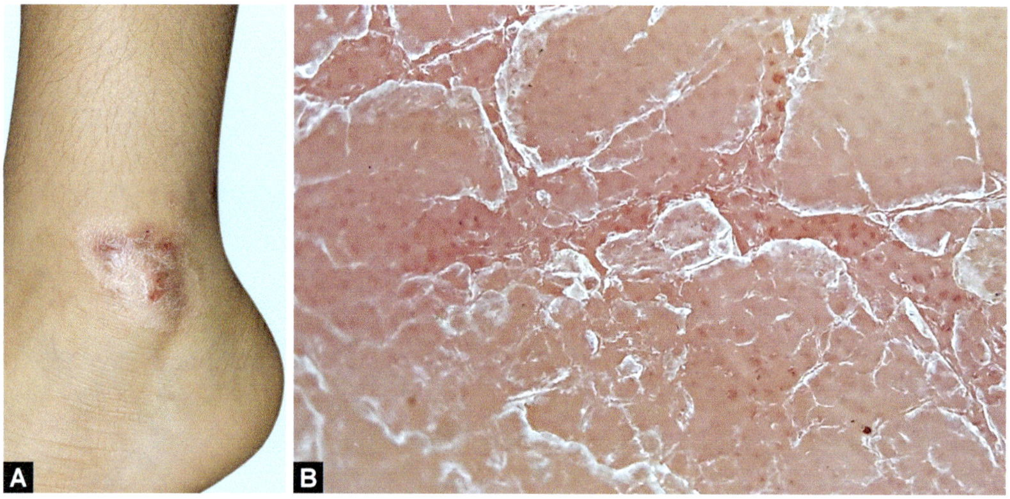

Figs. 4A and B: (A) Involvement of the lateral malleolar area in a 12-year-old boy in the form of a solitary, erythematous, and scaly plaque. Clinically, there was a dilemma between psoriasis and eczema; (B) Thick scales overlying a vascular pattern of regular red dots on a dull red background. Thus, a final diagnosis of psoriasis could be made.

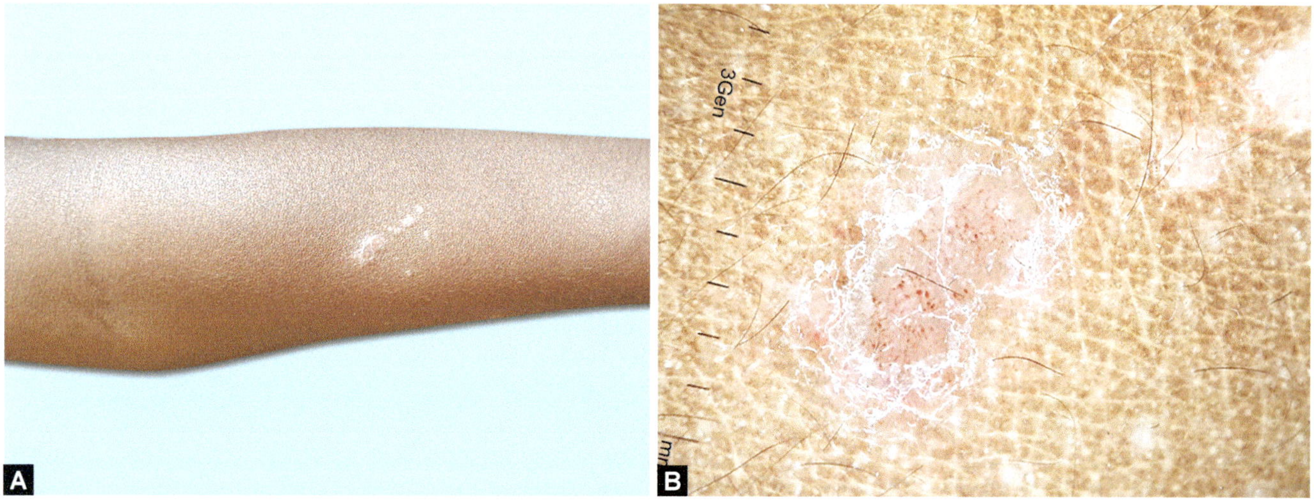

Figs. 5A and B: (A) Koebnerization seen in a case of psoriasis: presence of multiple erythematous, scaly papules arranged in a linear fashion; (B) Koebnerization noted dermoscopically. Multiple areas of red dots with scales can be appreciated.

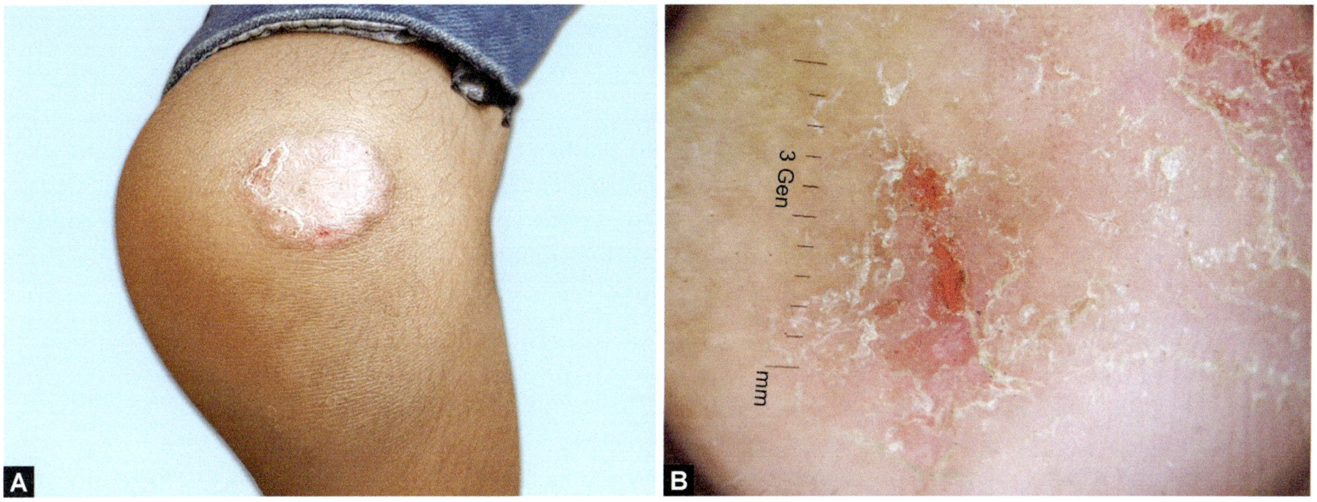

Figs. 6A and B: (A) Single scaly plaque over the left knee in a 14-year-old boy; (B) Thick white scales interspersed with regularly placed red dots.

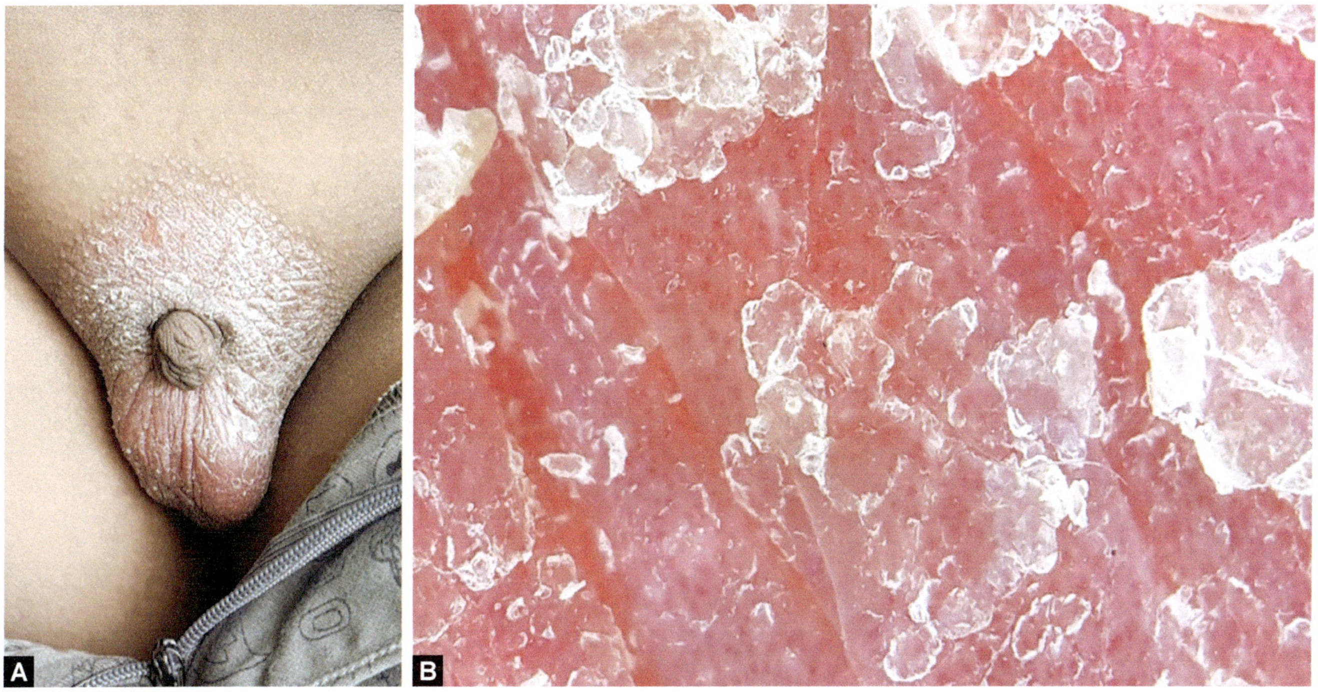

Figs. 7A and B: (A) A 7-year-old child presented with itchy lesions over the genital area of 8 months duration and was currently under treatment for a probable contact dermatitis; (B) Dermoscopy of the lesion in the above patient revealed silvery micaceous scales and sheets of red dots and globules.

REFERENCES

1. Lallas A, Kyrgidis A, Tzellos TG, et al. Accuracy of dermoscopic criteria for the diagnosis of psoriasis, dermatitis, lichen planus and pityriasis rosea. Br J Dermatol. 2012;166:1198-205.
2. Moscarella E, Longo C, Zalaudek I, et al. Dermoscopy and confocal microscopy clues in the diagnosis of psoriasis and porokeratosis. J Am Acad Dermatol. 2013;69:e231-3.
3. Vasquez Lopez F, Gonzalez-Lara L, Martin JS, et al. Holubar (1936-2013). Teaching with dermoscopy: Revealing the subsurface morphology of Auspitz 's sign and psoriasis. Int J Dermatol. 2014;53:e322-4.
4. S Malakar. Papulosquamous disorders. In: Dermoscopy Text and Atlas. New Delhi: Jaypee Brothers Medical Publishers; 2019. pp. 132-47.

LICHEN PLANUS

INTRODUCTION

Lichen planus in children is relatively common dermatoses in the Indian subcontinent. Studies have shown that the mean age of onset varies between 5 years and 9 years with a slight male predominance. Diagnosis of lichen planus (LP) is mainly clinical although histologic confirmation may be needed in few cases. The use of immersion oil to wet the lesion followed by visualization under magnifying lens helps in better appreciation of Wickham's striae (WS).

KEY DERMOSCOPIC FEATURES

- Wickham's striae
- Dotted/linear vessels at the periphery of the lesion
- Structureless homogeneous brown-gray areas or gray dots in regressing lesions of LP
- Comedo-like structures and "Bouquet of white roses" in hypertrophic LP.

DISCUSSION

The characteristic finding of LP is WS. It is a highly specific and sensitive pointer for LP. WS are seen as pearly whitish structures and they develop thin or broad arboriform projections. They are usually surrounded by dotted or linear vessels. The common morphological pattern of WS is reticular; the other patterns include linear, round, and annular. Some may display a "radial streaming" pattern, "starry sky" pattern, or "leaf venation". Histopathologically, WS corresponds to compact orthokeratosis atop the zones of wedge-shaped hypergranulosis.

Dotted and linear vessels are the predominant vascular pattern seen in LP. They are present on a commonly violet, pink, or reddish background, and frequently localized to the periphery of the lesion.

The two dermoscopic patterns invaluable in monitoring and follow-up of the disease are structureless homogeneous brown-gray areas and gray dots. The gray dots correspond histopathologically to melanophages in the dermis and are a sign of persisting lesions whereas the homogeneous pattern tends to be self-limiting and transient.

Hypertrophic LP has distinct findings of corn pearls and a rippled surface on dermoscopy.

KEYNOTE

Dermoscopy helps in conclusively differentiating LP from other papulosquamous dermatoses like psoriasis and eczema owing to their specific features. It also serves as an important tool in monitoring treatment efficacy in LP **(Figs. 8 to 12)**.

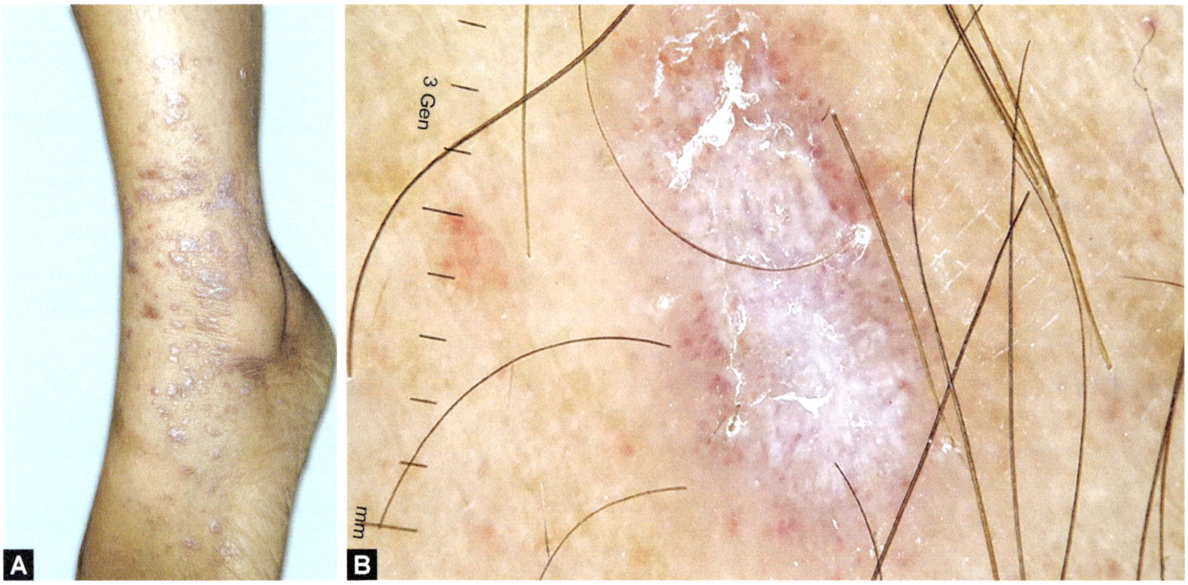

Figs. 8A and B: (A) A 10-year-old female with numerous, flat topped, violaceous papules, and plaques over left lower limb; (B) Dermoscopy of the lesions showed presence of Wickham's striae and peripheral vascular pattern of dotted vessels. A violaceous hue of the background is also noted.

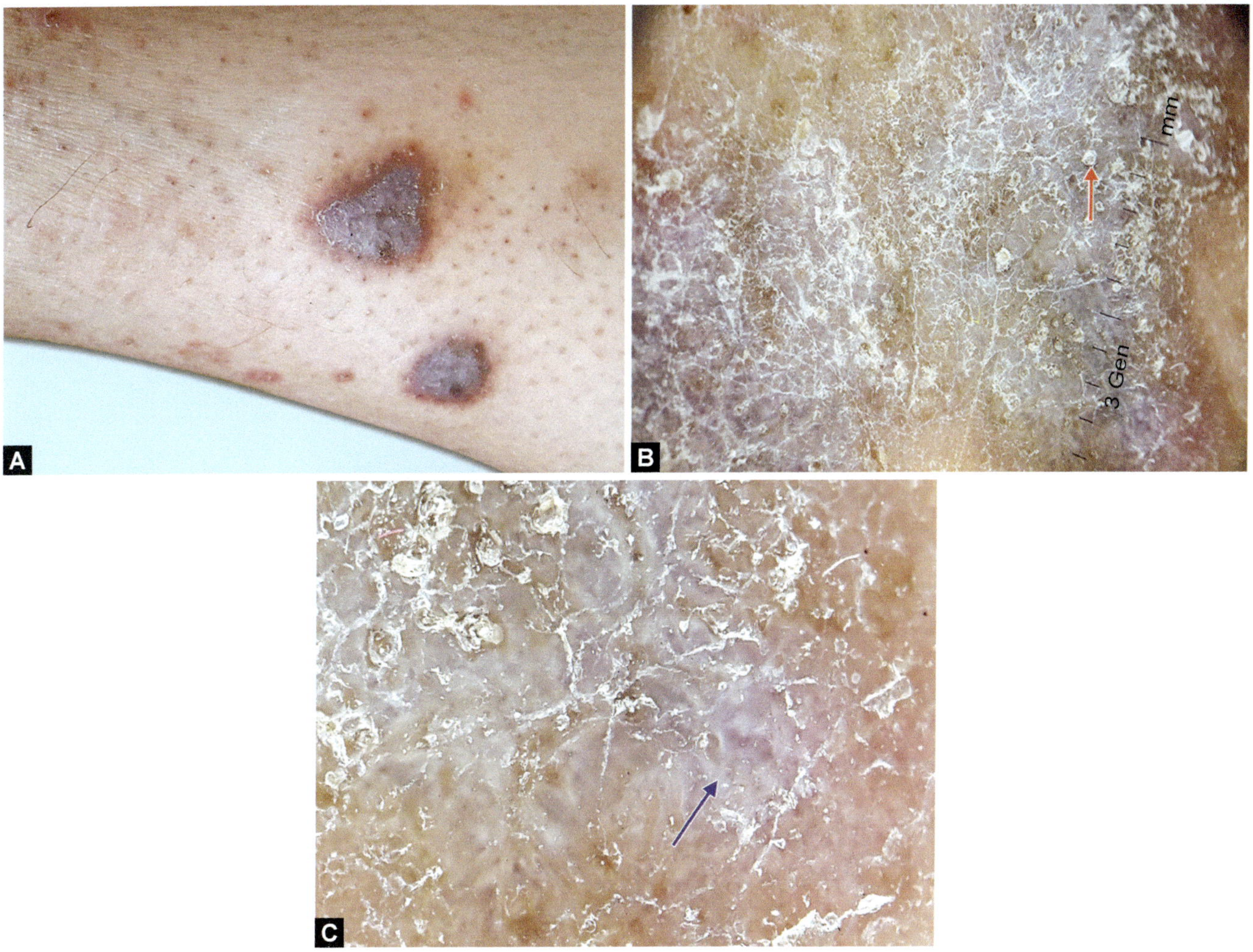

Figs. 9A to C: (A) Hypertrophic lichen planus: thick, violaceous papules, and plaques on the lower limb; (B) Dermoscopically, the lesion exhibits Wickham's striae (WS) in variable configurations, on a violaceous background. Here, corn pearls can be appreciated, thus aiding a diagnosis of hypertrophic lichen planus; (C) Wickham's striae, corn pearls can be seen distinctly. In the upper left corner, a "bouquet of roses" appearance is evident.

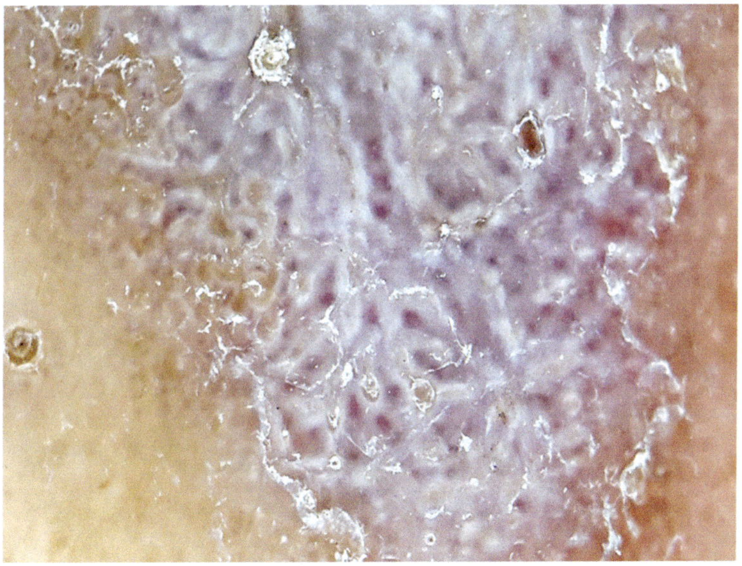

Fig. 10: A classical case of lichen planus showing reticular pattern of Wickham's striae.

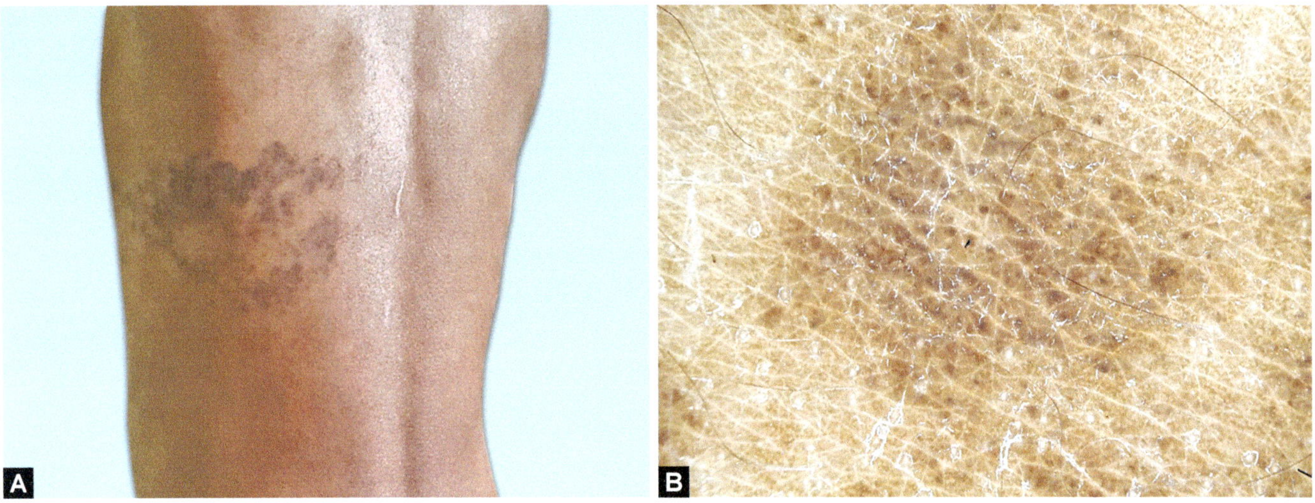

Figs. 11A and B: (A) Zosteriform lichen planus: presence of hyperpigmented macules and a few papules in a dermatomal pattern in a 15-year-old boy; (B) Zosteriform LP: Dermoscopy shows brown dots on a background of diffuse pigmentation. In presence of only diffuse hyperpigmentation, resolution is earlier. In case there are predominantly dots and globules, the disease tends to persist. The pathogenesis of zosteriform LP has many theories but the immunological hypothesis is widely accepted.

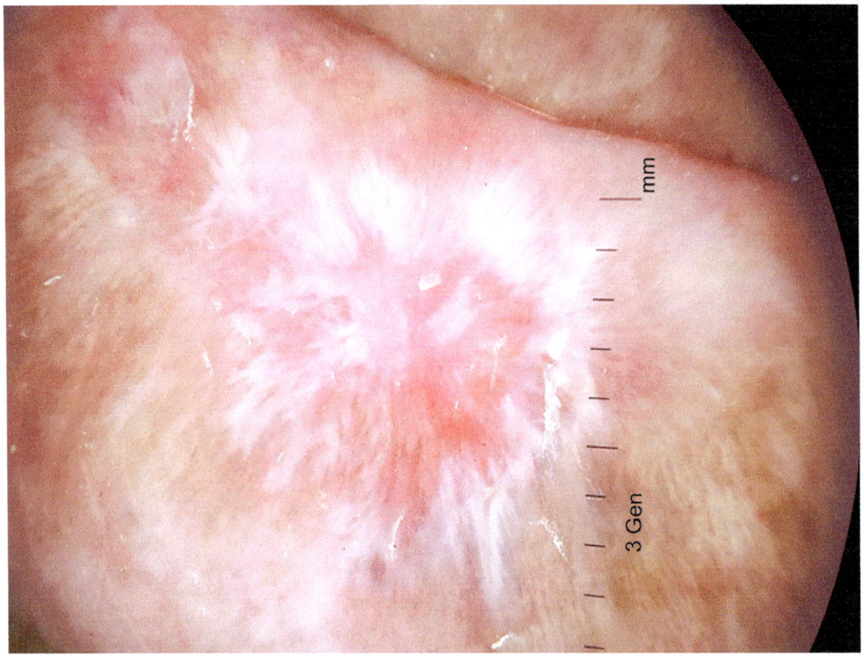

Fig. 12: Oral mucosal lichen planus, demonstrating radiating Wickham's striae.

SUGGESTED READING

1. Cho S, Whang KK. Lichen planus pigmentosus presenting in zosteriform pattern. J Dermatol. 1997;24:193-7.
2. Chuong CM, Dhouailly D, Gilmore S, et al. What is the biological basis of pattern formation of skin lesions? Exp Dermatol. 2006;15:547-64.
3. Frank G, Happle R. Cutaneous mosaicism: Right before our eyes. J Clin Invest. 2007;117:1216.
4. Friedman P, Sabban EC, Marcucci C, et al. Dermoscopic findings in different clinical variants of lichen planus. Is dermoscopy useful? Dermatol Pract Concept. 2015;5:51-5.
5. Gungor S, Topal IO, Goncu EK. Dermoscopic patterns in active and regressive lichen planus and lichen planus variants: A morphological study. Dermatol Pract Concept. 2015;5(2):6.
6. Gupta S, Thomas M, Mahendra A. Unilateral lichen planus along the lines of Blashko: A rare clinical presentation. Acta Med Indones. 2012;44:163-4.

7. Kanwar AJ, Dogra S, Handa S, et al. A study of 124 Indian patients with lichen planus pigmentosus. Clin Exp Dermatol. 2003;28: 481-5.
8. Knackstedt TJ, Collins LK, Li Z, et al. Squamous cell carcinoma arising in hypertrophic lichen planus: A review and analysis of 38 cases. Dermatol Surg. 2015;41(12):1411-8.
9. Lallas A, Giacomel J, Argenziano G, et al. Dermoscopy in general dermatology: Practical tips for the clinician. Br J Dermatol. 2014;170(3):514-26.
10. Lallas A, Kyrgidis A, Tzellos TG, et al. Accuracy of dermoscopic criteria for the diagnosis of psoriasis, dermatitis, lichen planus and pityriasis rosea. Br J Dermatol. 2012;166:1198-205.
11. Malakar S, Saha A. Successful treatment of resistant lichen planus pemphigoides with cyclosporine: A new hope. Indian J Dermatol. 2016;61:112-4.
12. Monteagudo B, Suarez-Armor O, Cabanillas M, et al. Superimposed lichen planus pigmentosus. Dermatol Online J. 2014;20(5):22639.
13. Sachdeva S, Sachdeva S, Kapoor P. Wickham striae: Etiopathogenesis and clinical significance. Indian J Dermatol. 2011;56:442-3.
14. Vasquez F, Vidal AM, Zalaudek I. Dermoscopic subpatterns of ashy dermatosis related to lichen planus. Arch Dermatol. 2010;146:110.
15. Vasquez-Lopez F, Alvarez-Cuesta C, Hidalgo-Garcia Y, et al. The handheld dermatoscope improves the recognition of Wickham striae and capillaries in lichen planus lesions. Arch Dermatol. 2001;137:1376.
16. Vasquez-Lopez F, Manjon Haces JA, Maldonado-Seral C, et al. Dermoscopic features of plaque psoriasis and lichen planus: new observations. Dermatology. 2003;207:151-6.
17. Vazquez F, Maldonado C, Lopez M, et al. Dermatoscopy of pigmented lichen planus lesions. Clin Exp Dermatol. 2003;28:554-5.
18. Vazquez-Lopez F, Gomez-Diez S, Sanchez J, et al. Dermoscopy of active lichen planus. Arch Dermatol. 2007;143(8):1092.
19. Zalaudek I, Argenziano G. Dermoscopy subpatterns of inflammatory skin disorders. Arch Dermatol. 2006;142(6):808.
20. Zalaudek I. Dermoscopy in general dermatology. In: Marghoob A, Malvehy J, Braun R (Eds). Atlas of Dermoscopy, 2nd edition. London: Informa Healthcare; 2012. pp. 329.

PITYRIASIS ROSEA

INTRODUCTION

Pityriasis rosea (PR) is an acute, self-limiting, and papulosquamous dermatosis with a duration of about 8–10 weeks. It commonly affects children, following an upper respiratory illness. It usually begins with a solitary, scaly plaque that heralds the onset of the disease, referred to as "herald patch". Then, crops of round to oval erythematous scaly patches appear arranged along Blaschko's lines.

Atypical presentations may be seen in one-fifth of the cases; the pattern of distribution may be altered as in inverse PR or localized PR in a single area like abdomen, distal extremities, palms and soles, or even a unilateral distribution. Sometimes herald patch may be absent. In other cases, double herald patch or presence of herald patch without crops of lesions may also be seen.

It has been reported that approximately 50% of the cases occur before the age of 20 years and there is a tendency to lifelong immunity in 98% of the cases.

It may mimic other conditions such as tinea corporis, secondary syphilis, guttate psoriasis, nummular eczema, seborrheic dermatitis, etc.[1-3]

In these circumstances, dermoscopic examination may point to the exact diagnosis.

KEY DERMOSCOPIC FEATURES[4-6]

- *Collarette of scale*: Arrangement of peripheral scaling along the border of the annular lesion represents the collarette seen clinically
- Occasionally, scaling may be diffuse and irregular instead of collarette
- Peripheral brown pigmentation, arranged in an annular fashion
- Irregularly distributed dotted vessels
- Yellow-orange structureless areas
- Accentuation of central melanocytic network of the lesion (personal observation).

DISCUSSION

Dermoscopy of both the herald patch and the secondary lesions may classically show "collarette sign" that consists of fragments of scales that from the border into the center of the lesion, like a curtain. Scaling at the periphery may often not show collarette but may instead be in the form of a diffuse irregular arrangement at the border.

In contrast to the regularly distributed dotted vessels in psoriasis, vessels in PR are distributed in an irregular or focal fashion; though they are quite uncommon in darker skin.

Localized or diffuse yellowish-orange structureless areas may also be observed specially in Caucasians whereas in darker skin, this dermoscopic structure is rarely visible. On the contrary, in darker skin, peripheral brown patch is frequently associated with the peripheral scale (personal observation).

KEYNOTE

Dermoscopy may be highly helpful to differentiate PR from other close differentials such as tinea corporis, psoriasis, seborrheic dermatitis, erythema annulare centrifugum, granuloma annulare, porokeratosis, and nummular eczema; as all of them have characteristic dermoscopic features **(Figs. 13 to 17)**.

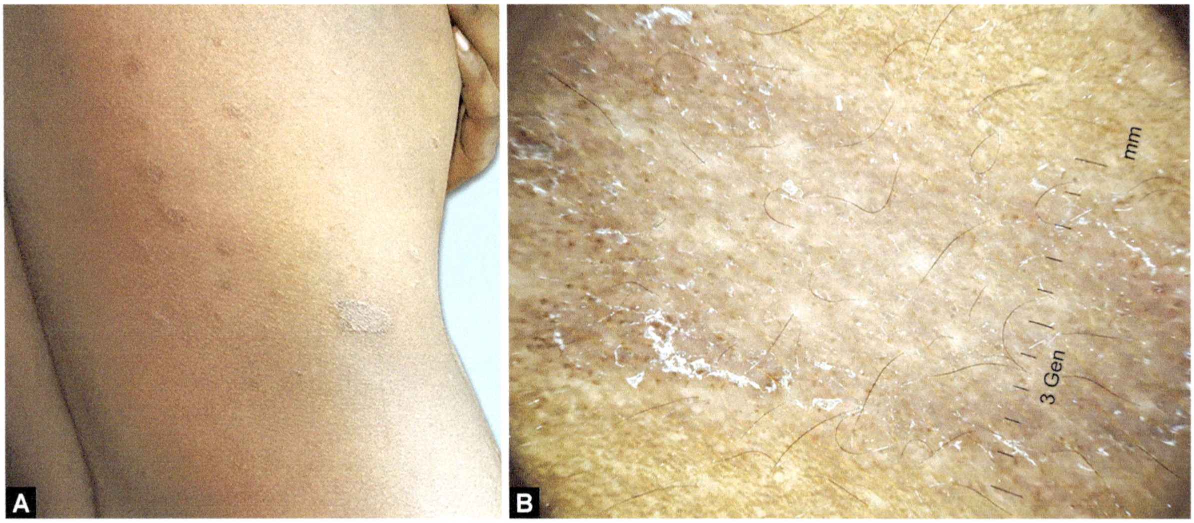

Figs. 13A and B: (A) A classical case of PR with herald patch and a crop of scaly papules, arranged along Blaschko's lines; (B) Typical findings of pityriasis rosea include peripheral and annular brown patch. Here, irregular scaling can also be appreciated at the periphery of the lesion.

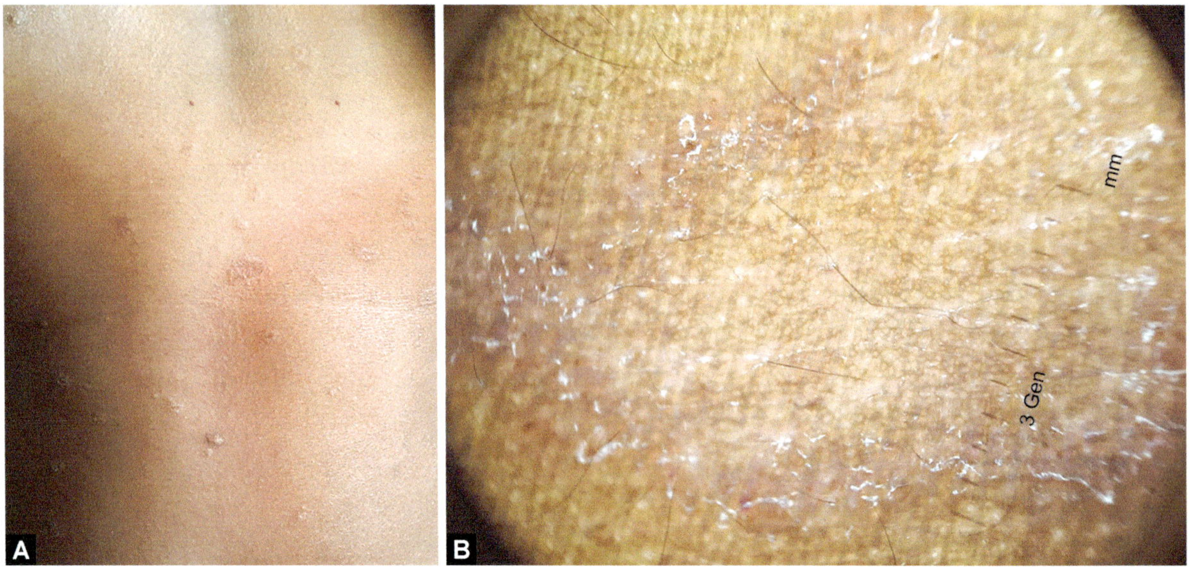

Figs. 14A and B: (A) Herald patch of PR along with multiple hyperpigmented to erythematous, scaly papules in a 16-year-old boy. Clinically, a fine collarette of scale can be appreciated; (B) A typical patch of PR sometimes shows diffuse and irregular scales instead of the classical collarette scale. Note the peripheral brown patch and also accentuation of central pigment network.

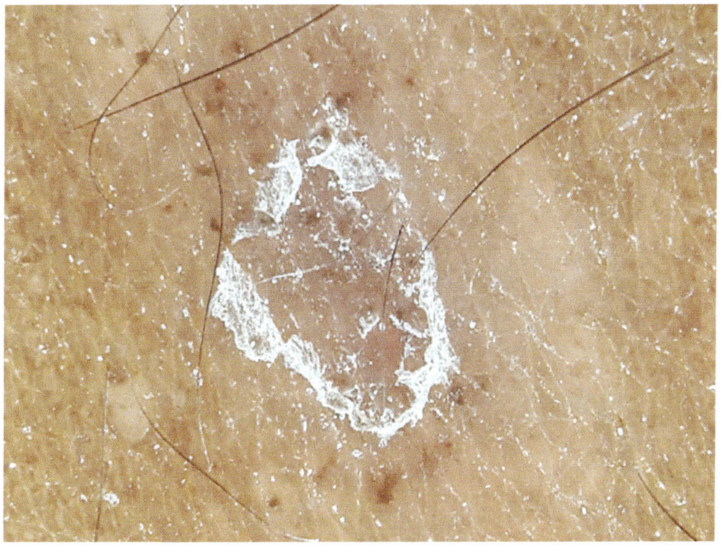

Fig. 15: A typical PR lesion showing a well-defined collarette of scale, attached at the periphery, hanging inward toward the center of the lesion.

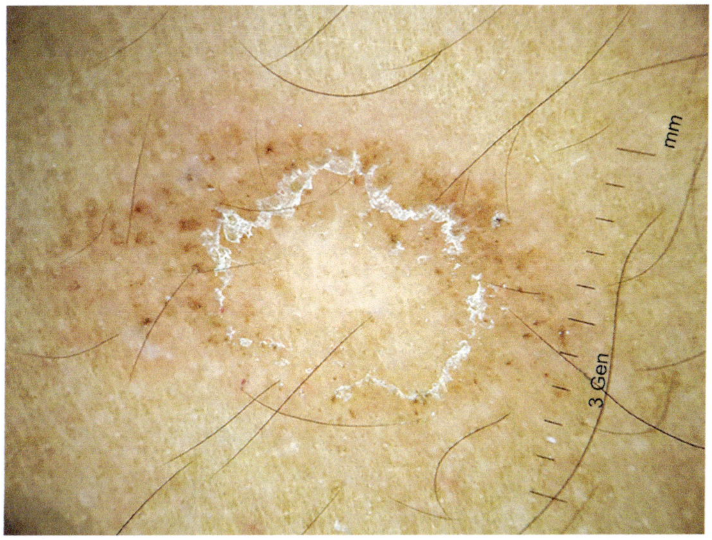

Fig. 16: Peripheral scales, hanging inward. Few dotted vessels in patchy distribution and red/orange color are seen peripherally.

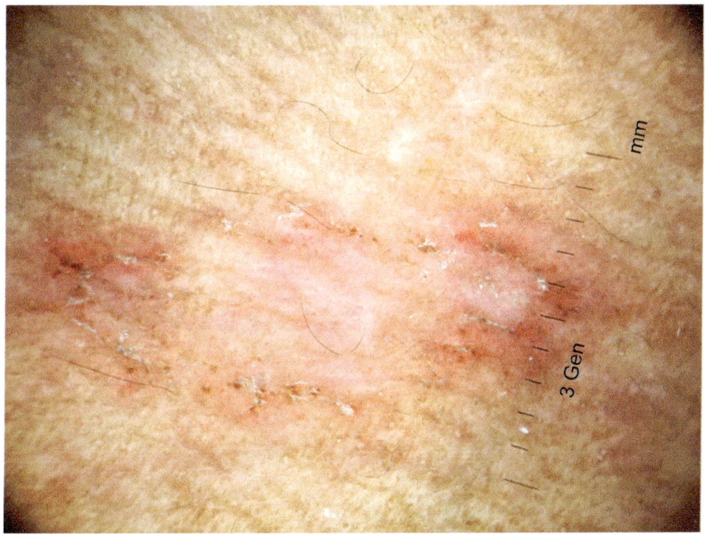

Fig. 17: Dermoscopy of PR showing irregular and sparse scaling at the periphery of an oblong plaque. In addition, orange color along with irregular red dots can be appreciated.

REFERENCES

1. Allen RA, Janniger CK, Schwartz RA. Pityriasis rosea. Cutis. 1995;56(4):198-202.
2. González LM, Allen R, Janniger CK, et al. Pityriasis rosea: An important papulosquamous disorder. Int J Dermatol. 2005;44(9): 757-64.
3. Browning JC. An update on pityriasis rosea and other similar childhood exanthems. Curr Opin Pediatr. 2009;21(4):481-5.
4. Tognetti L, Sbano P, Fimiani M, et al. Dermoscopy of Biett's sign and differential diagnosis with annular maculo-papular rashes with scaling. Indian J Dermatol Venereol Leprol. 2017;83:270-3.
5. Lallas A, Kyrgidis A, Tzellos TG, et al. Accuracy of dermoscopic criteria for the diagnosis of psoriasis, dermatitis, lichen planus and pityriasis rosea. Br J Dermatol. 2012;166:1198-205.
6. S Malakar. Papulosquamous disorders. In: Dermoscopy Text and Atlas. New Delhi: Jaypee Publishers Medical Publishers; 2019. pp. 128-31.

LICHEN NITIDUS

INTRODUCTION

Clinical diagnosis of lichen nitidus can be challenging as it mimics various conditions like polymorphous light eruption, lichen striatus, lichen sclerosus, etc. thus posing a diagnostic challenge. Dermoscopy demonstrates diagnostic findings, which help delineate lichen nitidus from other similar conditions obviating the need for biopsy.

Recent reports of linear lichen nitidus have intrigued many. In this discussion, we have included a similar case of linear lichen nitidus, which was confirmed on clinico-dermoscopic-histopathological evaluation.

KEY DERMOSCOPIC FEATURES

- Multiple, white, well-circumscribed circular areas, 1–2 mm in diameter with a smooth surface.
- An indistinct brown ghost shadow reflects through the center of each of these white circles.

DISCUSSION

White circles on dermoscopy are known to correspond to epidermal acanthosis on histopathology. The brownish ghost shadow at the center of each of these white circles, is a reflection of the underlying dense granulomatous foci of lymphocytes and epithelioid cells in the dermal papilla. This deduction concurs with the observation of the "peripilar sign" in cases of early androgenetic alopecia, wherein the superficial perifollicular lymphocytic infiltrate is seen as a brown halo around the hair follicles.

Hence, in lichen nitidus, the epidermal acanthosis corresponds to white circles and the central brownish shadow reflected through the white circles correspond to the inflammatory infiltrate enveloped by the acanthotic rete ridges.

KEYNOTE

Ghost shadow on dermoscopy establishes a strong dermoscopic and histopathological correlation in lichen nitidus, which enables us to differentiate it from other conditions mimicking it, such as polymorphous light eruption, lichen sclerosus, etc. **(Figs. 18 to 20)**.

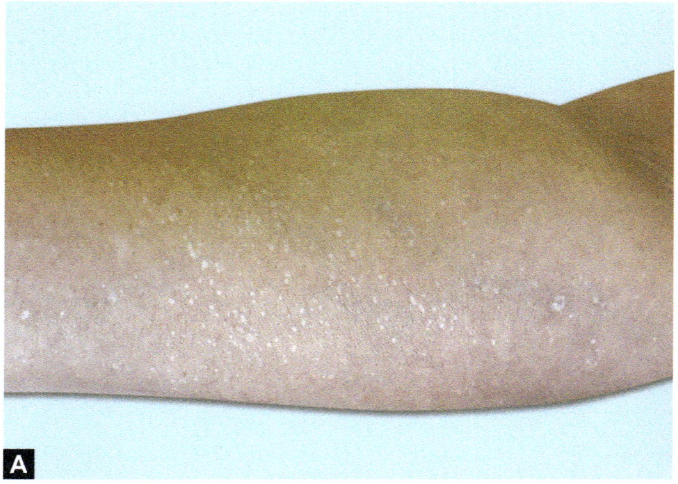

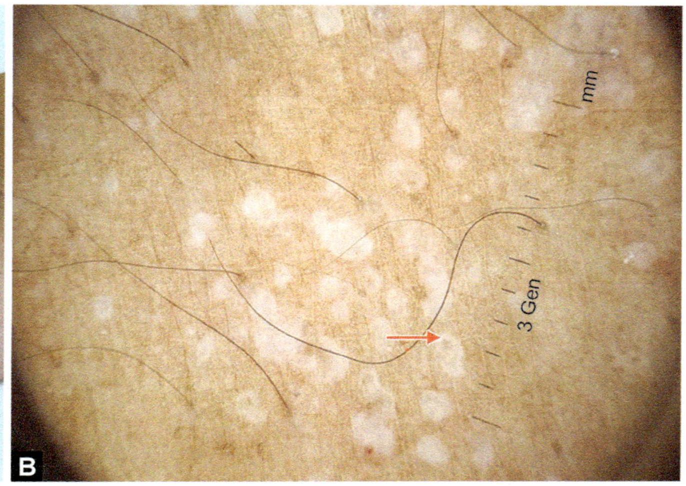

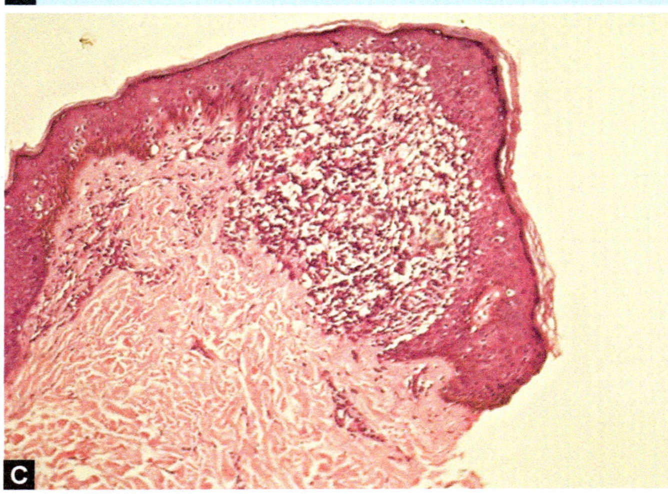

Figs. 18A to C: (A) A 10-year-old child with multiple white colored flat-topped papules over both the forearms; (B) Multiple, white, well-circumscribed circular areas, 1–2 mm in diameter with a smooth surface. An indistinct brown ghost shadow (red arrow) was reflected through the center of each of these white circles; (C) Histopathology revealed a circumscribed subepidermal dense focal lymphohistiocytic infiltrate along with occasional Langhans giant cells, flanked by collarettes of epidermal acanthosis on either sides which gave the "ball-in-clutch" appearance confirming the diagnosis of lichen nitidus. The overlying epidermis shows evidence of acanthosis and focal parakeratosis.

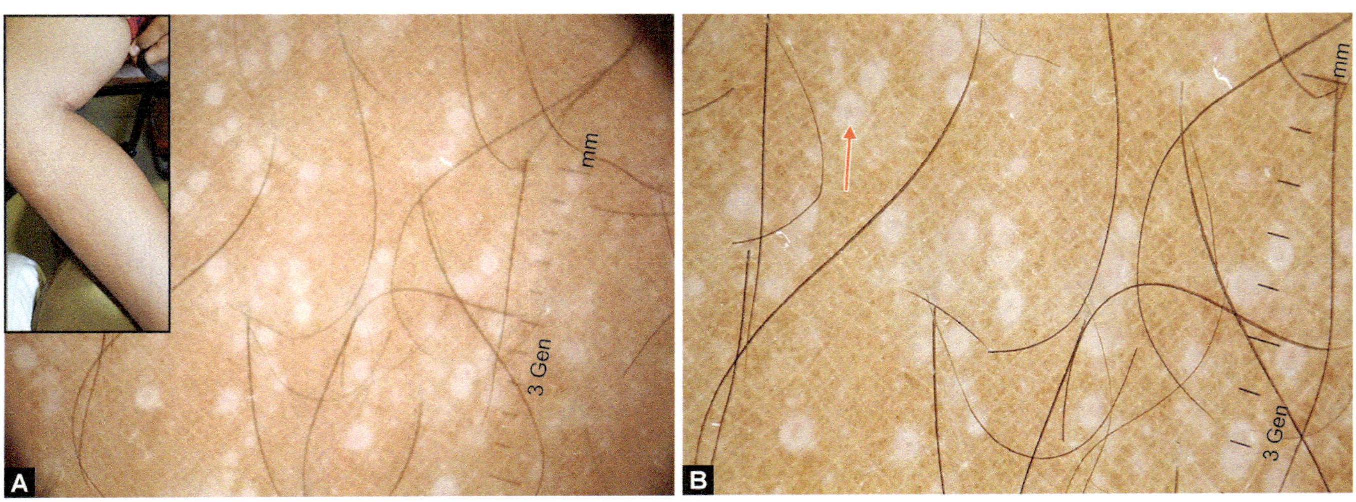

Figs. 19A and B: (A) A 9-year-old child with multiple shiny skin colored to hypopigmented papules arranged in a linear fashion in the right lower limb (Inset). Clinical differentials considered were lichen striatus and linear lichen nitidus. Dermoscopy shows multiple white, well-circumscribed circular areas with a smooth surface; (B) Dermoscopy (zoomed in view) of the same child showing indistinct brown ghost shadow (red arrows) in the center of all the white areas. Further histopathology done from these lesions demonstrated typical features of lichen nitidus thus confirming the dermoscopic diagnosis.

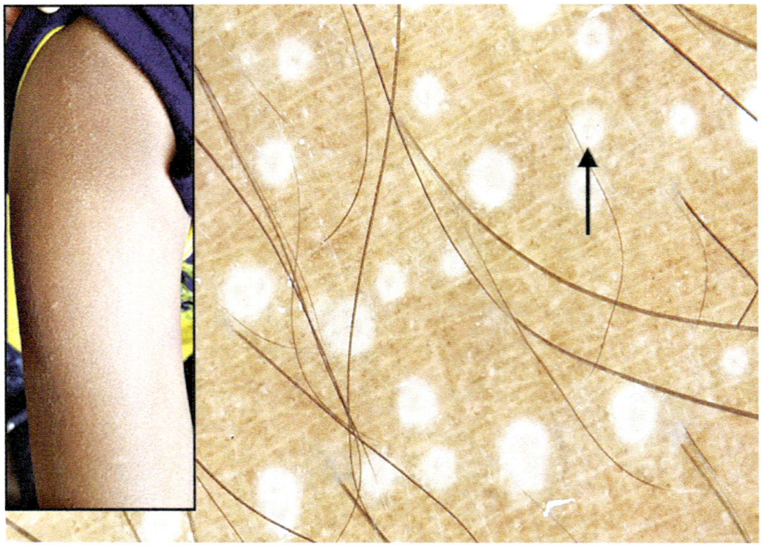

Fig. 20: Another child with similar lesions on the right forearm (inset). Dermoscopy of the lesions showed multiple well circumscribed whitish areas with a brown shadow in the center (black arrow), pointing to a diagnosis of lichen nitidus.[1]

REFERENCE

1. Malakar S, Save S, Mehta P. Brown shadow in lichen nitidus: A dermoscopic marker!. Indian Dermatol Online J. 2018;9: 479-80.

CHAPTER 6

Hereditary Disorders of Cornification

Subrata Malakar, Rashmi Agarwal, Seujee Das, Harshal Ranglani, Surit Malakar

DARIER'S DISEASE (KERATOSIS FOLLICULARIS)

INTRODUCTION

It is an autosomal dominant disorder, which first manifests in children of around 8–15 years of age[1] as dirty warty papules, mainly in the seborrheic areas. Characteristic palmar pits and punctate keratosis along with nail changes are present in most of the cases. Atypical presentations like linear pattern, freckle like lesions, blistered papules, etc. can also be seen. The use of dermoscopy, in addition to being a possible diagnostic tool, highlights the recognition of subtle but important features of Darier's disease (DD).

KEY DERMOSCOPIC FEATURES

- Polygonal star-like or round oval shaped yellow-brown areas with a collar of yellowish scales (pseudocomedones). A whitish halo surrounds the pseudocomedones
- Whitish scaling over a reddish-yellow background
- Dotted/linear/irregular vessels
- "Dermoscopic dirty scalp".

DISCUSSION

The central polygonal brownish star-shaped areas of the pseudocomedones on dermoscopy correspond histopathologically to compact hyperkeratosis and the whitish halo to acanthosis. The pinkish background along with the presence of vessels of different patterns indicates dermal inflammation.

On trichoscopic examination, the scalp shows a dirty look because of the presence of excess scales and excess sebum trapping the dirt from the environment. So, we have coined the term "dermoscopic dirty scalp" for the appearance of the scalp in Darier's disease.

KEYNOTE

Pseudocomedones seen on dermoscopy is a characteristic feature of Darier's disease corresponding to hyperkeratosis histopathologically. This feature is highly helpful in cases of diagnostic dilemma to rule out other dermatoses with similar presentations like seborrheic dermatitis **(Figs. 1 to 11)**.

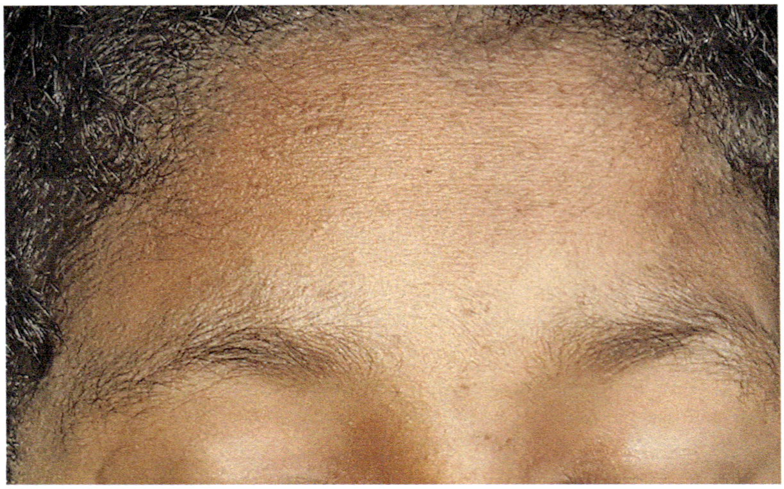

Fig. 1: Dirty warty papules over the forehead of a 13-year-old girl with Darier's disease. Similar lesions were present over other seborrheic areas.

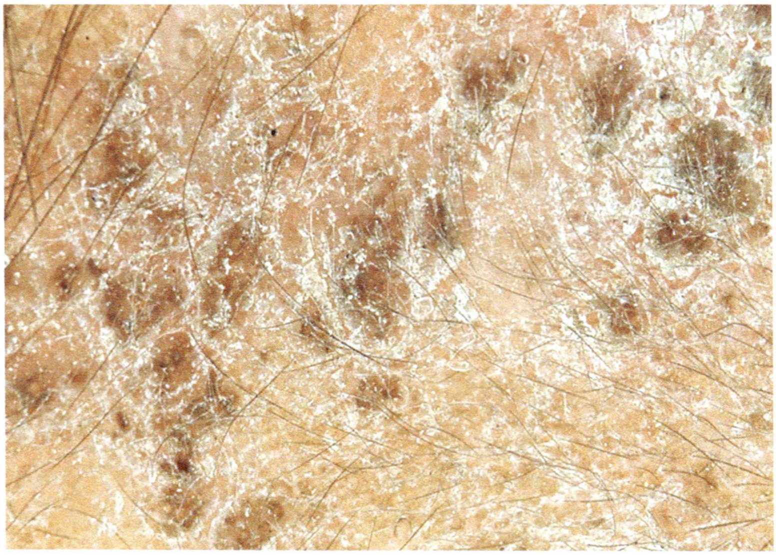

Fig. 2: Dermoscopy showing pseudocomedones. They are polygonal and oval brownish areas often surrounded by whitish halo. In this field, peudocomedones appear conglomerated.

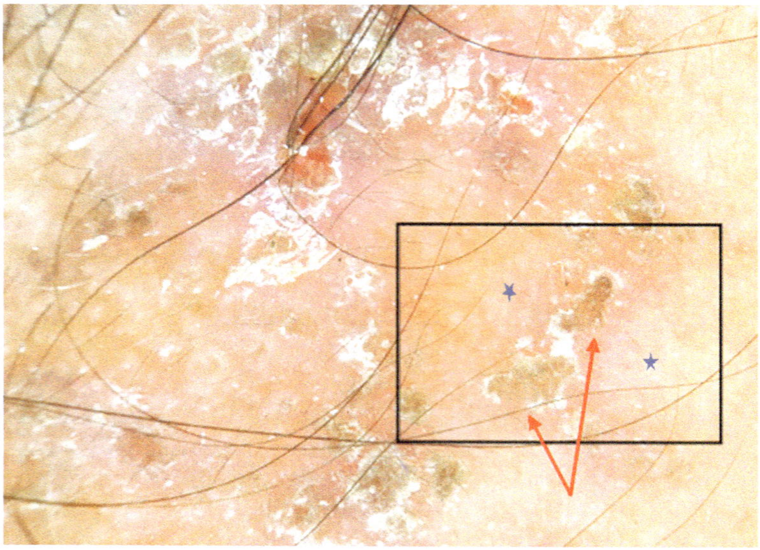

Fig. 3: Dermoscopy showing two pseudocomedones (red arrows) surrounded by whitish halo (blue stars) in the marked field.

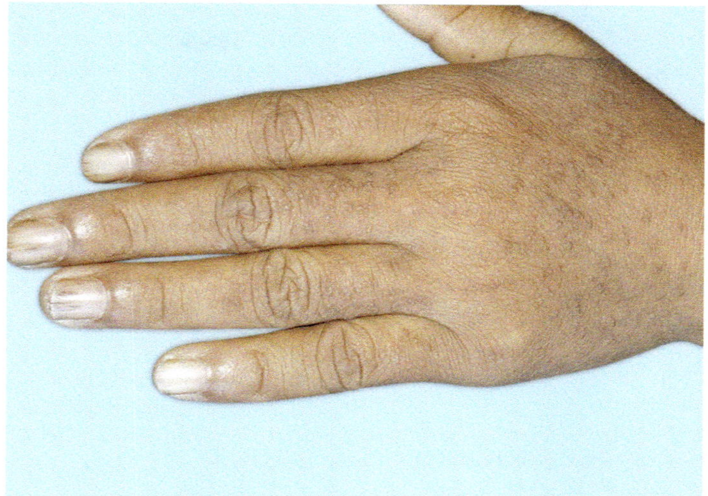

Fig. 4: Hyperkeratotic papules present over the dorsum of the hand and fingers.

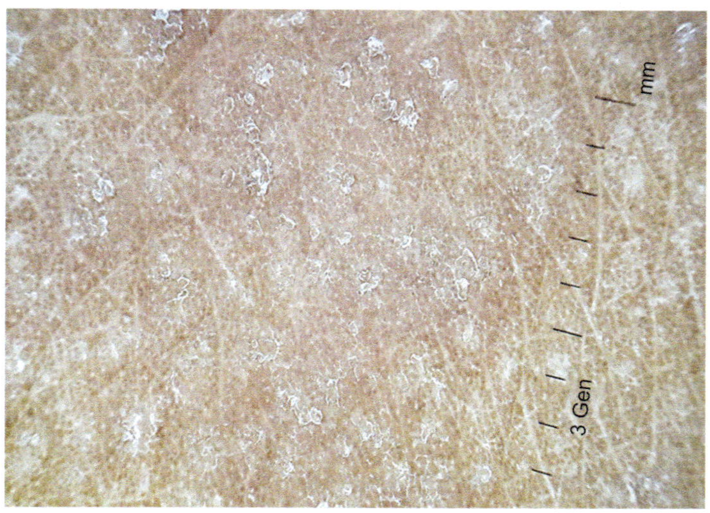

Fig. 5: Dermoscopy of the dorsum of hand showing plenty of pseudocomedones in yellowish red background which appears brownish in skin of color.

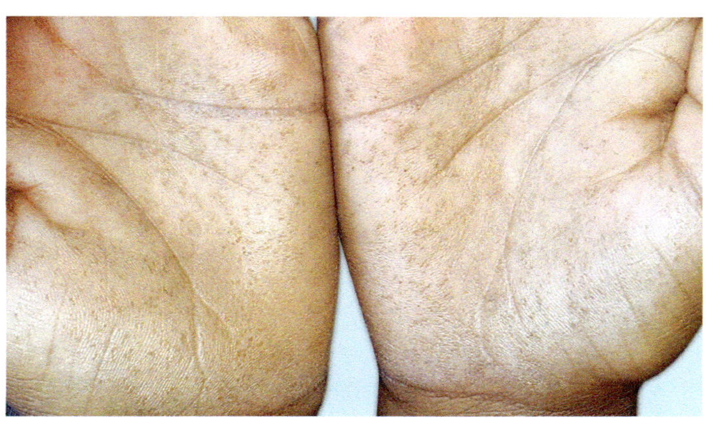

Fig. 6: Multiple palmar pits and punctate keratosis.

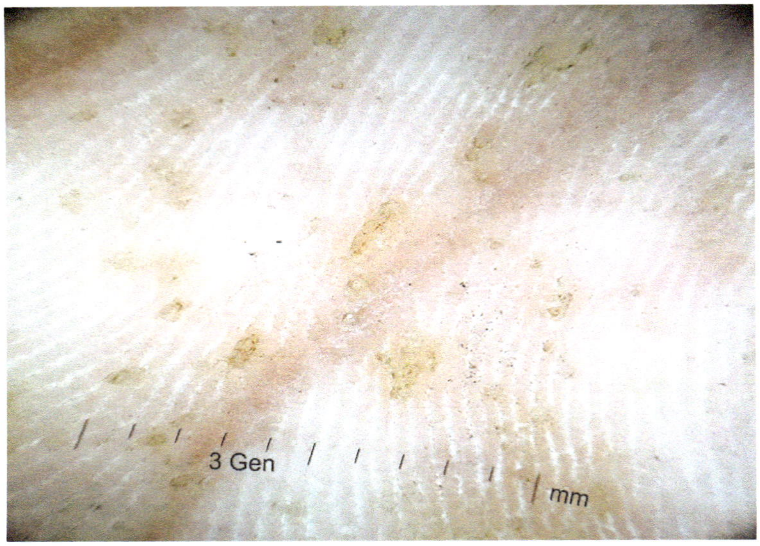

Fig. 7: Dermoscopy of palm enhancing the pits and punctate keratosis.

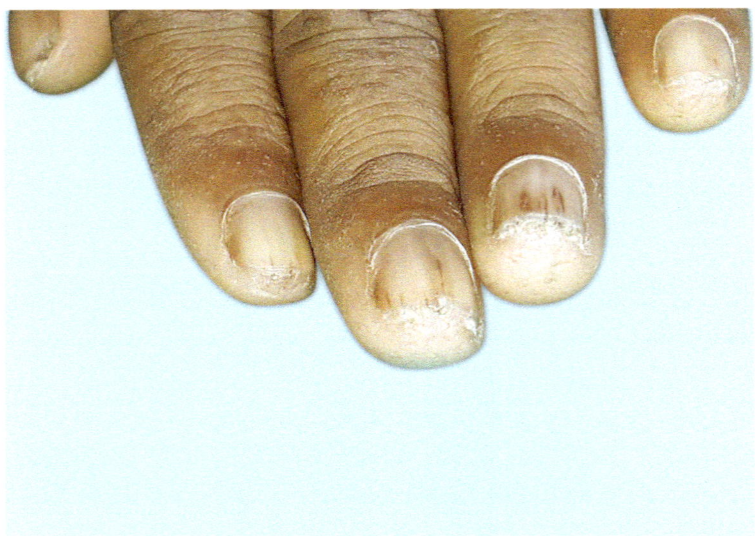

Fig. 8: Nail examination reveals V-shaped nick, splinter hemorrhages, alternating red and white bands, and subungual hyperkeratosis.

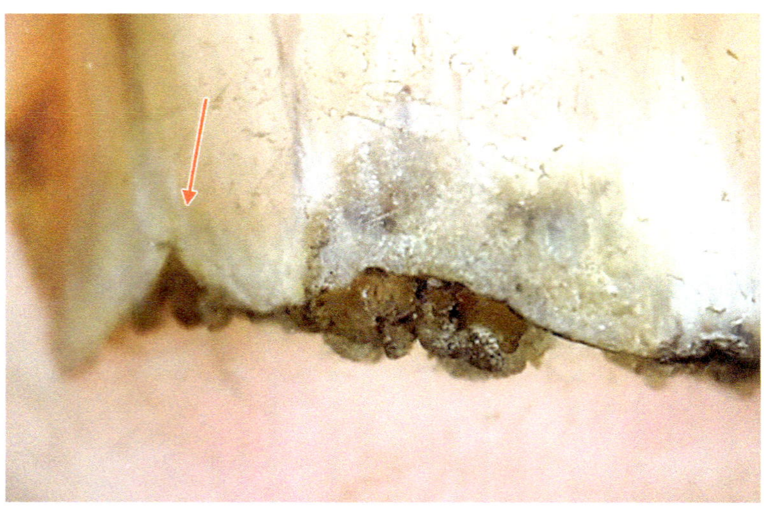

Fig. 9: Onychoscopy enhancing the V-shaped nick (red arrow) at the free margin of the nail. Note the obvious subungual hyperkeratosis.

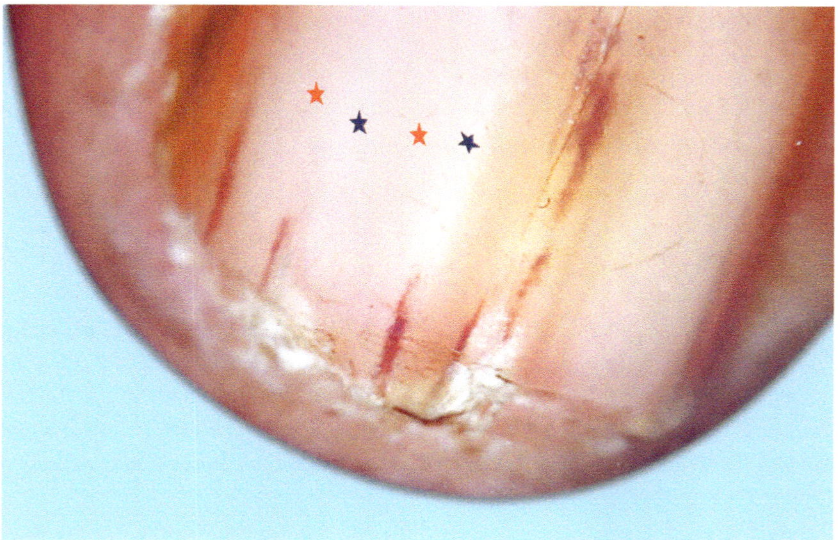

Fig. 10: Onychoscopy enhancing all the nail changes of Darier's disease—V-shaped nick, splinter hemorrhages, alternate red (red stars), and white (black stars) bands.

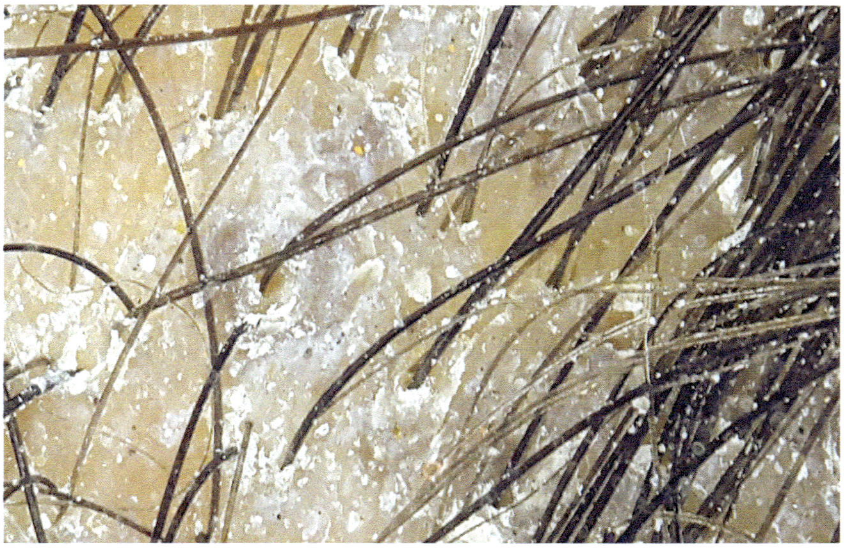

Fig. 11: "Dermoscopic dirty scalp" of Darier's disease.

REFERENCE

1. Amy PS, Mancini AJ. Hereditary disorders of cornification. Hurwitz Clinical Pediatric Dermatology: A Textbook of Skin Disorders of Childhood and Adolescence, 5th edition. Edinburgh: Elsevier; 2016. pp. 111-2.

POROKERATOSIS

INTRODUCTION

Porokeratosis is a disorder of epidermal keratinization characterized by annular plaques with a hyperkeratotic rim, which corresponds to its typical histopathologic feature, i.e. the cornoid lamella.

KEY DERMOSCOPIC FEATURES[1-8]

- "White track" structure—annular peripheral whitish hyperkeratotic structure
- The center of the lesion is atrophic which typically shows whitish or brownish color and may exhibit dotted or linear vessels according to the disease subtype and stage of progression
- Dark-brown globules/dots
- Hyperpigmented border.

DISCUSSION

The hallmark dermoscopic feature of all subtypes of porokeratosis is "white track" structure, which appears as a well-defined, whitish, peripheral, and annular hyperkeratotic structure. "Cornoid lamella" the histopathological hallmark of porokeratosis corresponds to this "white track" structure. The "white track" structure is somewhat identical to the outlines of a volcanic crater as observed from above. It may be hyperpigmented in disseminated superficial actinic porokeratosis.

The center of the lesion is typically whitish or brownish and may reveal circular or linear whitish and/or hyperpigmented tracks, blue-gray dots, and dotted or linear vessels.[4-10]

Yucel et al. reported hyperpigmented border and dark brown dots and globules on a brownish background in the center on dermoscopy of a case of linear porokeratosis **(Figs. 12 to 15)**.[2]

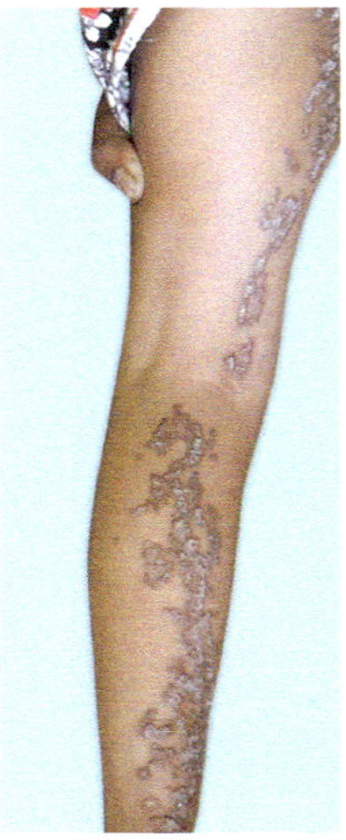

Fig. 12: A 9-year-old child presented with dirty looking warty papules over the lower limb in a linear fashion slowly increasing in extent since 3 years of age.

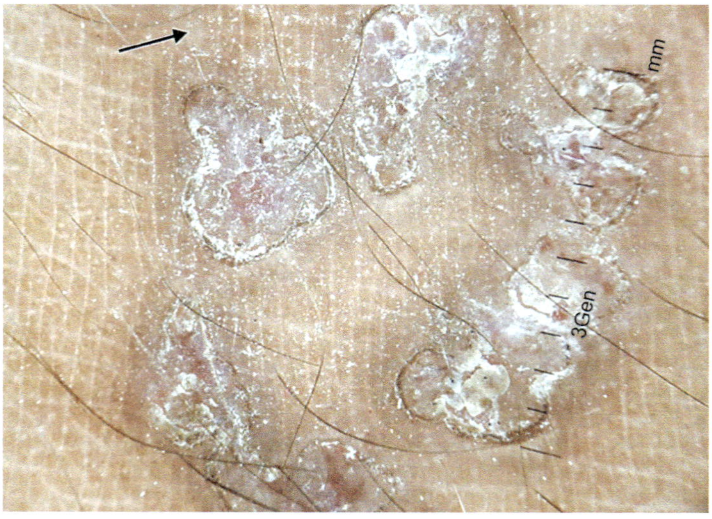

Fig. 13: Dermoscopy shows multiple annular lesions with hyperpigmented border, white track appearance, and atrophic center.

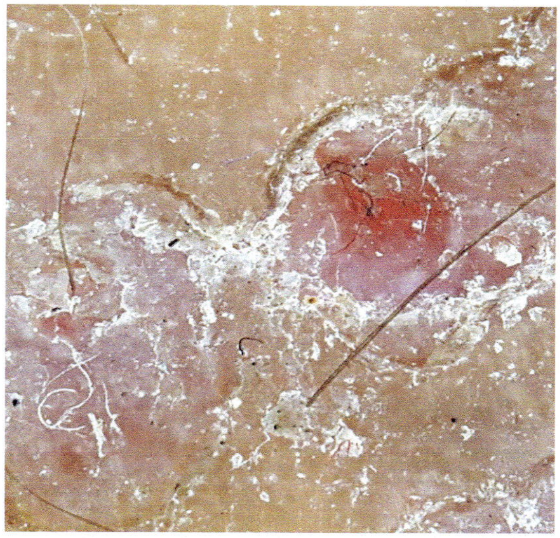

Fig. 14: A close-up view shows central erosion with sticky fiber sign along with other features of porokeratosis.

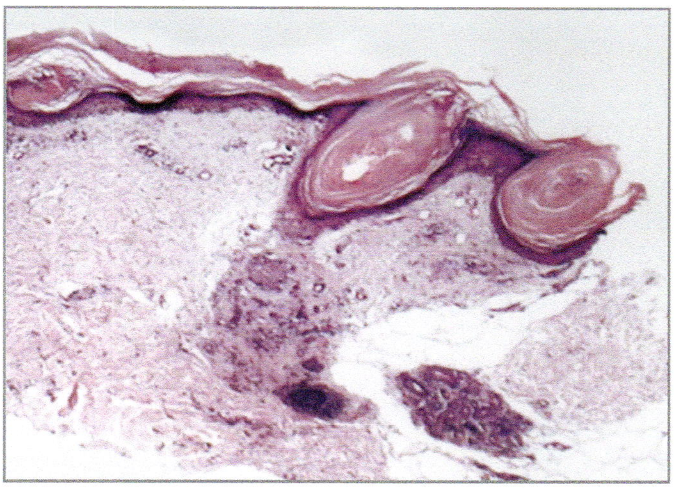

Fig. 15: Biopsy shows a sparse superficial perivascular patchy lichenoid lymphocytic infiltrate with focal interface vacuolar change. In two to three small foci, the epidermis shows deep invaginations of the floor which lacks granular layer. Rising from the center of these invaginations is a tiny column of parakeratotic cells (cornoid lamella). At the bottom of this, are seen scattered dyskeratotic cells.

REFERENCES

1. Delfino M, Argenziano G, Nino M. Dermoscopy for the diagnosis of porokeratosis. J Eur Acad Dermatol Venereol. 2004;18:194-5.
2. Yücel A, Günaştı S, Maraklı SS, et al. A case of linear porokeratosis: Dermoscopic and immunofluorescence findings. J Turk Acad Dermatol. 2008;2(2):82202c.
3. Pizzichetta MA, Canzonieri V, Massone C, et al. Clinical and dermoscopic features of porokeratosis of Mibelli. Arch Dermatol. 2009;145:91-2.
4. Zaballos P, Puig S, Malvehy J. Dermoscopy of disseminated superficial actinic porokeratosis. Arch Dermatol. 2004;140:1410.
5. Panasiti V, Rossi M, Curzio M, et al. Disseminated superficial actinic porokeratosis diagnosed by dermoscopy. Int J Dermatol. 2008;47:308-10.
6. Oiso N, Kawada A. Dermoscopic features in disseminated superficial actinic porokeratosis. Eur J Dermatol. 2011;21: 439-40.
7. Uhara H, Kamijo F, Okuyama R, et al. Open pores with plugs in porokeratosis clearly visualized with the dermoscopic furrow ink test: Report of 3 cases. Arch Dermatol. 2011;147:866-8.
8. Moscarella E, Longo C, Zalaudek I, et al. Dermoscopy and confocal microscopy clues in the diagnosis of psoriasis and porokeratosis. J Am Acad Dermatol. 2013;69:e231-3.
9. Hayashi Y, Ozeki M, Ishizaki S, et al. Inguinal porokeratosis in a Japanese man. Dermatol Pract Concept. 2013;3:29-31.
10. Vargas-Laguna E, Nagore E, Alfaro A, et al. Monitoring the evolution of a localized type of porokeratosis using dermatoscopy. Actas Dermosifiliogr. 2006;97:77-8.

NETHERTON SYNDROME

INTRODUCTION

Netherton syndrome (NS)—an autosomal recessive condition that is characterized by ichthyosis linearis circumflexa (ILC), atopy, and hair shaft deformities.

In some patients, the sole presentation may be ILC without the other features of NS. ILC is characterized by migratory polycyclic scaly lesions with a peripheral double-edged scale.[1] Routine histologic examination is not helpful to diagnose ILC.[1]

The classic hair shaft abnormality is trichorrhexis invaginata (bamboo hairs). Dermoscopy shows "match-stick" hair defect.[2]

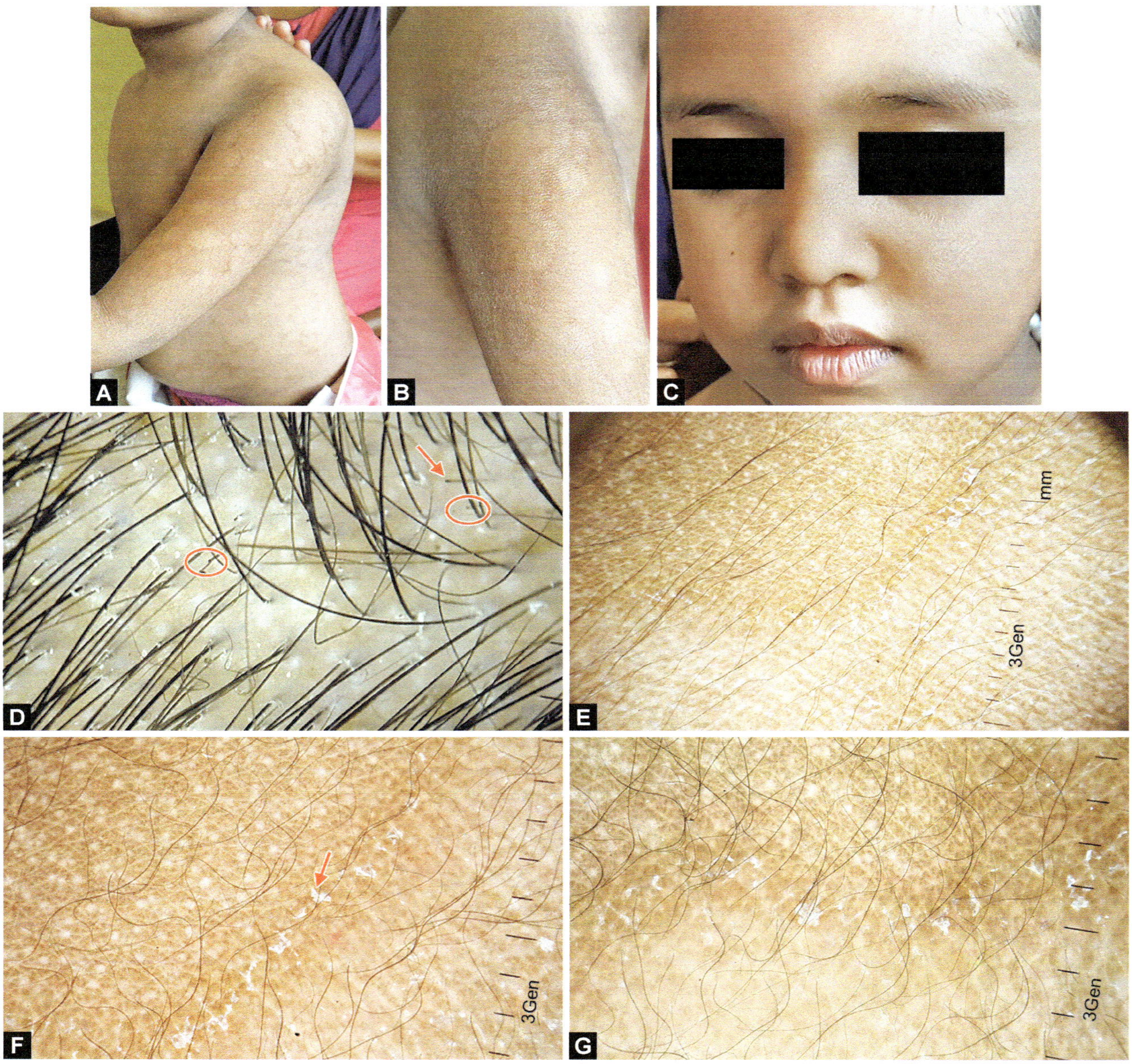

Figs. 16A to G: (A) Netherton syndrome in a 4.5-year-old girl showing polycyclic lesions of ILC; (B) Close-up view showing polycyclic lesions and double-edged scales; (C) Polycyclic lesions involving face and eyelids. Note the eyebrow involvement; (D) Trichoscopy shows multiple match-stick hairs (red circles and arrow); (E) Compare the normal and lesional skin. Note the prominent pinpoint white dots of normal skin in comparison to lesional skin; (F) Dermoscopy shows double-edged scales (red arrow); (G) Trichoscopy of another field showing double-edged scales.

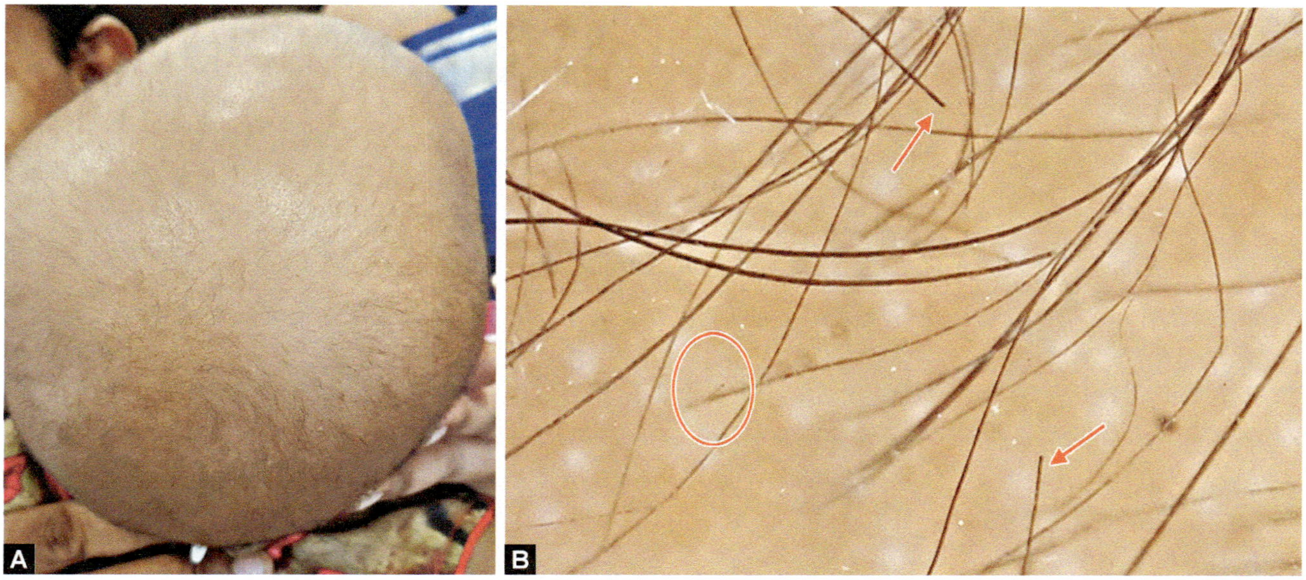

Figs. 17A and B: (A) Scalp showing sparse and short hairs in Netherton syndrome of a 1.5-year-old child; (B) Trichoscopy shows "match-stick" hair defect (red circle and arrows).

KEY DERMOSCOPIC FEATURES

- It highlights the peripheral double-edged scales.
- Pinpoint white dots are much less apparent in lesional skin in comparison to normal uninvolved skin (probably the scales in the lesional skin obscures the sweat glands).
- Melanocytic network appears blunted in comparison to the normal skin.
- Subtle erythema along the polycyclic border.

KEY TRICHOSCOPIC FEATURES

- Hair shaft deformities—shows "match-stick" hair.
- Scalp—mostly perifollicular scales are observed.

KEYNOTE

Trichoscopy of the eyebrow and scalp hair should be done in all cases of erythroderma in children as bamboo hair/match-stick hair is very specific of NS and helps in early diagnosis of this fatal condition **(Figs. 16 and 17)**.

REFERENCES

1. Amy PS, Mancini AJ. Hereditary disorders of cornification. Hurwitz Clinical Pediatric Dermatology: A Textbook of Skin Disorders of Childhood and Adolescence, 5th edition. Edinburgh: Elsevier; 2016. pp. 104-5
2. Meltem Akkurt Z, Tuncel T, Ayhan E, et al. Rapid and easy diagnosis of Netherton syndrome with dermoscopy. J Cutan Med Surg. 2014;18(4):280-2.

CHAPTER 7

Infections and Infestations

Subrata Malakar, Seujee Das, Rashmi Agarwal

INFECTIONS

FUNGAL INFECTIONS

PITYRIASIS VERSICOLOR

Introduction

Pityriasis versicolor (PV) is a common superficial fungal infection of the skin mostly affecting young adults but, it can also affect children, adolescents, and older adults. It is usually asymptomatic, but may be mildly pruritic in a few. It is clinically characterized by hyperpigmented or hypopigmented, round to oval macules and patches commonly found on the trunk, upper arms, and face.[1]

Pityriasis versicolor usually occurs in the summer months as the causative organism has a propensity to grow in hot and humid climate. It is caused by mycelial growth of fungi of the genus *Malassezia*.

Key Dermoscopic Features[2,3]

Fine scales in a net-like distribution in the skin furrows.

Discussion

Pityriasis versicolor is mainly a clinical diagnosis, characterized by thin patches and fine scaling and can be confirmed by skin scraping and microscopy of potassium hydroxide (KOH) preparation, which shows spaghetti and meatball appearance.[4]

However, the fine scales on the affected lesion cannot always be easily observed; and require scratching or scraping to make it apparent. These fine scales with a net-like distribution can easily be observed by a dermoscope which not only obviates the need of scratching but, also prevents unnecessary side laboratory procedures.

Keynote

Dermoscopy may serve as an essential tool for the diagnosis of hyperpigmented and erythematous variant of PV **(Figs. 1 to 4)**.

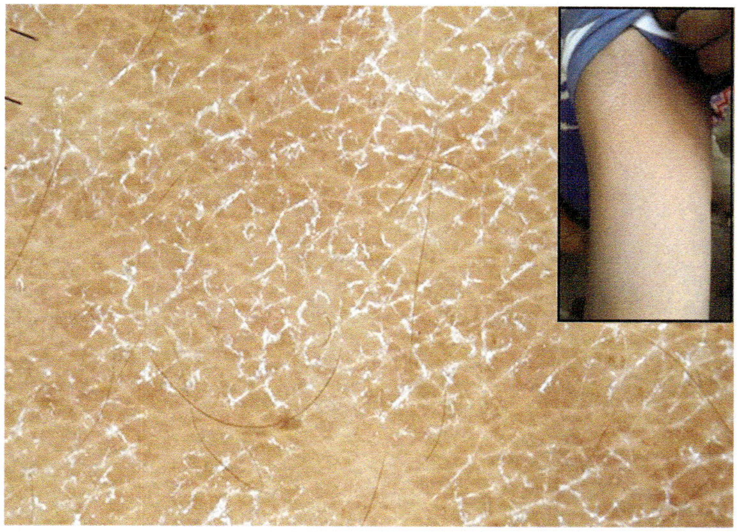

Fig. 1: Net-like scaling confined to the skin furrows.

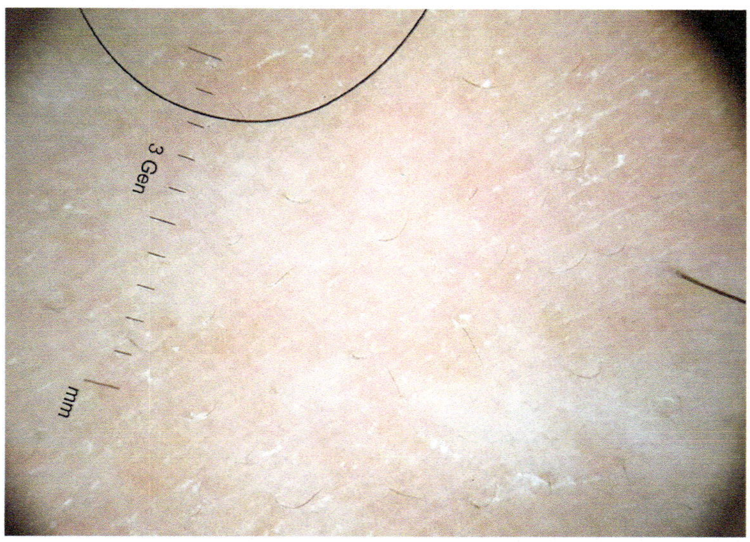

Fig. 2: Dermoscopy of the erythematous variety of PV: erythematous background with net-like scaling.

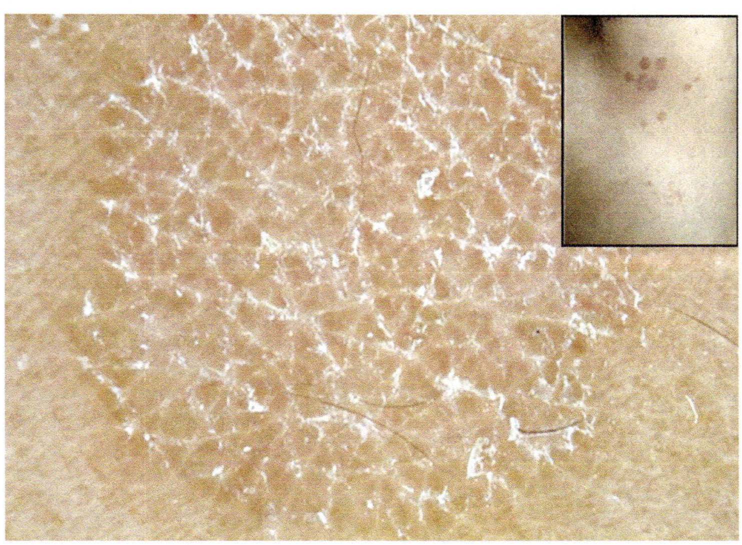

Fig. 3: Dermoscopy of the hyperpigmented variant of PV reveals a brownish background with net-like scales.

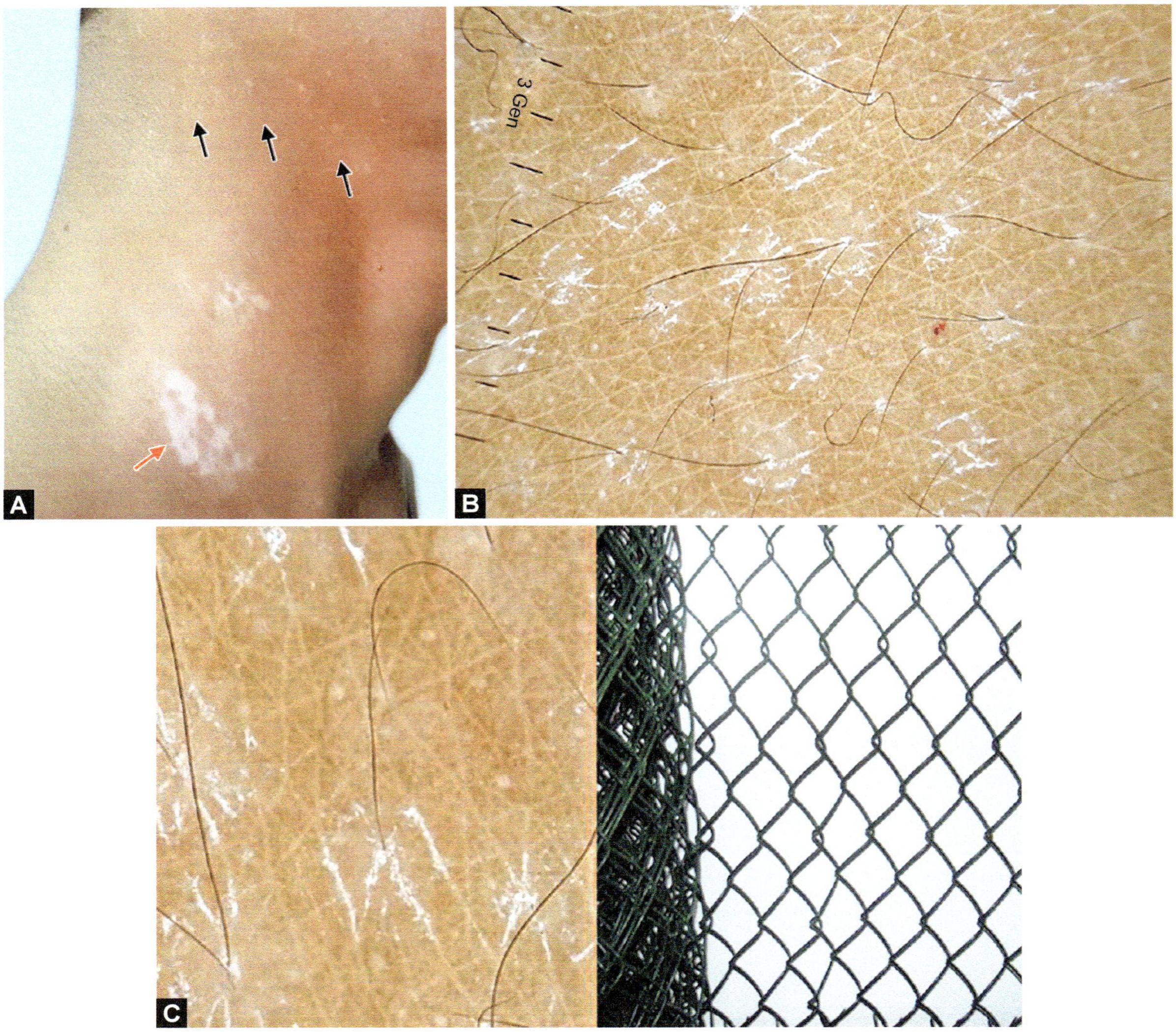

Figs. 4A to C: (A) Patient with vitiligo (red arrow) showing multiple hypopigmented to depigmented macules (black arrows) on the neck; (B) Dermoscopic picture showing fine scales along the skin markings with sparing of the skin between the markings; (C) Magnified dermoscopic picture showing scales arranged along diamond-shaped skin markings giving a "wire fence" or "fish net appearance".

References

1. Pedrosa AF, Lisboa C, Rodrigues AG. Malassezia infections: a medical conundrum. J Am Acad Dermatol. 2014;71(1):170-6.
2. Zhou H, Tang XH, De Han J, et al. Dermoscopy as an ancillary tool for the diagnosis of pityriasis versicolor. J Am Acad Dermatol. 2015;73(6):e205-6.
3. Erichetti E, Stinco G. The practical usefulness of dermoscopy in general dermatology. G Ital Dermatol Venereol. 2015;150:533-46.
4. Thomas N, Malakar S. Dermoscopy: an easy way to solve the diagnostic puzzle in pityriasis versicolor. Indian J Dermatol Venereol Leprol. 2019;85:664-5.

VIRAL INFECTIONS

HPV Infections

COMMON WART (VERRUCA VULGARIS)

Introduction

Verruca vulgaris is characterized by hyperplasia of all the layers of the epidermis caused by the human papilloma virus (HPV). They present as hyperkeratotic papules with a rough, verrucous surface. They can occur in any part of the body but, mostly involve the dorsum of hands and fingers and the knees in children. Dermoscopy not only helps in diagnosing the condition but also in therapeutic monitoring after treatment to evaluate a possible recurrence.

Key Dermoscopic Features[1-3]

- Multiple densely packed papillae, each containing a central red dot or loop
- Whitish keratotic halo.

Discussion

Dermoscopy of a common wart reveals numerous densely packed papillae each containing a central red or black dot or loop, surrounded by a whitish halo. These features altogether give the appearance of a frogspawn. The red dots and black dots correspond to normal and thrombosed vessels, respectively, while the keratotic whitish halo corresponds to papillomatosis on histopathology. The halo may not be visible in case of significant vascular occlusion **(Figs. 5 to 8)**.

The central vessels are usually larger in comparison to plane warts and frequently associated with hemorrhages. This feature helps when the diagnosis is in doubt such as in cases of irritated or periungual warts.[1]

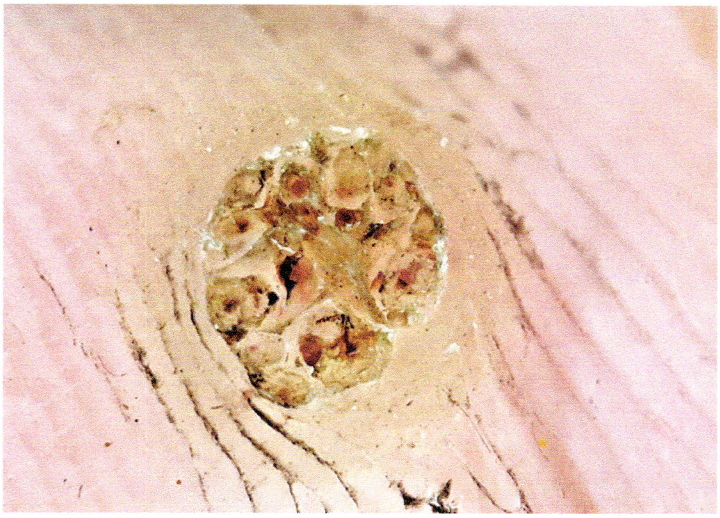

Fig. 5: Dermoscopy reveals red dots and keratotic halos.

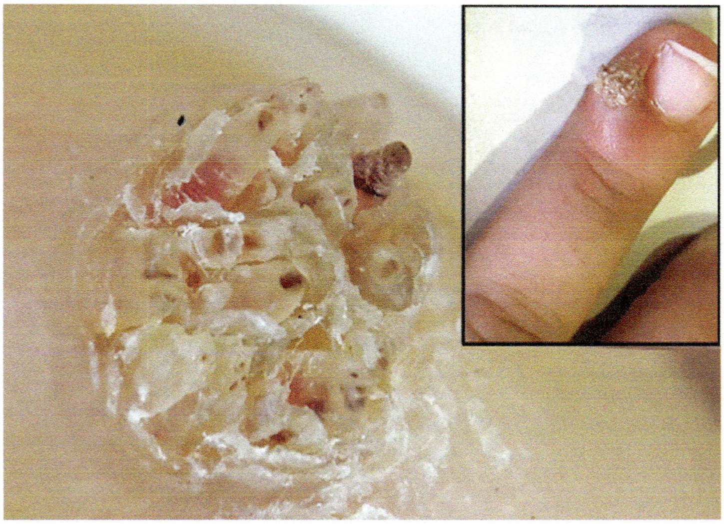

Fig. 6: Clinical and dermoscopic picture of verruca vulgaris on the fingers (common in children with easy transmission through fomites/direct contact, therefore early diagnosis and treatment is imperative).

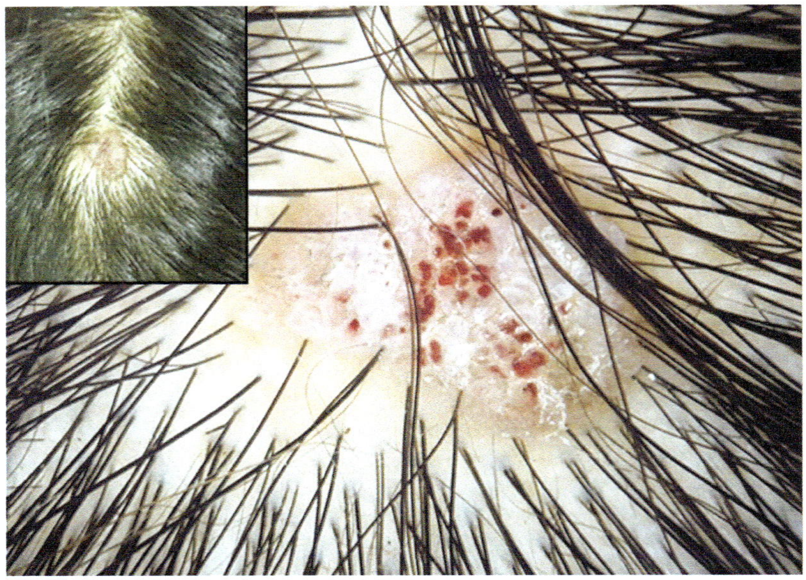

Fig. 7: Verruca on the scalp.

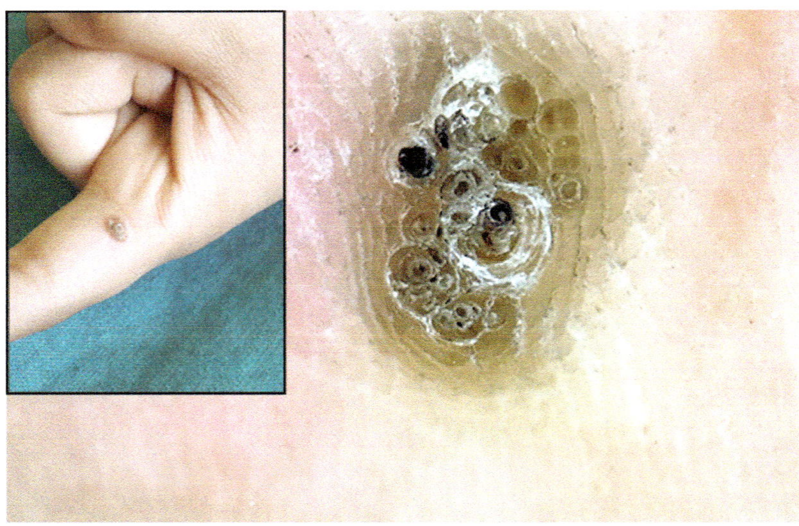

Fig. 8: Wart on the finger.

References

1. Zalaudek I, Giacomel J, Cabo H, et al. Entodermoscopy: a new tool for diagnosing skin infections and infestations. Dermatology. 2008;216:14-23.
2. Tanioka M, Nakagawa Y, Maruta N, et al. Pigmented wart due to human papilloma virus type 60 showing parallel ridge pattern in dermoscopy. Eur J Dermatol. 2009;19:643-4.
3. Yoong C, Di Stefani A, Hofmann-Wellenhof R, et al. Unusual clinical and dermoscopic presentation of a wart. Australas J Dermatol. 2009;50:228-9.

PLANE WARTS (VERRUCA PLANA)

Introduction

Plane warts (verruca plana) are smooth, flesh-colored to slightly pink or brown flat topped papules ranging in size from 2 mm to 5 mm in diameter. The common sites of involvement include face, neck, arms, and legs.

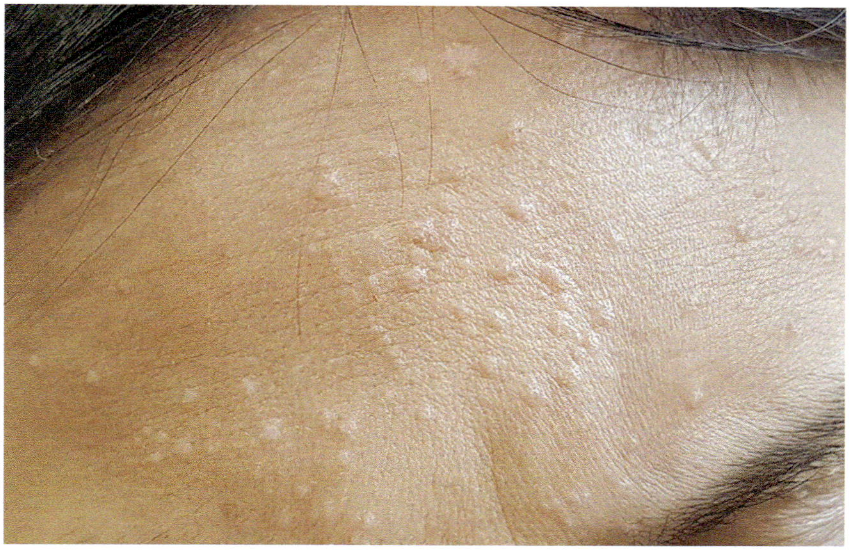

Fig. 9: Fleshy skin-colored macules of verruca plana.

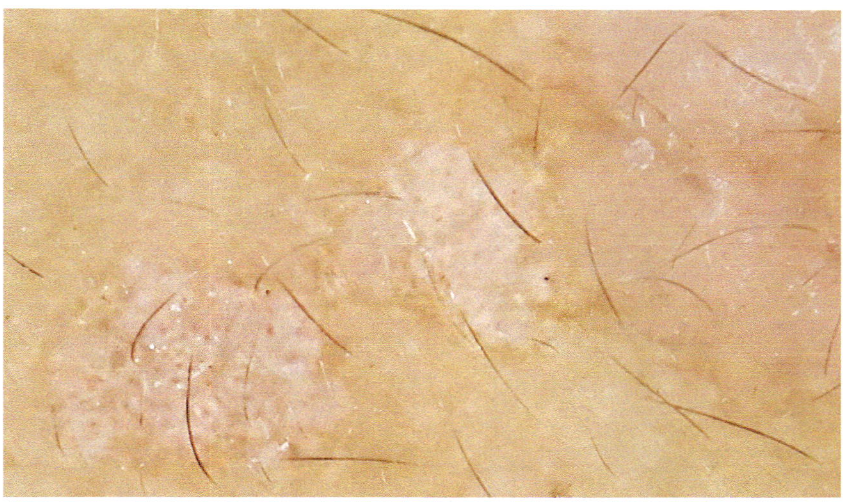

Fig. 10: Dermoscopy shows tiny red dots with central homogeneous pattern.

Key Dermoscopic Features[1]

- Regularly distributed tiny red dots intermingled by whitish lines
- Light brown or yellow background.

Discussion

The hallmark dermoscopic sign of verruca plana reveals regularly distributed red dots on a light brown or flesh colored background. The red dots represent apices of capillaries in the papillary dermis **(Figs. 9 and 10)**.

Reference

1. Zalaudek I, Giacomel J, Cabo H, et al. Entodermoscopy: a new tool for diagnosing skin infections and infestations. Dermatology. 2008;216(1):14-23.

PLANTAR WART

Introduction

Verruca plantaris (plantar wart) manifests on the plantar surfaces of the feet, especially on the weight-bearing areas of the heels, toes, and mid-metatarsal areas.

Key Dermoscopic Features

- Irregularly distributed red/brown/black dots, loops or linear streaks
- Keratotic halo
- Verrucous yellowish structureless area
- Disruption of dermatoglyphics.

Discussion

The dermoscopic picture of plantar wart is slightly modified in comparison to warts of other region, due to pressure effect on vessels of weight bearing area. Dermoscopically, they appear as verrucous yellowish structureless area showing irregularly distributed red/brown/black dots, globules, loops, or linear streaks representing hemorrhages that are caused due to high pressure on plantar vasculature. These characteristic hemorrhages differentiate plantar warts from callus which is devoid of hemorrhage. Keratotic halos surround the hemorrhagic dots which histologically correspond to papillomatosis.[1]

Corns are painful localized hyperkeratosis that forms over interphalangeal joints due to pressure and friction. Calluses are hyperkeratotic lesions resulting from excess friction. Corns develop from localized forces, whereas calluses develop from forces distributed over a broad area of skin.

Sometimes, it is difficult to differentiate plantar warts from corns or calluses clinically. Dermoscopy plays an important role in differentiating them. Corn shows a translucent central core that is more visible dermoscopically after trimming; whereas callus demonstrates homogeneous opacity.[2] Dermatoglyphics are maintained in corns, whereas they are disrupted in plantar warts **(Figs. 11 to 16)**.

Keynote

Dermoscopy proves to be a promising tool in differentiating plantar warts from corns and calluses whenever clinical diagnosis is in doubt.

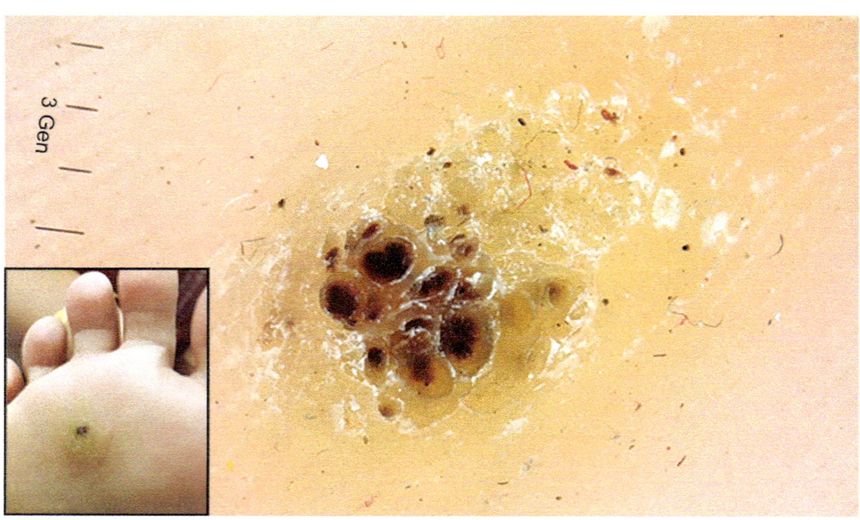

Fig. 11: A case of plantar wart dermoscopically showing red dots, black dots, and keratotic halos. Note the disruption of dermatoglyphics.

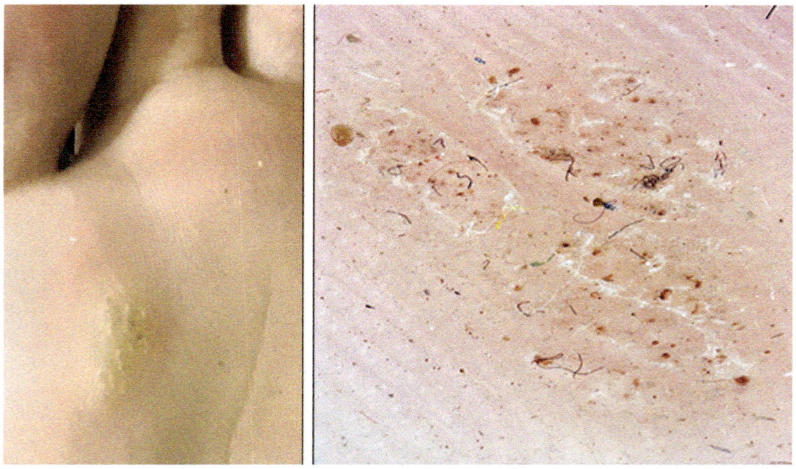

Fig. 12: Mosaic wart. A case of conglomeration of warts in a mosaic pattern showing extensive red dots, few black dots, and tiny keratotic halos.

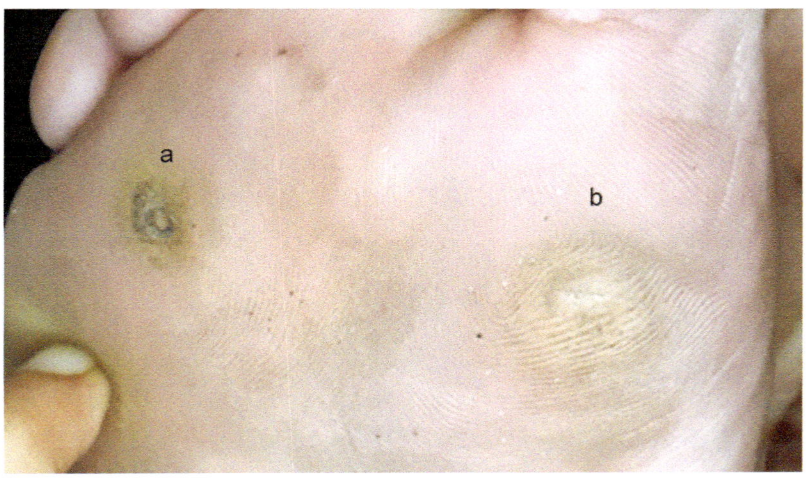

Fig. 13: Both (a) corn and (b) callus, which may at times be difficult to differentiate clinically.

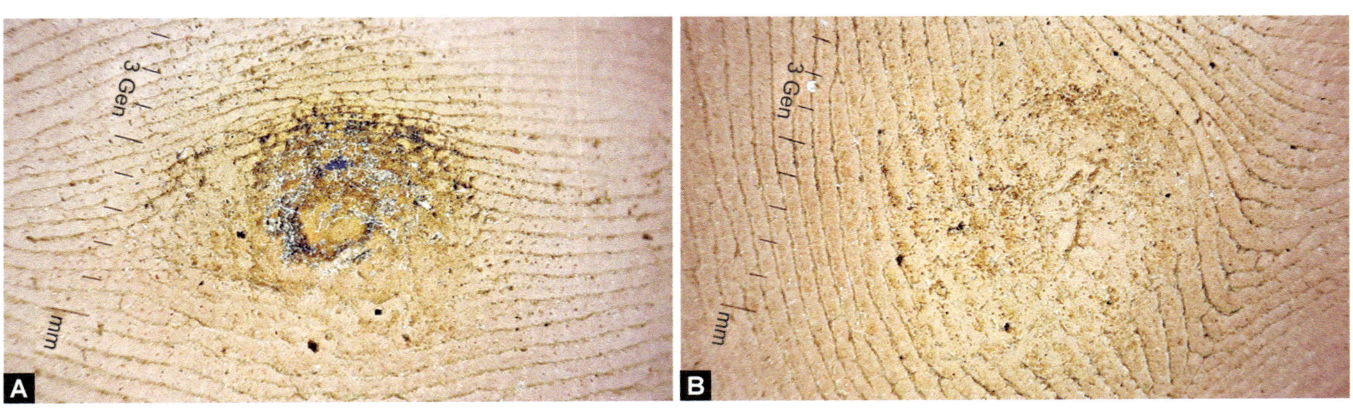

Figs. 14A and B: (A) On dermoscopy corn shows a central core with maintained dermatoglyphics; (B) Dermoscopy of callus showing homogeneous opacity.

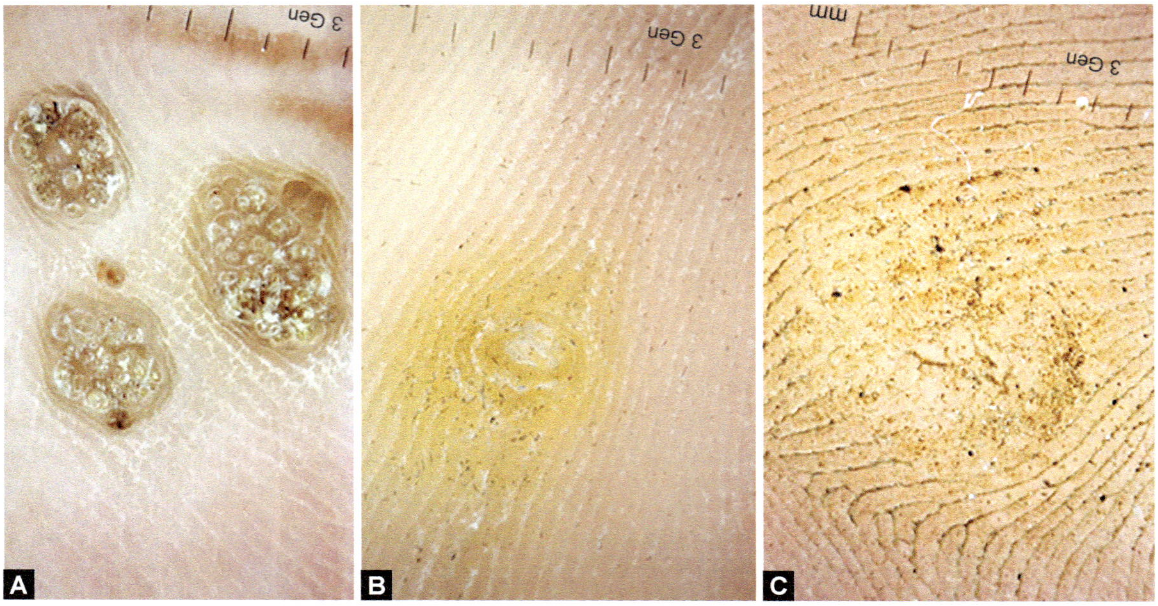

Figs. 15A to C: A comparative picture showing dermoscopic features of (A) wart—red dots and black dots surrounded by keratotic halo along with disruption of dermatoglyphics, (B) corn—central core with intact dermatoglyphics, and (C) callus—homogeneous opacity.

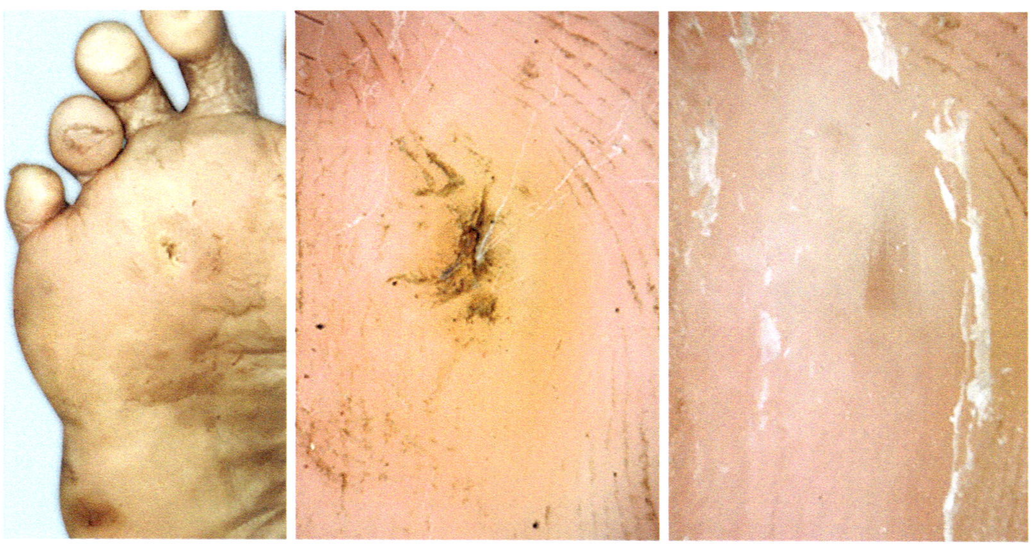

Fig. 16: Superficial paring of a corn revealed central black core. On enucleation, homogeneous opacity is seen.

References

1. Martín JM, Bella-Navarro R, Jordá E. Vascular patterns in dermoscopy. Actas Dermosifiliogr. 2012;103(5):357-75.
2. Bae JM, Kang H, Kim HO, et al. Differential diagnosis of plantar wart from corn, callus and healed wart with the aid of dermoscopy. Br J Dermatol. 2009;160(1):220-2.

MOLLUSCUM CONTAGIOSUM

Introduction

Molluscum contagiosum (MC) is a common benign viral infection of children causing characteristic skin lesions. Skin lesions are single or often multiple shiny, pearly white, waxy, round or hemispherical papules with central umbilication that contain a caseous plug consisting of distorted and destroyed squamous epithelial cells; they form large hyaline bodies (molluscum bodies or Henderson-Paterson bodies) containing cytoplasmic masses of viral material.

Key Dermoscopic Features

- White-to-yellow polylobular amorphous structure is seen in association with central pore or umbilication.
- Crown vessels distributed radially that do not cross the center of the lesion.
- Rosettes are commonly observed in MC.

Discussion

The polylobular structure that is seen on dermoscopy, histologically corresponds to inverted lobules of hyperplastic squamous epithelium, at the center of which lies the molluscum bodies. As the disease progresses, the molluscum bodies expand displacing the dermis to reveal dermal vessels at the periphery of the papule.[1,2] They appear as crown vessels with a radial distribution resembling a crown under the dermoscope. These vessels do not cross the center of the lesion.[3,4]

Rosettes constitute another important dermoscopic feature of MC. They are rather a frequent dermoscopic finding in MC. Rosettes may be of great value in giving a clue to the diagnosis of MC when other dermoscopic features are less evident.[5]

Keynote

Molluscum contagiosum is mostly a clinical diagnosis but, sometimes a very early lesion may pose a diagnostic dilemma. Dermoscopy definitely helps in such a situation. Though rosettes are an additional dermoscopic finding yet provides a valuable clue to the diagnosis of MC **(Figs. 17 to 21)**.

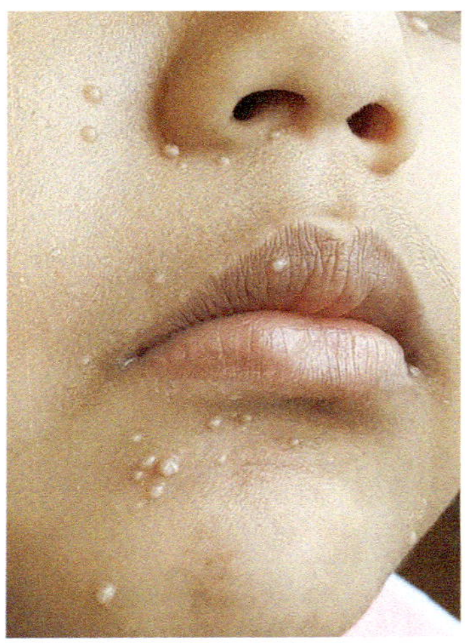

Fig. 17: A 6-year-old child with multiple molluscum contagiosum lesions over the face.

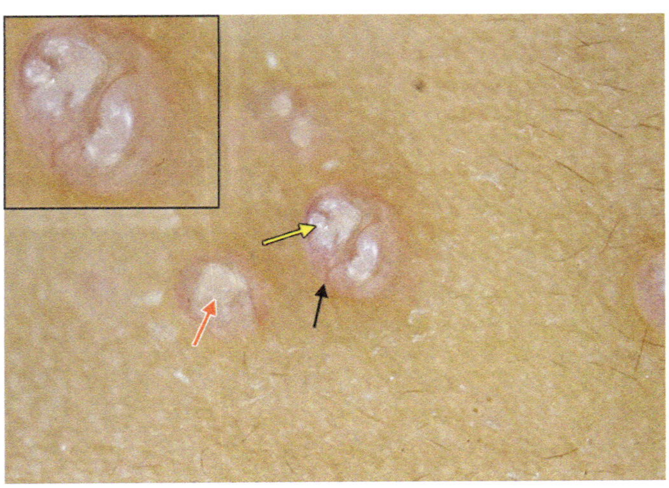

Fig. 18: In the center of the field, dermoscopy shows two closely set molluscum contagiosum with crown vessels (black arrow) and rosette (yellow arrow). Red arrow points toward amorphous globules. Inset showing the larger view of the dermoscopic findings.

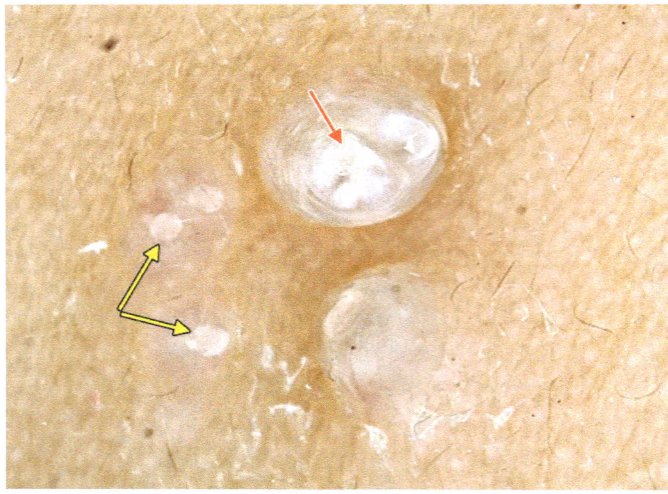

Fig. 19: Dermoscopy shows rosettes (yellow arrows) and amorphous globules (red arrow).

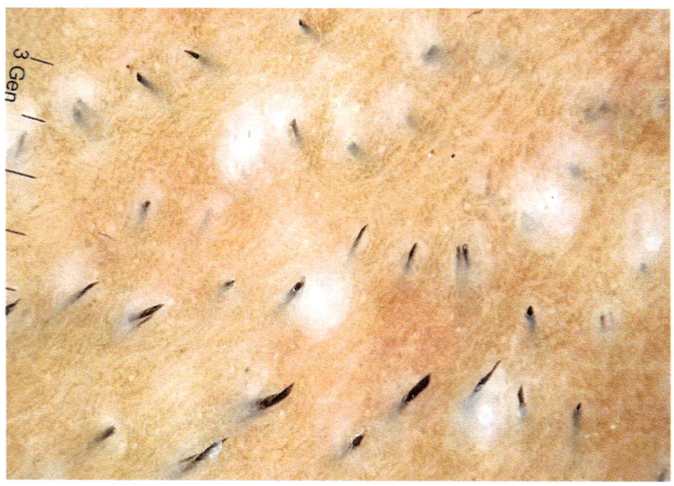

Fig. 20: Rosettes are important additional features of molluscum contagiosum. When other dermoscopic features are less evident, rosettes may be highly valuable clue to the diagnosis. Multiple rosettes are evident.

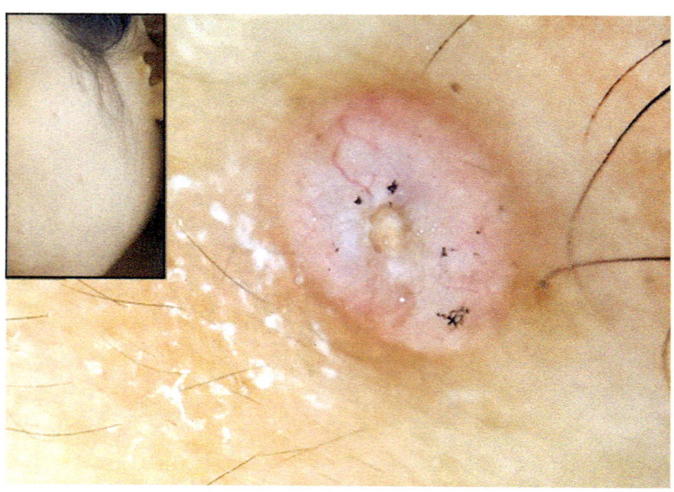

Fig. 21: Classical vascular pattern of molluscum contagiosum with crown vessels and central amorphous globules.

References

1. Morales A, Puig S, Malvehy J. Dermoscopy of molluscum contagiosum. Arch Dermatol. 2005;141(12):1644.
2. Zaballos P, Ara M, Puig S, et al. Dermoscopy of molluscum contagiosum: a useful tool for clinical diagnosis in adulthood. J Eur Acad Dermatol Venereol. 2006;20(4):482-3.
3. Malvehy J, Puig S. Principios de dermatoscopia, 2nd edition. Barcelona: Cege editores; 2010.
4. Zalaudek I, Kreusch J, Giacomel J, et al. How to diagnose nonpigmented skin tumors: a review of vascular structures seen with dermoscopy. Part II. Nonmelanocytic skin tumors. J Am Acad Dermatol. 2010;63:377-86.
5. Malakar S, Mukherjee SS. Rosette: an additional in vivo dermoscopic finding in molluscum contagiosum. Indian J Paediatr Dermatol. 2019;20:349-50.

INFESTATIONS

PARASITIC INFECTIONS

DEMODICOSIS

Introduction

It results from infestation with the *Demodex* mite, an obligate human parasite having two species, *D. folliculorum* and *D. brevis*. *Demodex* can only live in the human hair follicle.[1] *Demodex* is an ectoparasite of pilosebaceous follicle and sebaceous gland, typically found on the face including cheeks, nose, chin, forehead, temples, eye lashes, brows, and also on the balding scalp, neck, and ears. Clinically, it may present as erythema, burning and stinging sensation, or a nonspecific rash over the face. Demodicosis is diagnosed when there is high density of *Demodex* mites (>5/cm^2).

Key Dermoscopic Feature

- *Demodex* tails—appear as white spicules at the root of the hair follicle
- Demodex follicular openings—appear as course follicular openings containing brownish/grayish plugs
- Subtle erythema with reticular dilated vessels
- Scaling and pustules.

A *Demodex* spicule is a protruding 3 dimensional structure, whereas the scale is a flattened structure that does not protrude.

Keynote

Dermoscope provides clinical diagnosis instantly and noninvasively. Routine dermoscopy is a must in patients with dry facial skin and erythematous rash to rule out demodicosis **(Figs. 22 to 26)**.[2]

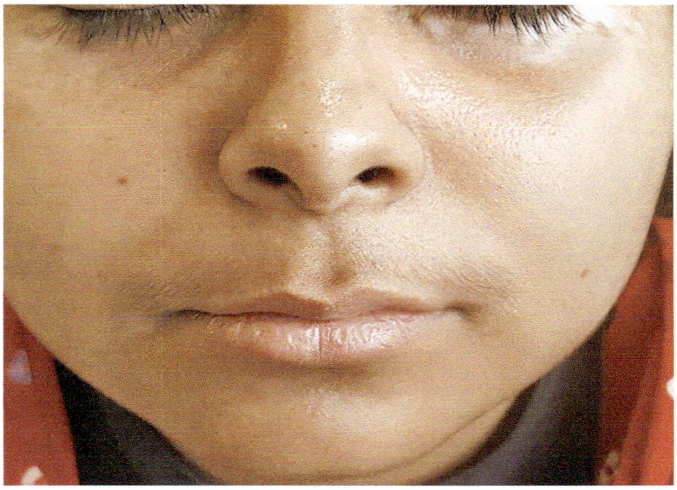

Fig. 22: Mild erythematous rash and burning sensation over face for last 7 months which was not responding to topical steroid or calcineurin inhibitors.

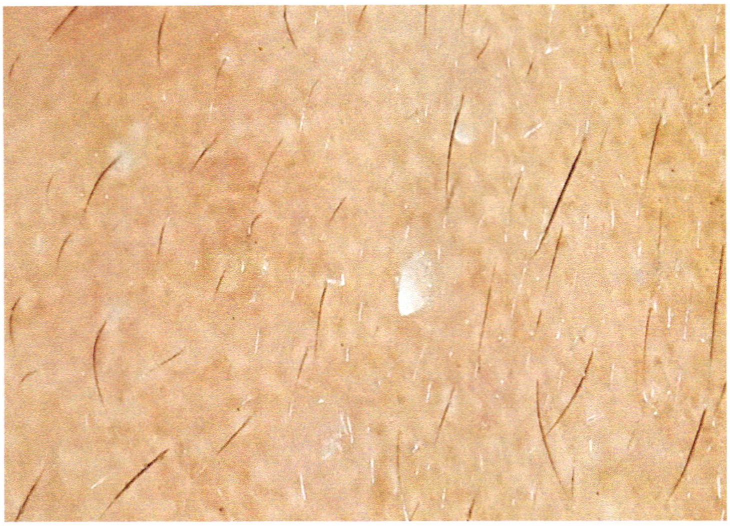

Fig. 23: On trichoscopy of facial hairs a prominent white spicule, a faint white spicule and a white globule is seen protruding from the follicular opening.

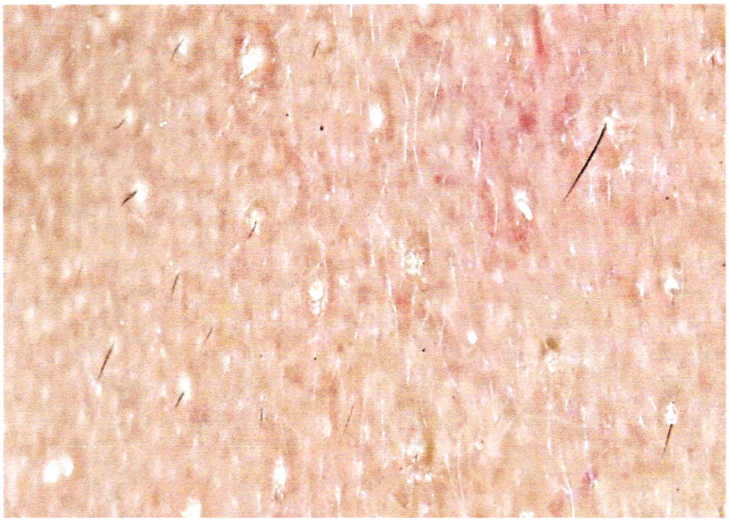

Fig. 24: More white spicules in another field and subtle reticular dilated vessels forming a pink network.

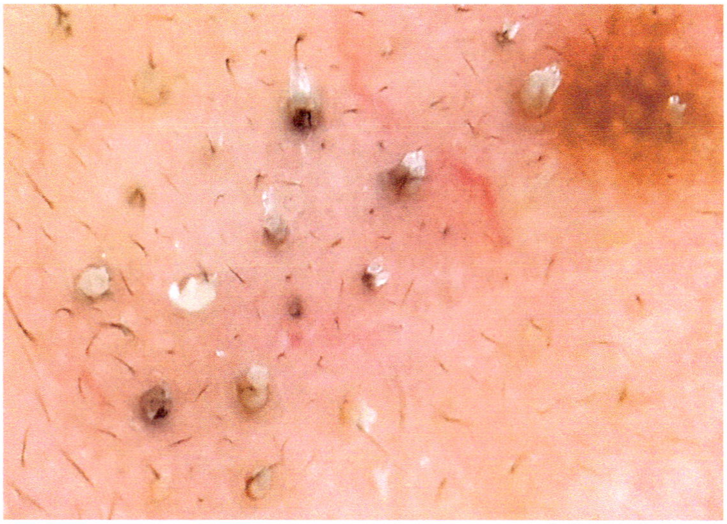

Fig. 25: Dilated pores containing amorphous brown/gray plugs can also be associated with this disorder.

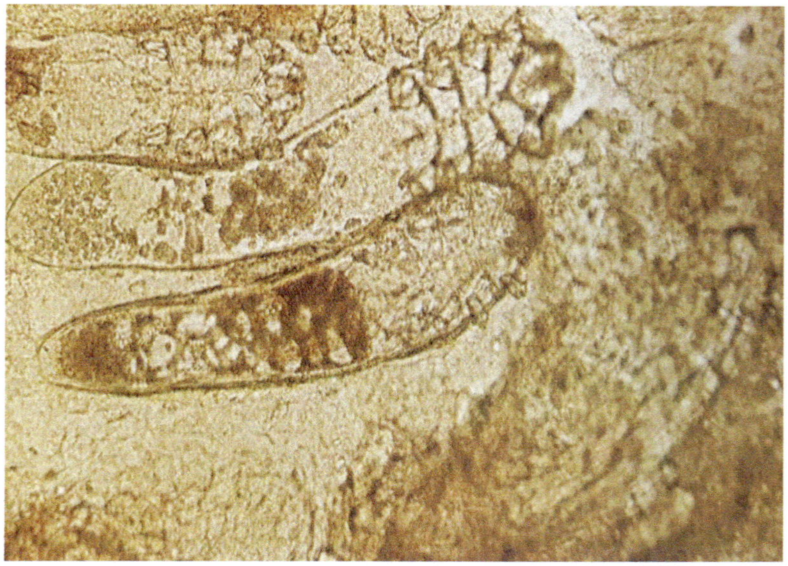

Fig. 26: Skin scrapings (KOH): live, cigar-shaped, and actively moving *Demodex* mite.

References

1. Forton F, Germaux MA, Brasseur T, et al. Demodicosis and rosacea: epidemiology and significance in daily dermatologic practice. J Am Acad Dermatol. 2005;52(1):74-87.
2. Mangold A, Swanson DL. Dermoscopy in general dermatology; In: Johr RH, Stolz W (Eds). Dermoscopy, 2nd edition. United States: McGraw-Hill; 2015. pp. 505-28.

PEDICULOSIS CAPITIS

Introduction

Infestation of pediculosis capitis (*pediculus humanus var capitis*) is common and can easily be diagnosed clinically upon close examination. Diagnostic signs of head lice infestation are lice and/or nits. Nonetheless, it may be time consuming and nits may be confused with pseudonits (scales of different origin).[1,2] Trichoscopy allows straightforward identification of head lice and nits and also can differentiate nit (louse egg) and nit cast (empty egg). As trichoscopy can assess the viability of the contents of the nits, it can be used to monitor the treatment efficacy.[3]

Key Features

- Nit—louse egg attached to hair shaft
- Nit cast—empty egg appearing as a translucent structure fixed to a hair shaft
- Head louse.

Discussion

Dermoscopy helps in diagnosing pediculosis capitis and differentiating nits from pseudonits. Pseudonits are basically scales of different origins. A pseudonit encircles the hair shaft, whereas a nit does not encircle the shaft but is attached to one side of the shaft, at an angle. On the other hand, single scales and yellowish background are clues to diagnosis of seborrhoeic capitis.

Keynote

Dermoscopy can help detect both live and dead nits on the scalp of infested children. Thus, response to treatment at follow-up can be assessed **(Figs. 27 to 30)**.

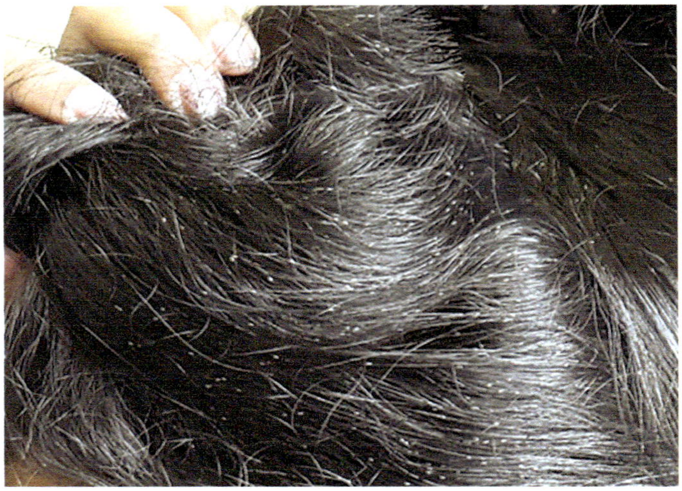

Fig. 27: Numerous nits on the hair shafts.

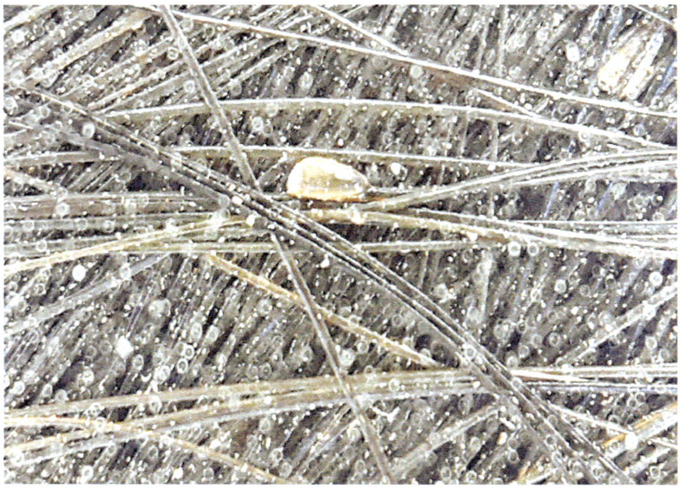

Fig. 28: Dermoscopy demonstrating nits which characteristically attached to one side of hair shaft at an angle.

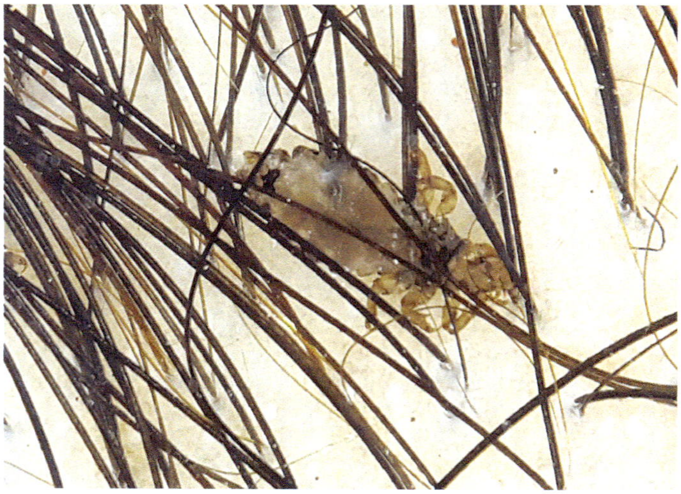

Fig. 29: Dermoscopy demonstrating a head louse after a blood meal.

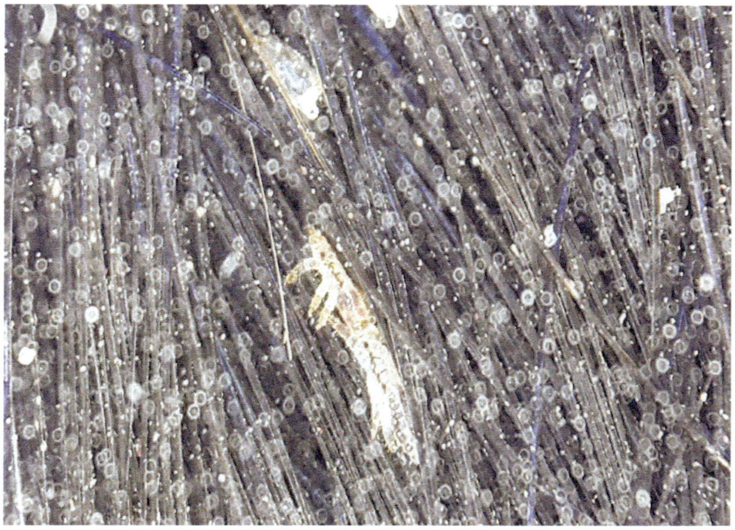

Fig. 30: Dermoscopy showing male and female head louse in addition to nits.

References

1. Micali G, Lacarrubba F, Massimino D, et al. Dermatoscopy: alternative uses in daily clinical practice. J Am Acad Dermatol. 2011;64:1135-46.
2. Bowling J. General dermatology. In: Bowling J (Ed). Diagnostic Dermoscopy. Oxford: Wiley; 2012. pp. 123.
3. Lacarrubba F, Dinotta F, Micali G. Parasitic scalp infections. In: Rudnicka L, Olszewska M, Rakowska A (Eds). Atlas of Trichoscopy. London: Springer; 2012. pp. 357.

SCABIES

INTRODUCTION

Since the introduction of dermoscopy scabies mite can be observed in-vivo very easily.

Pediatric scabies often presents with pruritus. Mostly the lesions consist of erythematous papules and burrows. It is a contagious cutaneous condition where the mites are transferred by direct contact, including sexual contact and indirect contact through fomites. Symptoms may be apparent after 2–6 weeks of acquiring infection. The rash is often most obvious in the interdigital web spaces, inner side of thighs, around the umbilicus, nipples, and genitals. The diagnosis can be confirmed by the microscopic examination of the contents of a burrow, however, that may be cumbersome and time consuming. The modern gadget, dermoscopy provides instant diagnosis of the condition without a diagnostic dilemma.

KEY DERMOSCOPIC FEATURES[1]

- Diagnostic clue by dermoscopy—pigmented triangle of the mouth parts and fore limbs at the end of the burrow. If the triangle is full, it is the ventral view of the mite whereas in case of partial triangle, it is the dorsal view.
- Burrows of different lengths and shapes.
- Delta wing jet, translucent scabies body, and scabious eggs.

DISCUSSION

Dermoscopically the mite and burrow are represented by a delta-shaped jet airplane followed by its whitish condensation trail, respectively. Burrows are a pathognomonic sign and this intradermal tunnel is created by the movement of the female mite. Sometimes a burrow filled with eggs can also be demonstrated under dermoscopy which appear as "string of pearls".

The sensitivity of dermoscopy for the diagnosis of scabies when compared with that of conventional microscopic examination of skin scrapings or adhesive tape test is reported to be either equal to or greater than for the other two modalities.[2,3] Dermoscopy has also been used to monitor treatment response and it has been shown that the mites begin to decompose and become indistinct after 2 weeks of treatment.

KEY MESSAGE

In case of diagnostic dilemmas with atopic dermatitis and other closer mimics, dermoscopy serves as an important tool for instant differentiation by finding the scabies mite in-vivo **(Figs. 31 to 35)**.

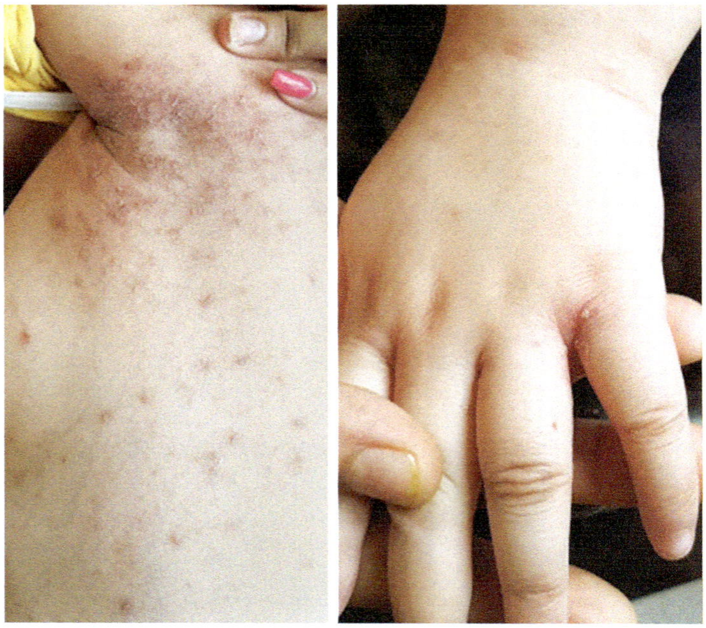

Fig. 31: The classical presentation of scabies on the web space and armpit in a 3-year-old child. Note the excoriated erythematous papules and vesicles.

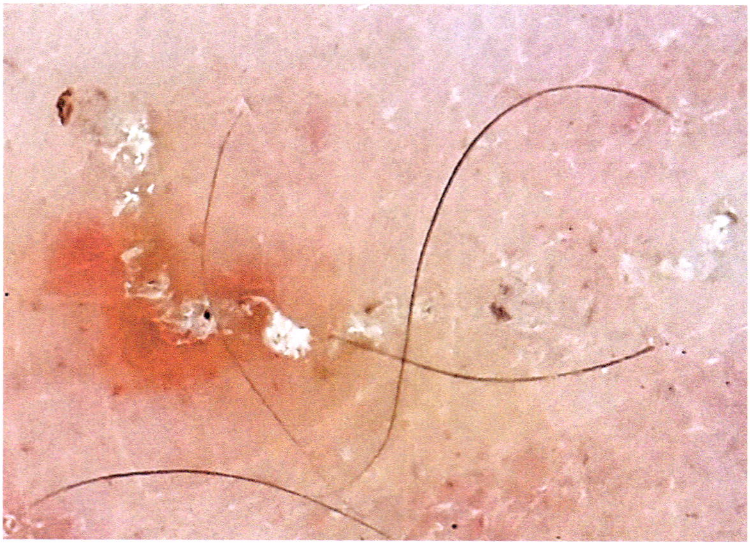

Fig. 32: Dermoscopy shows a scabetic mite (magnified) with pigmented triangle at the end of the burrow represented by a triangular tip giving rise to the jet with contrail appearance.

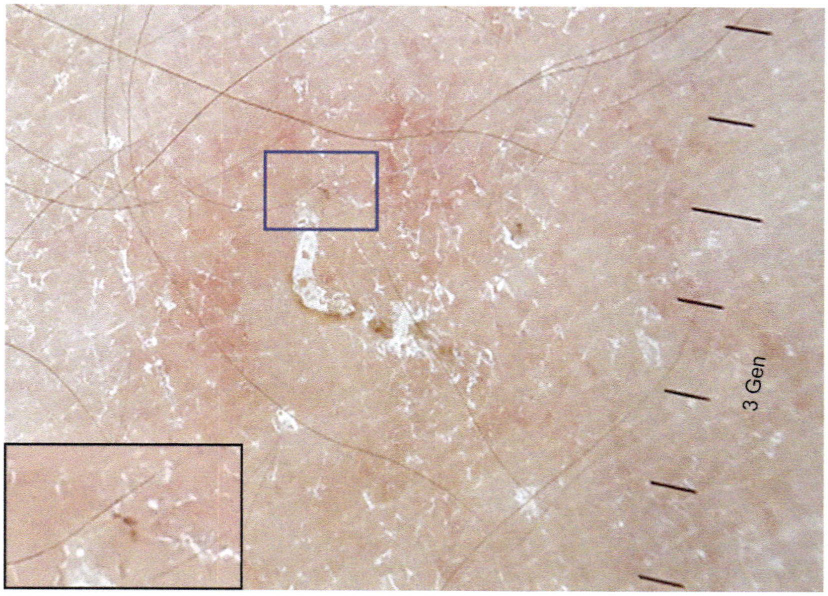

Fig. 33: Pigmented triangle at the end of the burrow represents head and a classic delta wing jet. *Inset* showing the more prominent view of the triangular scabetic mite.

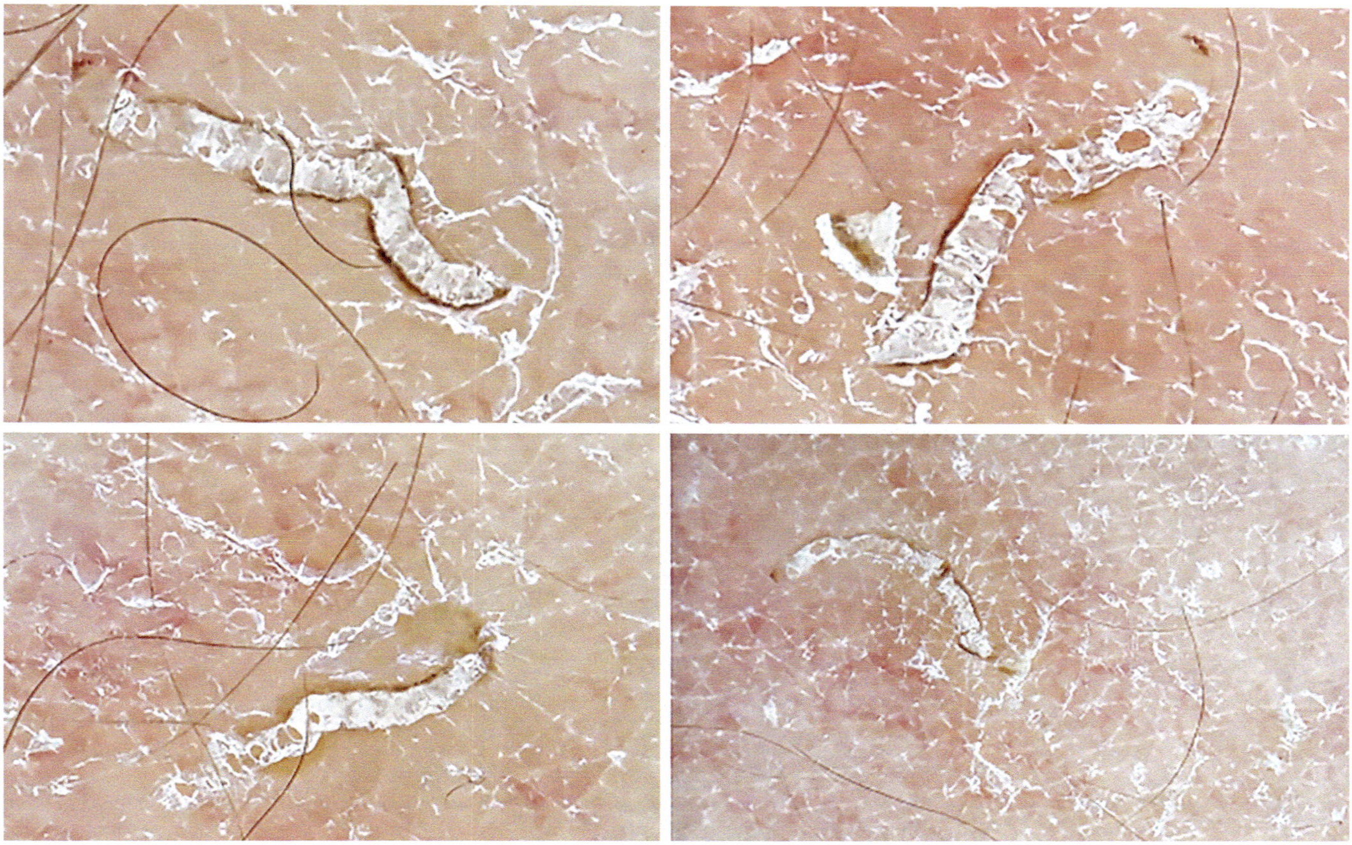

Fig. 34: The classical jet and contrail appearance of the scabetic burrows along with the mites from different patients.

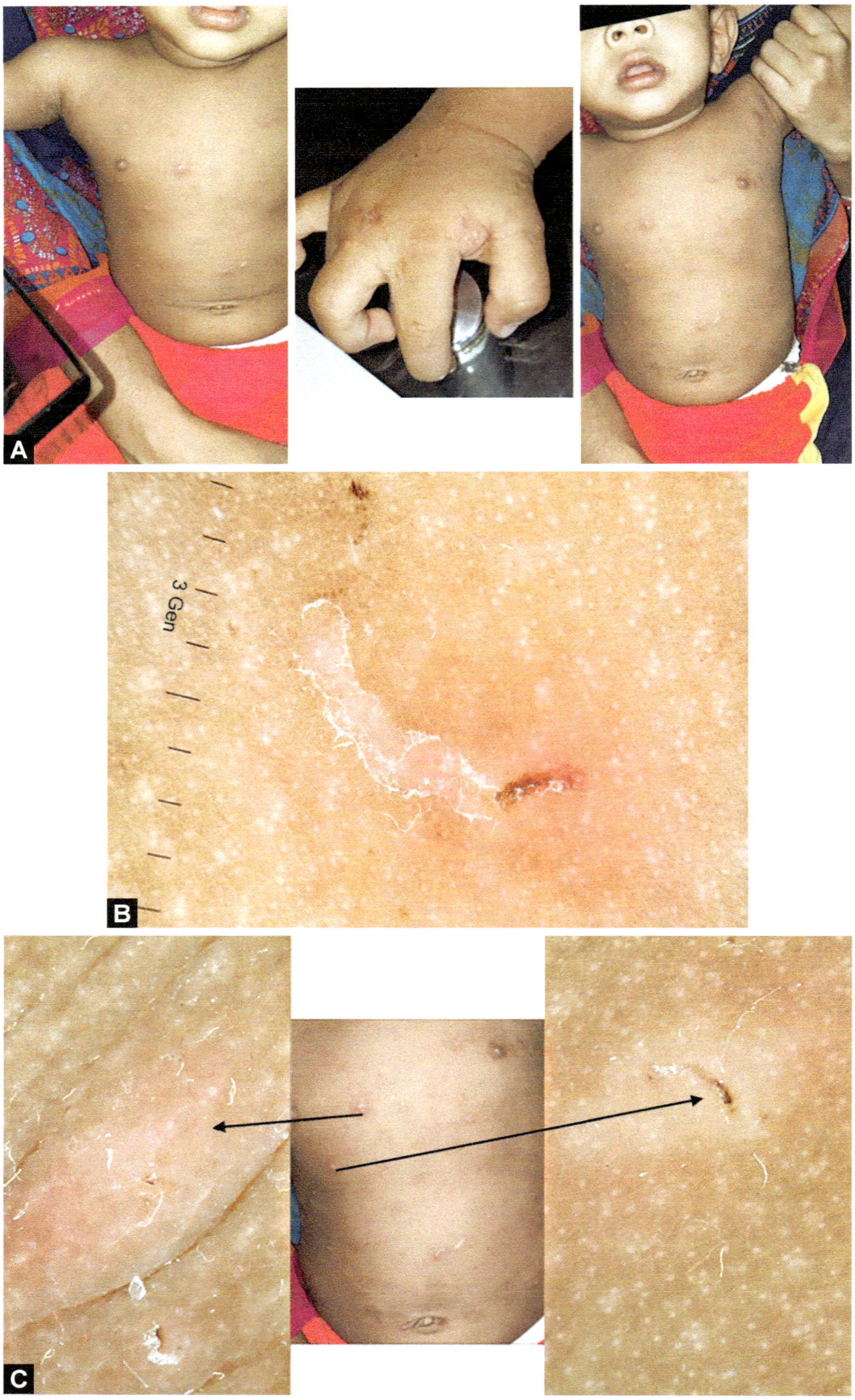

Figs. 35A to C: (A) A case of scabies in a 2-year-old boy, having a few nodular lesions in addition to the papulovesicles; (B) A serpiginous burrow is demonstrated here; (C) On dermoscopy, scabies mites have been demonstrated in nodular lesions of nodular scabies as well.

REFERENCES

1. Park JH, Kim CW, Kim SS. The diagnostic accuracy of dermoscopy for scabies. Ann Dermatol. 2012;24(2):194-9.
2. Walter B, Heukelbach J, Fengler G, et al. Comparison of dermoscopy, skin scraping, and the adhesive tape test for the diagnosis of scabies in a resource-poor setting. Arch Dermatol. 2011;147:468-73.
3. Dupuy A, Dehen L, Bourrat E, et al. Accuracy of standard dermoscopy for diagnosing scabies. J Am Acad Dermatol. 2007;56:53-62.

CHAPTER 8

Developmental Anomalies of the Newborn

Subrata Malakar, Seujee Das, Rashmi Agarwal, Surit Malakar

APLASIA CUTIS CONGENITA

INTRODUCTION

Aplasia cutis congenita (ACC) is characterized by the localized absence of skin at birth. The most common site is the scalp but other regions such as the limbs and trunk may also be involved occassionally.[1] The clinical findings include a shiny, atrophic, alopecic patch, and frequently occurring over the vertex.

While the diagnosis is usually clinical, dermoscopic examination may be needed to differentiate it from nevus sebaceous and post-traumatic lesion of the scalp, which are the other common differentials in this age group.

KEY DERMOSCOPIC FEATURES

Scalp

- Elongated, pigmented hair bulbs, clearly visible through the translucent membrane.
- Radial arrangement of hair shafts around the central patch of aplasia—so called "collar hypertrichosis/hair collar sign".[2,3]
- Prominent vessels.
- Lack of follicular openings.

Nonscalp Areas

- Healing areas show thinned out whitish membrane, linear vessels of increased caliber and perceptible erythema.
- Healed areas show intensified melanin pigment network.
- No hair collar sign.

DISCUSSION

Visualization of elongated, darkly pigmented hair bulbs are suggestive of anagen hair follicles visible through the translucent membrane. The radial arrangement of these bulbs (so-called collar hypertrichosis) suggests a neural tube defect, producing an aberrant shearing force during formation of the follicles, pulling them outward from the defect. Prominent vessels of increased caliber and absence of follicular openings both correspond to scarring.

For areas other than the scalp, dermoscopic findings of translucent membrane with background erythema, linear vessels and lack of follicular and eccrine openings point to the diagnosis of ACC. The thick, linear vessels correspond to the superficial vascular plexus of the upper dermis. The peripheral pigment network signifies the healing of the lesion from the periphery.

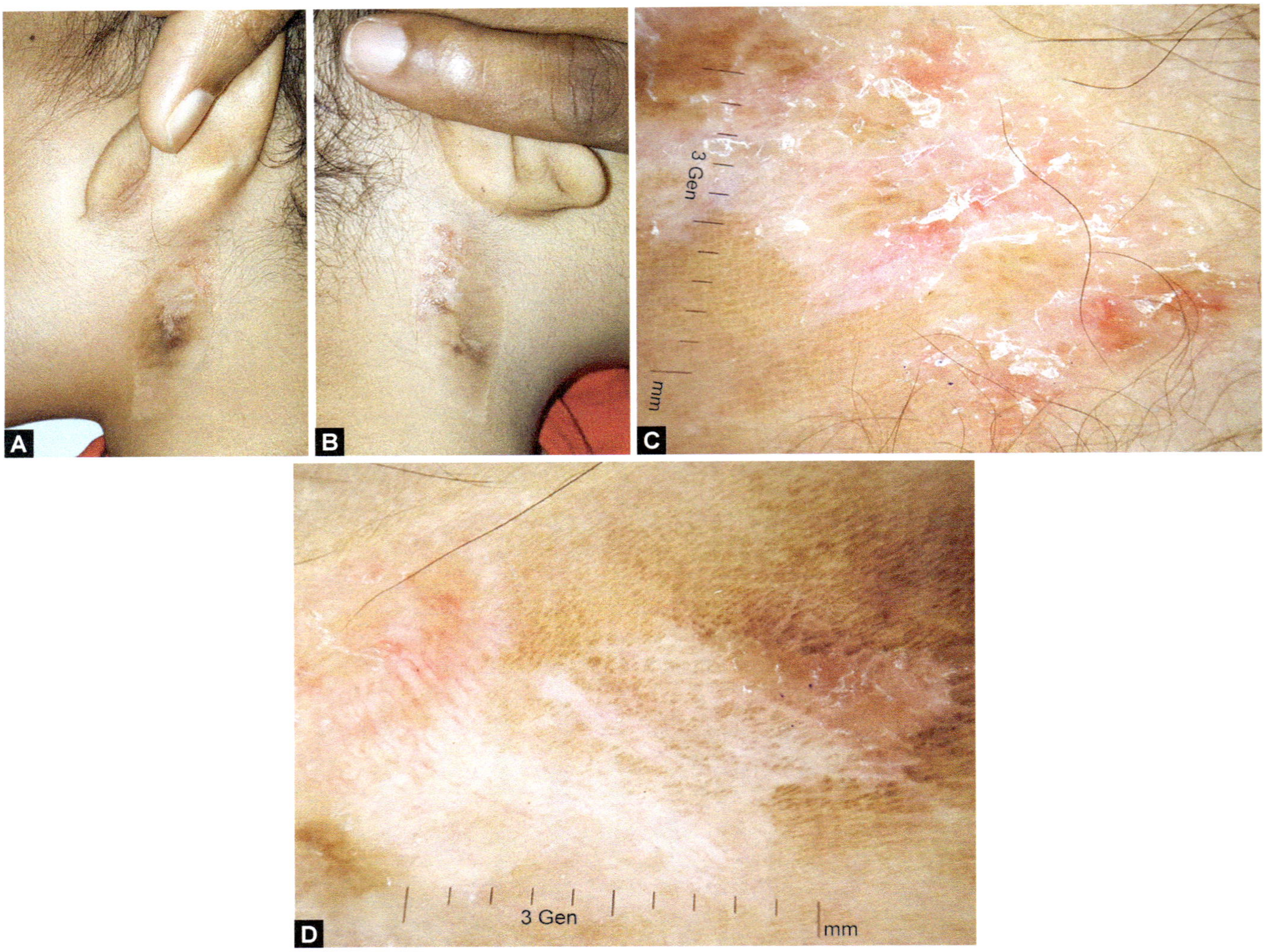

Figs. 1A to D: (A and B) This 4-year-old boy presented with symmetrical lesions below the ears, since birth. These were in the form of discolored patches with a smooth surface and visible erythema (more on the right side than the left). There were signs of healing present in both the lesions at their lower ends, as evidenced by hyperpigmentation and reduced erythema. (C) Dermoscopy of the right-sided lesion: Presence of a whitish membrane along with a few linear vessels and erythema in the healing part of the lesion. Note the lack of hair in the aplastic patch, whereas the surrounding skin shows presence of hair. Peripherally, increased melanin pigment can be seen. (D) Dermoscopy of the left-sided lesion: Whitish membrane with linear vessels of increased caliber in association with erythema is present in the healing areas. The healed areas show marked melanin pigment network encroaching the center of the lesion from the periphery, suggestive of postinflammatory hyperpigmentation.

KEYNOTE

- Radially arranged hair bulbs seen through a translucent membrane are the trichoscopic hallmark of scalp ACC. Trichoscopy is thus invaluable in differentiating aplasia cutis from nevus sebaceous and post-traumatic scarring.
- Dermoscopic findings of nonscalp ACC mainly include translucent membrane and thickened vessels with signs of healing in the form of melanin pigment network **(Figs. 1A to D)**.

REFERENCES

1. Malakar S, Mukherje SS. Defining the dermoscopic characteristics of aplasia cutis congenita on the body. Indian J Paediatr Dermatol. 2019;20:347-9.
2. Damiani L, Aguiar FM, Da Silva MV, et al. Dermoscopic findings of scalp aplasia cutis congenita. Skin Appendage Disord. 2017;2(3-4):177-9.
3. Pinheiro AM, Mauad EB, Fernandes LF, et al. Aplasia cutis congenita: trichoscopic findings. Int J Trichol. 2016;8:184-5.

BRANCHIAL FISTULA

INTRODUCTION

Branchial cleft cysts are congenital epithelial cyst, located on the lower one-third of the neck at the anteromedial border of sternocleidomastoid muscle, resulting from failure of closure of one of the four branchial clefts, with or without a sinus tract to the overlying skin.[1] It presents as a solitary painless papule on the neck with occasional mucoid discharge from the anterior aspect of the neck during the first and the second decade of life. It can rarely be confused with a thyroglossal cyst or dermoid cyst, cervical abscess, lymphadenopathy, cystic hygroma and ectopic thyroid, or salivary tissue.

It is usually a clinical diagnosis, but dermoscopy helps in highlighting its features, thereby avoiding the need of imaging studies and other invasive diagnostic procedures.

KEY DERMOSCOPIC FEATURES[2]

- Pale circular area with central horizontal slit.
- On pressing the papule, transparent mucus may be expressed making the area hazy and oval in shape due to contact with the lens of the dermoscope.

DISCUSSION

On dermoscopy, the tiny papule appears as pale area surrounding the slit that probably corresponds to the branchial cyst. Secretion of mucous on pressing the cyst makes the area hazy with the borders extending to form an oval shape; this is due to contact with the lens of dermoscope.

Imaging studies such as sinogram, ultrasonography, and computed tomography scan help in identifying the nature of the lesion whereas fine-needle aspiration may be helpful in differentiating branchial cleft cysts from malignant neck masses **(Figs. 2 to 4)**.[3,4]

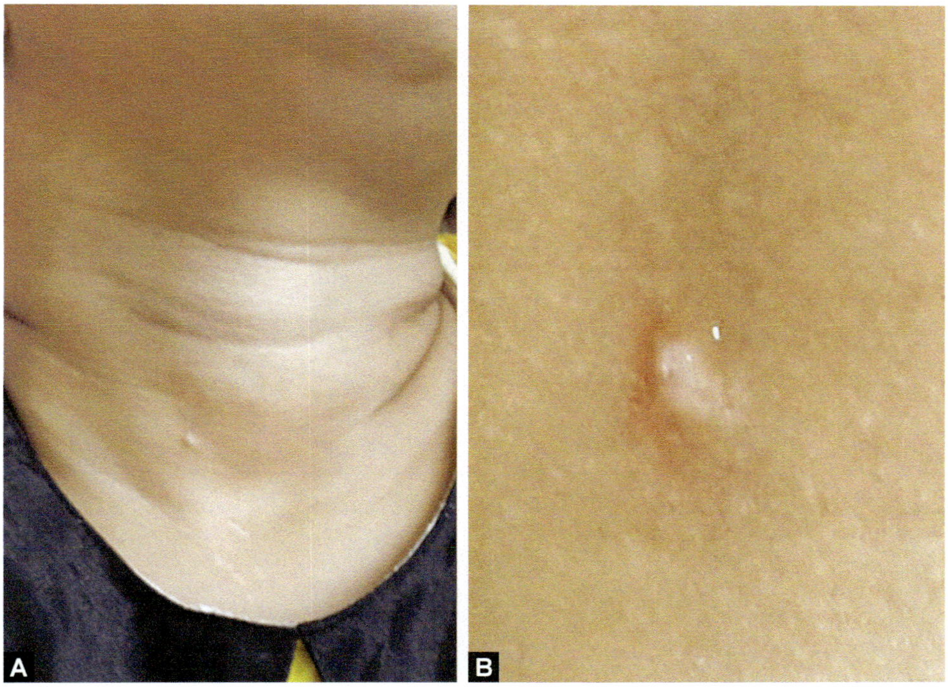

Figs. 2A and B: (A) Tiny skin colored papule (branchial cyst) at the right side of the neck along the border of the sternocleidomastoid muscle in a 3-year-old girl; (B) Close-up view of the branchial cyst.

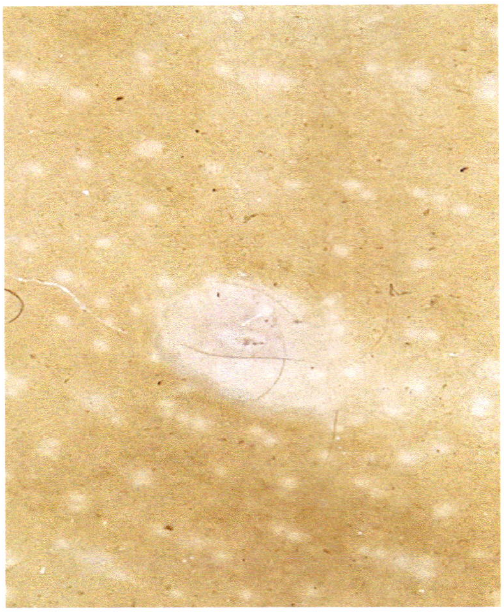

Fig. 3: Dermoscopy showing a pale circular area with central horizontal slit.

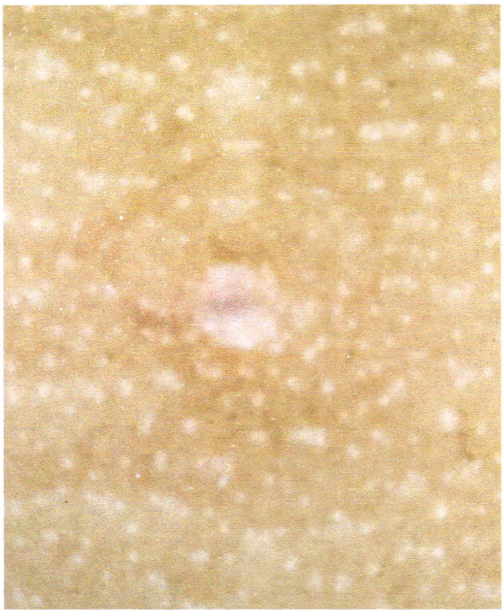

Fig. 4: On pressing the papule, transparent mucus was expressed, which made the area hazy and was oval in shape due to contact with the lens of the dermoscope.

REFERENCES

1. Wagner AM, Hansen RC. Neonatal skin and skin disorders. In: Schachner LA, Hansen RC (Eds). Pediatric Dermatology. 2nd edition, Vol. 1. New York: Churchill Livingston; 1995. pp. 291-3.
2. Malakar S, Diwaker P, Pradhan P. Dermoscopy of branchial fistula. Indian J Paediatr Dermatol. 2018;19:342-3.
3. Bloch R. Images in emergency medicine. Branchial cleft cyst. Ann Emerg Med. 2006;47:291,308.
4. Rosa PA, Hirsch DL, Dierks EJ. Congenital neck masses. Oral Maxillofac Surg Clin North Am. 2008;20:339-52.

CHAPTER 9

Genodermatoses

Subrata Malakar, Seujee Das, Rashmi Agarwal, Surit Malakar

TUBEROUS SCLEROSIS COMPLEX

Tuberous sclerosis is an autosomal dominant disorder characterized by the development of hamartomas of the skin, brain, eye, heart, kidneys, lungs, and bones. Cutaneous features of this complex include hypopigmented macules, angiofibromas, fibrous tumors and periungual, and gingival fibromas.[1,2]

HYPOPIGMENTED MACULES

Introduction

Three or more hypopigmented macules measuring 5 mm or more in diameter is characteristic of tuberous sclerosis complex (TSC). They usually present at birth or shortly thereafter, being the first sign of the disease to appear. They can vary in shape from confetti like macules (pretibial area) to thumbprint and lanceolate (ash leaf macules) shaped. These lesions are most difficult to distinguish from nevus depigmentosus, which has also been reported in children with TSC. Dermoscopy shows characteristic patterns in ash leaf macules and thus helps in its accurate diagnosis.

Key Dermoscopic Feature

- White areas
- Zones of total loss of pigment
- Zones of faint pigment network **(Figs. 1A and B)**.

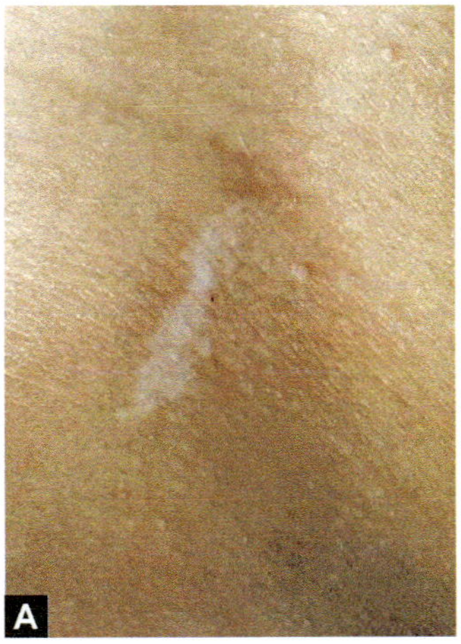

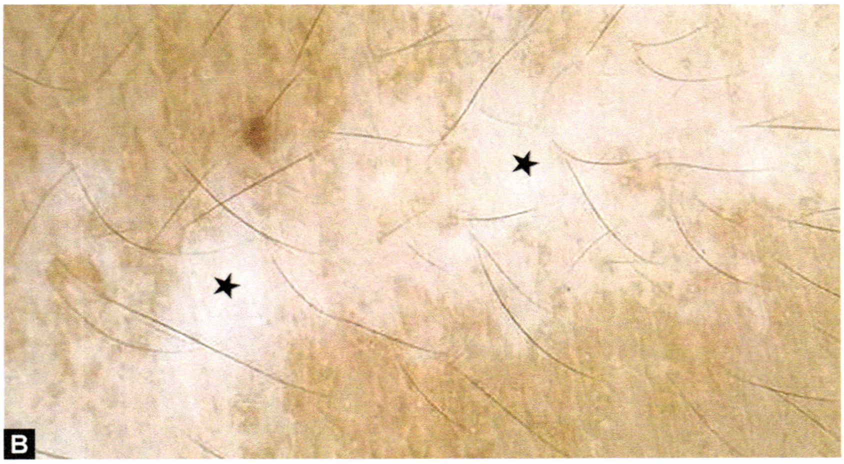

Figs. 1A and B: (A) Hypopigmented macule on the anterior neck of a patient with tuberous sclerosis; (B) Dermoscopy of the macule showing white with zones of total loss of pigment network (stars) among the areas of faint pigment network.

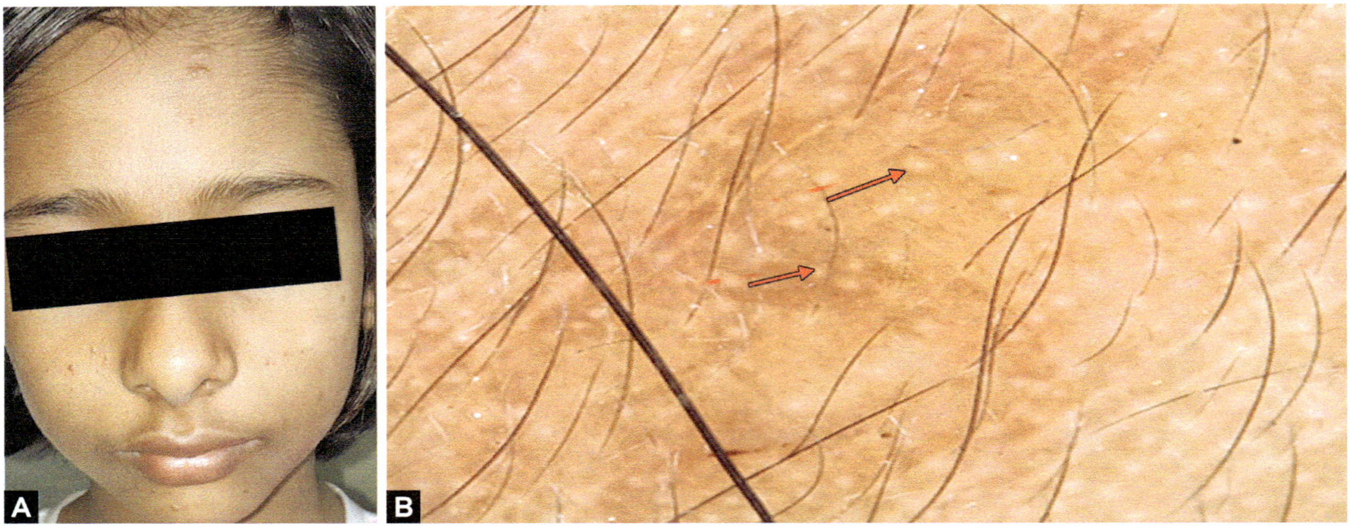

Figs. 2A and B: (A) An 8-year-old girl presenting with multiple facial angiofibromas and fibrous cephalic plaque; (B) Dermoscopy of angiofibroma showing multiple yellowish white dots (red arrows) on a pinkish background.

ANGIOFIBROMAS

Introduction

In TSC, multiple facial angiofibromas are a characteristic feature which often starts to appear within the first 2–3 years of life with augmentation of growth by puberty. Clinically, they present as reddish brown papulonodules with a smooth, glistening surface distributed symmetrically on the face. Fibrous cephalic plaques presenting as raised firm plaques on the forehead or scalp are also a variant of angiofibromas. Facial angiofibromas can be confused with multiple trichoepitheliomas, acne vulgaris, trichofolliculomas, and syringomas. In doubtful cases, dermoscopy can prove to be an important noninvasive tool for confirmation of the diagnosis.

Key Dermoscopic Features

- Multiple yellowish-white dots
- Pinkish gray background
- Crypts.

Discussion

Dermoscopy of angiofibromas reveal multiple yellowish white dots on a pinkish gray background with few papules also showing crypts over the surface. Histopathologically, the yellowish white dots represent the follicular hyperkeratosis with sebum while the pinkish gray areas correspond to the proliferating blood vessels along with pigmentary incontinence and dermal melanophages. The crypts represent the pseudofollicular openings **(Figs. 2A and B)**.

SHAGREEN PATCH

Introduction

A shagreen patch is a form of collagenoma seen as part of the TSC. It is a hamartomatous proliferation characterized by increase in collagen associated with its haphazard arrangement.

Key Dermoscopic Features

Multiple, whitish, and bulbous areas.

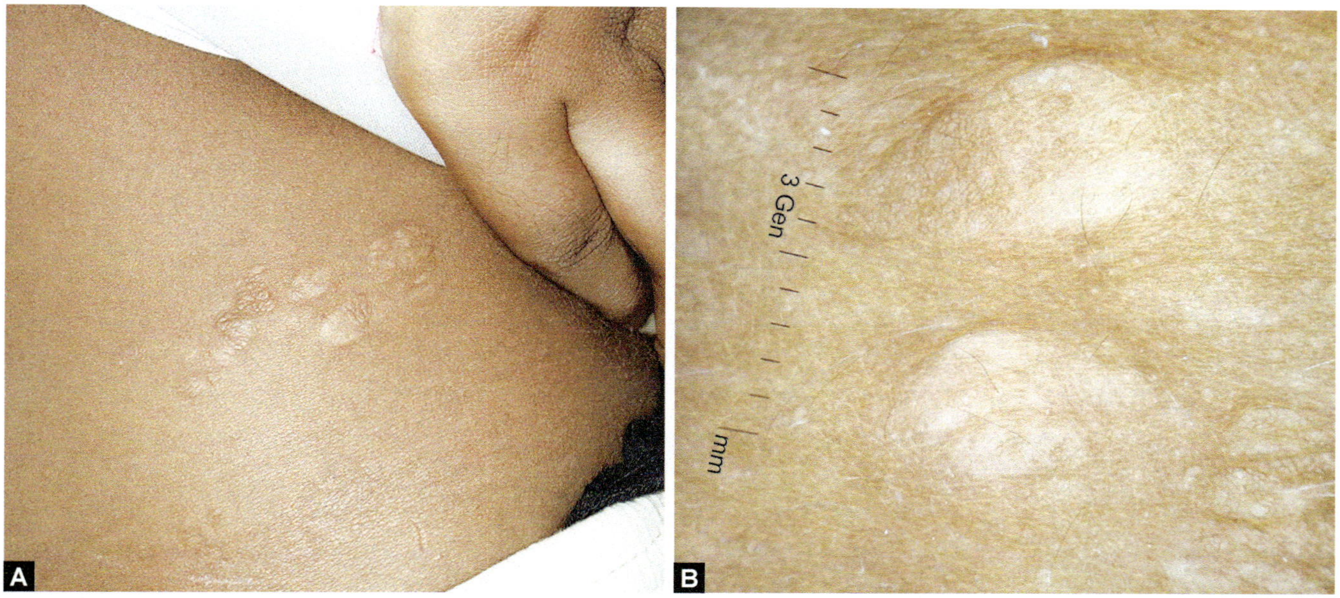

Figs. 3A and B: (A) Shagreen patch over the waist; (B) Multiple, white bulbous areas are seen on dermoscopic evaluation of a shagreen patch.

Discussion

On dermoscopy of a shagreen patch, multiple, white, and bulbous areas are noted. These correspond histopathologically to the increased collagen **(Figs. 3A and B)**.

References

1. Paller A, Mancini AJ. Disorders of pigmentation. Hurwitz Clinical Paediatric Dermatology, 5th edition. Netherlands: Elsevier; 2016. pp. 245-78.
2. Malakar S, Mukherjee SS, Malakar S. Uniform faint reticulate pigment network: a dermoscopic hallmark of nevus depigmentosus. Our Dermatol Online. 2018;9(2):225-6.

VERRUCOUS EPIDERMAL NEVUS

INTRODUCTION

Epidermal nevi are benign congenital lesions characterized by hamartomatous proliferation of the epidermis and can involve keratinocytes, sebaceous glands, hair follicles, eccrine, and apocrine glands. Epidermal nevi have different variants, of which verrucous epidermal nevus (VEN) is the most common.[1]

Clinically, VEN presents at birth or in early childhood. To begin with, it is an isolated benign, skin-colored lesion which over time becomes thicker, darker, and verrucous. Multiple such lesions coalescing to form large plaques may be seen. Rarely, it may be extensive and associated with abnormalities which involving internal organs and systems, when it is termed as "epidermal nevus syndrome".

Dermoscopy improves the specificity of the diagnosis thereby reducing the frequency of biopsy.

KEY DERMOSCOPIC FEATURES

- Large brown circles, which consist of a darker brown edge, surrounding a central lighter area
- In some cases, comedo-like openings
- Vascular pattern—dotted vessels
- White circles with white edge (personal observation).

DISCUSSION

The characteristic dermoscopic finding of VEN is large, brown circles surrounding a central light area. Histopathologically, this corresponds to the pigmented keratinocytes surrounding the central dermal papillae.

At the same time, there is absence of pigment network. This helps to distinguish these cases from melanocytic lesions.

Presence of large and white circles has been noted in the early, evolving lesions of VEN. This may be explained by the prominent hyperkeratosis on histopathology. In addition, of rete ridges are relatively less developed in these early lesions, explaining the white edge.

KEYNOTE

Large brown circles represent a specific finding on dermoscopy of VEN **(Figs. 4 and 5)**.[2,3]

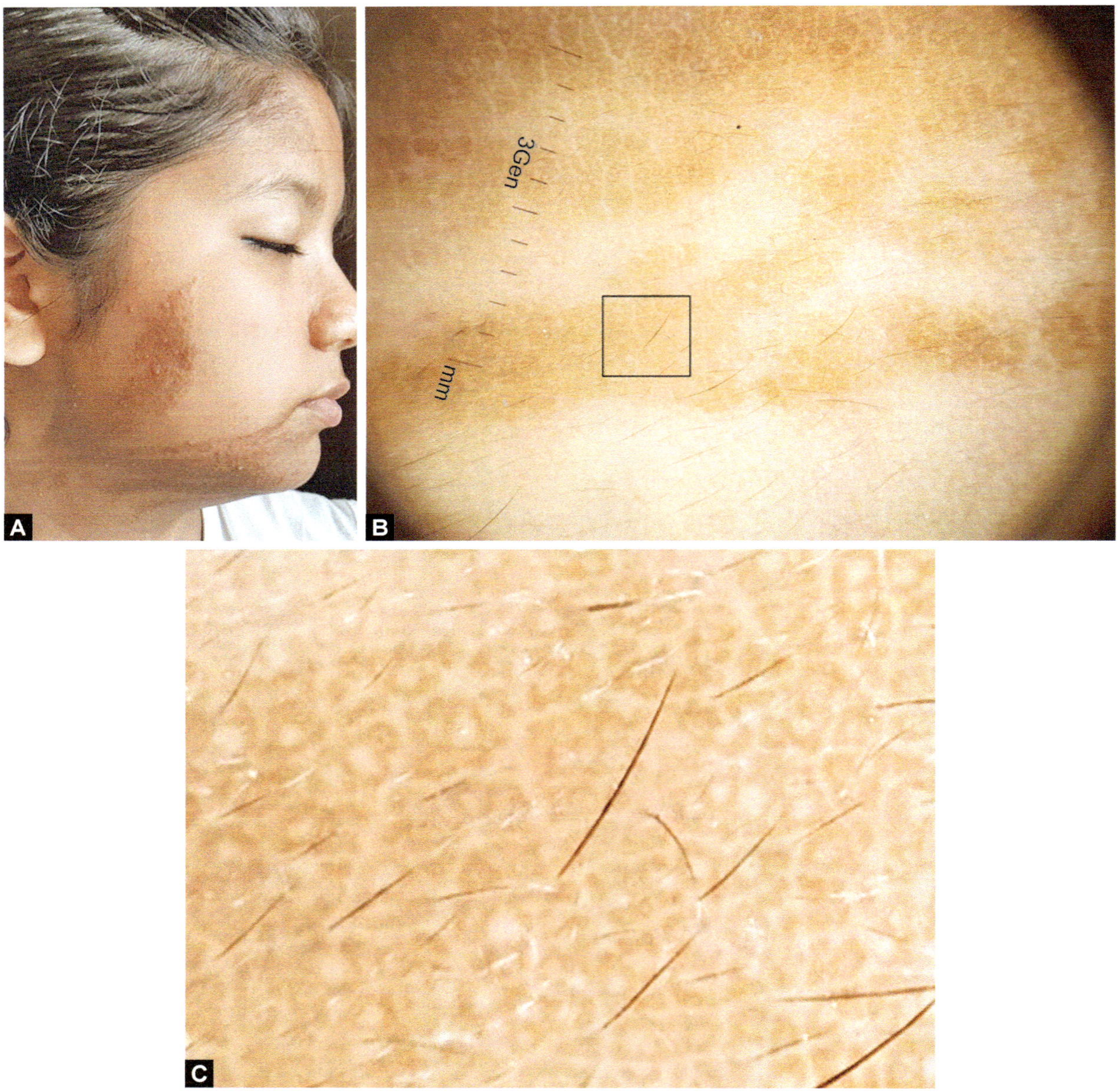

Figs. 4A to C: (A) Involvement of the right side of the face in a 12-year-old girl, in the form of linear, verrucous plaques arranged along Blaschko's lines; (B) Multiple large brown circles surrounding a central hypochromic area. The dark brown circles correspond to pigmented keratinocytes whereas the central hypochromic area represents the dermal papilla; (C) Magnified view of the box of the above lesion highlighting the presence of numerous large, brown circles.

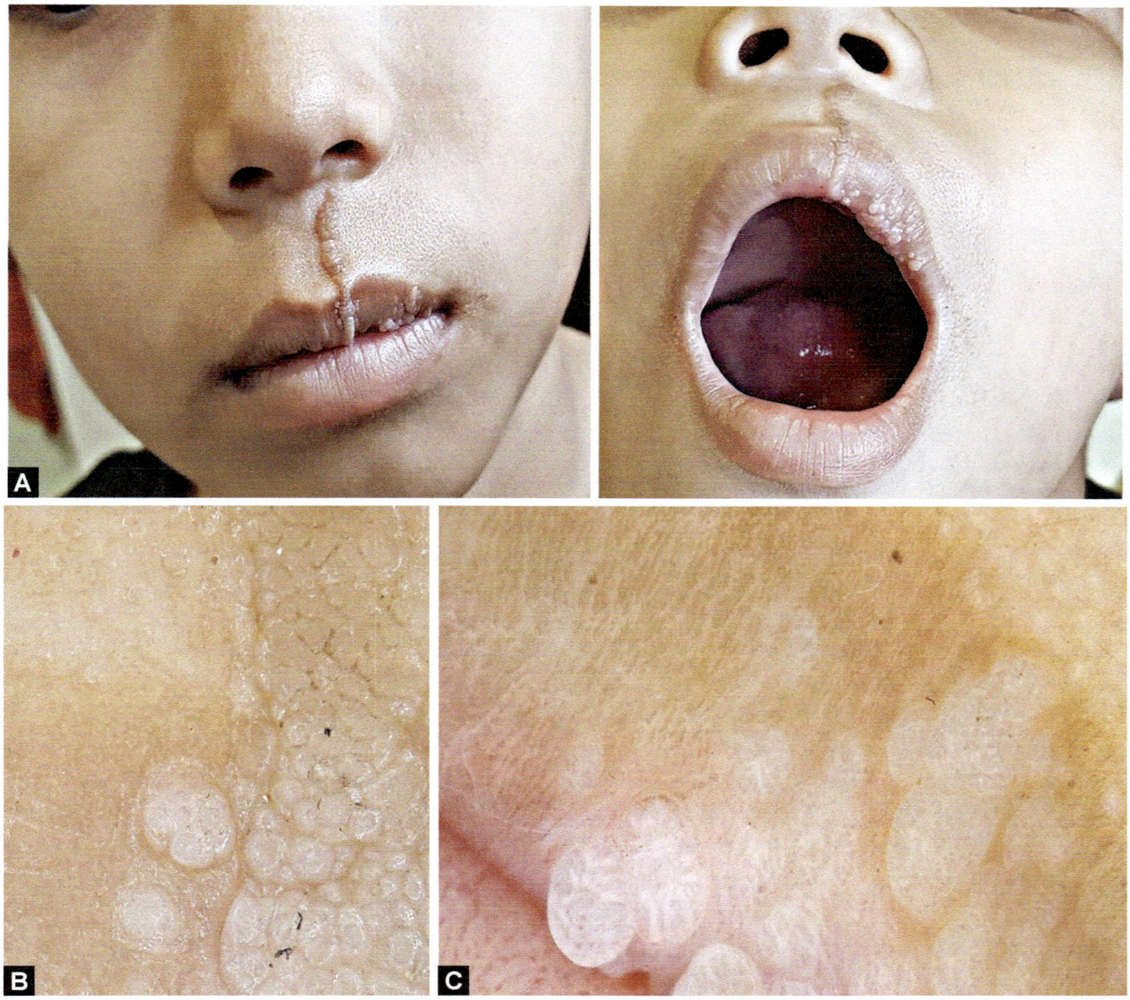

Figs. 5A to C: (A) A linear, verrucous, skin-colored plaque, running from the nose to the upper lip in a 6-year-old boy; (B) Numerous large, white circles with white rim can be appreciated on dermoscopy of the above lesion; (C) Higher magnification of the same lesion showing dotted vessels, in addition to large, white circles.

REFERENCES

1. Verzi AE, Lacarrubba F, Quattrocchi E, et al. Verrucous epidermal nevus: dermoscopy, reflectance confocal microscopy, and histopathological correlation. Dermatol Pract Concept. 2019;9(3):230-1.
2. Carbotti M, Coppola R, Graziano A, et al. Dermoscopy of verrucous epidermal nevus: large brown circles as a novel feature of diagnosis. Int J Dermatol. 2016;55(6):653-6.
3. Elmas OF, Akdeniz N. Dermoscopic aspect of verrucous epidermal nevi: new findings. Turk J Med Sci. 2019;49(3):710-4.

CHAPTER 10

Tumors

Subrata Malakar, Surit Malakar

NEVUS SEBACEOUS

INTRODUCTION

Nevus sebaceous of Jadassohn (NAJ) is a complex cutaneous hamartoma generally presenting on the head, neck, and face area. When present on the scalp, it may produce alopecia mimicking aplasia cutis congenital, while on face and neck verrucous epidermal nevus forms a close differential diagnosis. Clinically, it presents as a smooth yellowish hairless patch in childhood which increases during puberty to form lobulated/verrucous masses with greasy yellowish overlying scales. Dermoscopy is a noninvasive imaging technique useful for diagnosing a number of skin lesions through the in vivo observation of distinct structures that are considered highly disease specific.[1,2]

KEY DERMOSCOPIC FEATURES

- Yellowish or brown globules aggregated in clusters on a yellow background (present in the stage of alopecic patch)
- Whitish-yellow lobular aspect and grayish papillary appearance (lobulated and verrucous form)
- Homogeneous yellow-whitish pattern (nodular form).

DISCUSSION

- *First stage*: This stage shows yellowish globules aggregated in clusters on a yellow background.
- *Second stage*: This stage of elevated verrucous plaques demonstrates four dermoscopic features—(1) whitish-yellow lobular or papillary structures, (2) yellow-grayish papillary appearance, (3) brown globules on a yellow background, and (4) yellowish globules aggregated in clusters.
- *Tumoral stage*: In the final stage or the tumoral stage, a homogeneous yellowish hue can be seen.

In a study of 13 cases of nevus sebaceous, the authors also showed the presence of irregular linear vessel and arborescent vessels.

It is believed the yellowish hue emerges from the sebaceous secretions from the glands in this nevus.

KEYNOTE

Dermoscopy is also useful in differentiating NSJ in the first stage from aplasia cutis congenital, second stage from verrucous epidermal nevus, and tumoral stage from other sebaceous affections such as sebaceous adenoma and sebaceous hyperplasia owing to its specific dermoscopic characteristics **(Figs. 1 and 2)**.

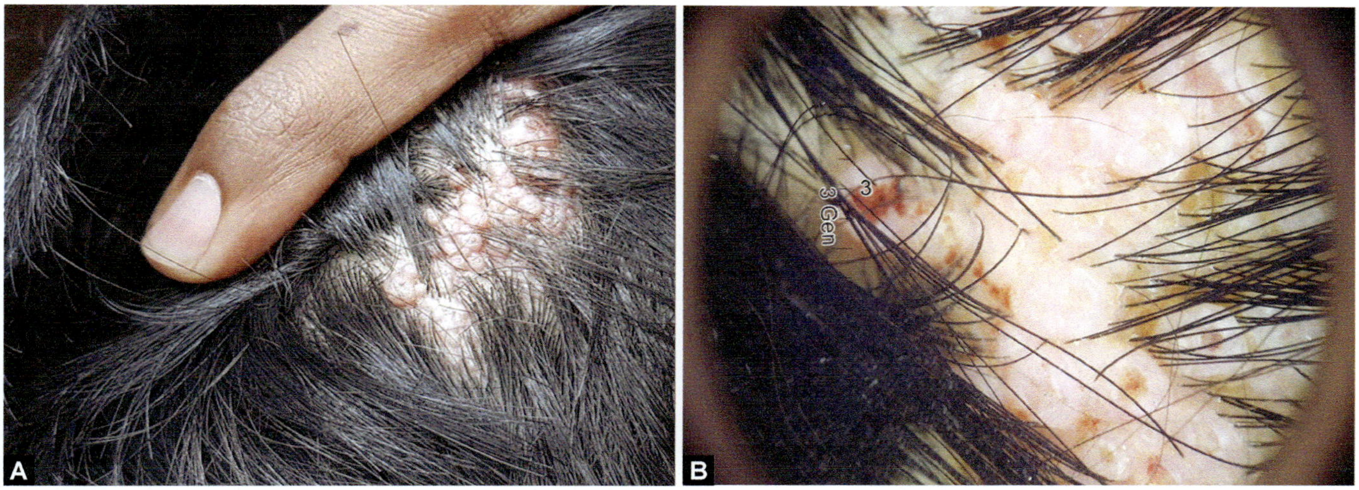

Figs. 1A and B: (A) Lobulated verrucous plaques over right temporal area in a 14-year-old male slowly progressing in size; (B) Whitish-yellow lobular appearance and grayish papillary appearance.

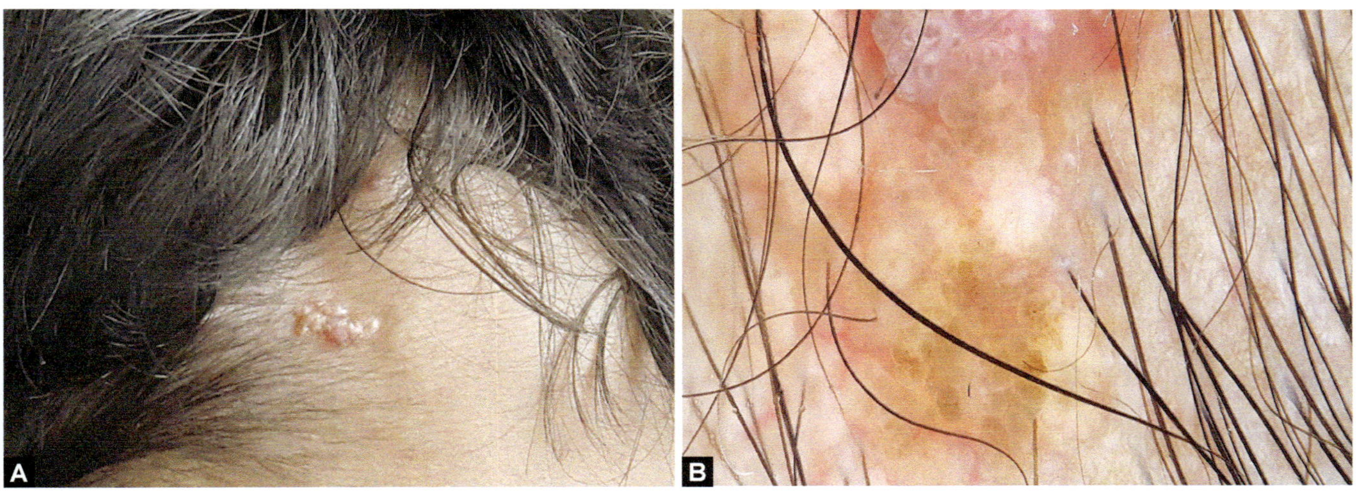

Figs. 2A and B: (A) A very small nevus sebaceous on the forehead; (B) Dermoscopy of the lesion shows yellow-brown globules aggregated in clusters on a yellow background, in an alopecic patch. The upper part of the lesion shows a grayish papillary appearance.

REFERENCES

1. Kelati A, Baybay H, Gallouj S, et al. Dermoscopic analysis of nevus sebaceous of Jadassohn: a study of 13 cases. Skin Appendage Disord. 2017;3(2):83-91.
2. Ankad B, Beergouder S, Domble V. Trichoscopy: the best auxiliary tool in the evaluation of nevus sebaceous. Int J Trichol. 2016;8(1):5-10.

TRICHOEPITHELIOMA

INTRODUCTION

Trichoepitheliomas in pediatric age group can occur either as multiple small lesions primarily on the face, inherited in an autosomal dominant fashion (Brooke-Spiegler syndrome and multiple familial trichoepitheliomas) or as a solitary nonhereditary lesion. Multiple trichoepitheliomas usually present during early childhood or at the time of puberty as small, flesh-colored firm papules with a translucent sheen on the mid-facial areas and occasionally the scalp, neck, trunk, scrotum, and perianal area. Although clinical diagnosis is usually straightforward by naked eye examination, it may pose a diagnostic

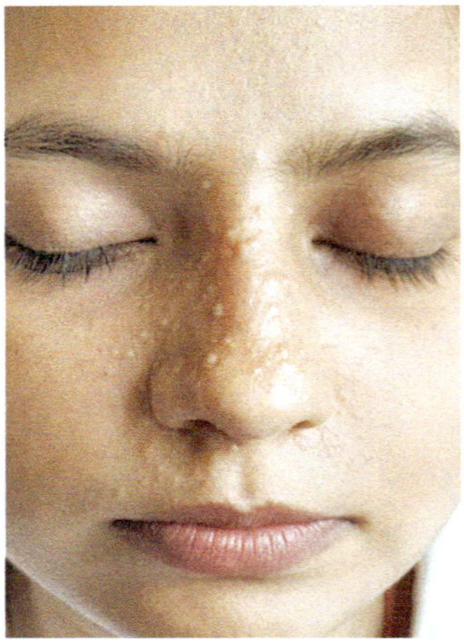

Fig. 3: Multiple shiny, flat topped, and firm papules in the central part of face of an adolescent girl suggestive of trichoepithelioma clinically.

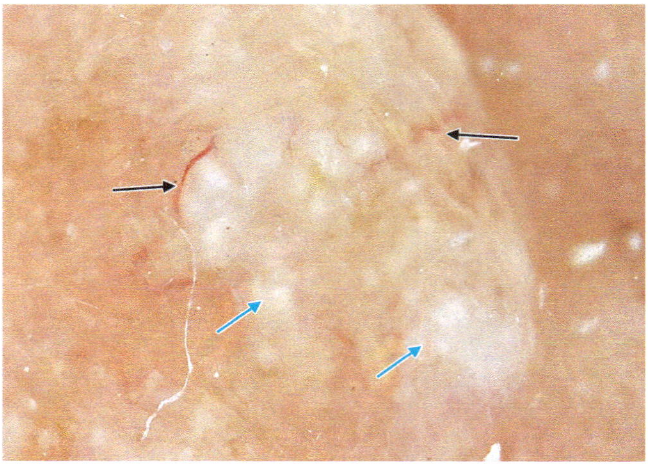

Fig. 4: Dermoscopy of a papular lesion of the previous patient shows multiple milia-like cysts (blue arrows) with arborizing vessels (black arrows).

dilemma to the treating physician in some cases presenting as flat-topped papules on the face, where dermoscopy may aid in its confirmation.

KEY DERMOSCOPIC FEATURES

- Arborizing vessels
- Milia-like cysts.

DISCUSSION

Classical dermoscopic features of trichoepithelioma include multiple arborizing vessels with milia-like cysts on a yellowish white background. Rosettes can also be seen in a few cases.

The milia-like cysts on dermoscopy correspond to the keratinous cysts on histopathology[1] while the whitish background corresponds to the proliferation of fibroblasts and presence of collagenous material. Presence of arborizing vessels suggests the lifting up of overlying skin with vascular proliferation **(Figs. 3 and 4)**.

REFERENCE

1. Dechent CV, Shirin B, Marghoob AA, et al. Multiple familial trichoepithelioma: confirmation via dermoscopy. Dermatol Pract Concept. 2016;6:10.

CHAPTER 11

Hypopigmented Lesions

Subrata Malakar, Surit Malakar

CONGENITAL HYPOPIGMENTARY DISORDERS

INTRODUCTION

Congenital hypopigmentary disorders include conditions such as nevus depigmentosus, piebaldism, hypomelanosis of Ito, ash leaf macules, and nevus anemicus. Though rare, these cases are not infrequently seen in clinical practice.

They have distinct pathophysiological mechanisms, ranging from defective melanoblast migration to defective melanosome transfer. However, they often closely mimic each other clinically, and thus pose a diagnostic challenge.

Some of these conditions are important as they may point to the presence of underlying systemic involvement, as in tuberous sclerosis or neurodevelopmental problems associated with hypomelanosis of Ito. Hence, an accurate diagnosis becomes vital in these cases.

However, in the pediatric age group, it is not always feasible or desirable to do a biopsy. A noninvasive diagnostic tool such as dermoscopy is thus invaluable and obviates the need for any invasive procedures.

In addition, acquired hypopigmentary disorders such as vitiligo and pityriasis versicolor are relatively easier to diagnose, as compared to the congenital ones. Moreover, specific diagnosis of congenital hypopigmentary disorders and confirmation of them being nonvitiliginous would put anxious parents at ease.

Hence, a focused assessment and understanding of the dermoscopic features of congenital hypopigmentary disorders are needed, for optimal management of pediatric cases **(Tables 1 and 2)**.

Table 1: Key features of the congenital hypopigmentary disorders.

Parameters	*Nevus depigmentosus*	*Hypomelanosis of Ito*	*Ash leaf macule*	*Piebaldism*
Background color	Light brown	Light brown	Light brown and white	White
Pigment network	Uniformly faint pigment network throughout the lesion	Uniform faint reticular pigment network with pigment blotches	Zones of faint pigment network with zones of total loss of pigment network	Distorted pigment network with absence at places
Perifollicular pigmentation	Mostly present	Absent	Absent	Absent
Islands of normal pigment network	Absent	Absent	Absent	Present
Margin of the patch	Serrated (accentuated) or wavy or pseudopod like extension	Irregular and cloudy	Ill-defined and irregular	Irregular
Leucotrichia	Absent	Absent	Absent	+/–

Note: Diascopy of nevus anemicus tis diagnostic. Hence, dermoscopy may not be needed.

Table 2: Hypopigmentary disorders.

Parameters	*Nevus depigmentosus*	*Hypomelanosis of Ito*	*Nevus anemicus*	*Piebaldism*	*Ash leaf macule*	*Vitiligo*	*LSEA*
Background color	Light brown	White	Light brown or erythematous	White	Light brown	White	Porcelain white
Pigment network	Faint pigment network with variable intensity of pigment	Uniform faint reticular pigment network		Distorted pigment network with absence at places	Faint pigment network with patchy absence of pigment network	Absent	Absent
Perifollicular pigmentation	Present	Absent				Absent	May be present
Islands of normal skin	Present	Absent	Absent	Present	Absent	May be present	Absent
Pseudopods at the margin	Present	Absent	Absent	Absent	Absent	Absent	Absent
Margin of the patch	Serrated					Convex	Irregular
Leucotrichia	Absent	Absent	Absent	Absent	Absent	Present	Absent
Special features							Follicular plugging, telangiectasia

ASH LEAF MACULE

INTRODUCTION

Ash leaf macules (ALM) are characterized by depigmented macules which are lanceolate in shape. Less than 3 ALM are considered as normal even though ALMs are specific for tuberous sclerosis.

Ash leaf macule appears even before the other clinical signs of tuberous sclerosis are evident. Three or more hypopigmented macules of tuberous sclerosis are seen in 97% of patients at birth or shortly after.[1] Once present, the hypopigmented macules tend to be persistent and stable in shape and size.[1] Sometimes, it can be mistaken for vitiligo or nevus depigmentosus. Hence, its diagnosis becomes an important aspect in clinical practice. Dermoscopy shows characteristic patterns in ALM.[2]

KEY DERMOSCOPIC PATTERNS[1]

- White areas
- Zones of total loss of pigment network
- Zones of faint pigment network.

DISCUSSION

On dermoscopy of ALM, the white areas correspond to areas of complete pigment loss, whereas in other zones, some faint pigmentation may be seen. The margins are typically irregular and ill-defined, with there being no evidence of perifollicular pigmentation or leucotrichia.

KEYNOTE

Ash leaf macule is a prime example of how a dermatological sign can lead to the diagnosis of an internal disease, in this case: tuberous sclerosis. In children with such lesions, diagnostic tests including skin biopsy may not be practical. Thus, the knowledge of dermoscopic patterns in ALM can help in its early diagnosis and management. It also greatly alleviates the apprehension associated with hypopigmented lesions such as vitiligo **(Figs. 1A and B)**.

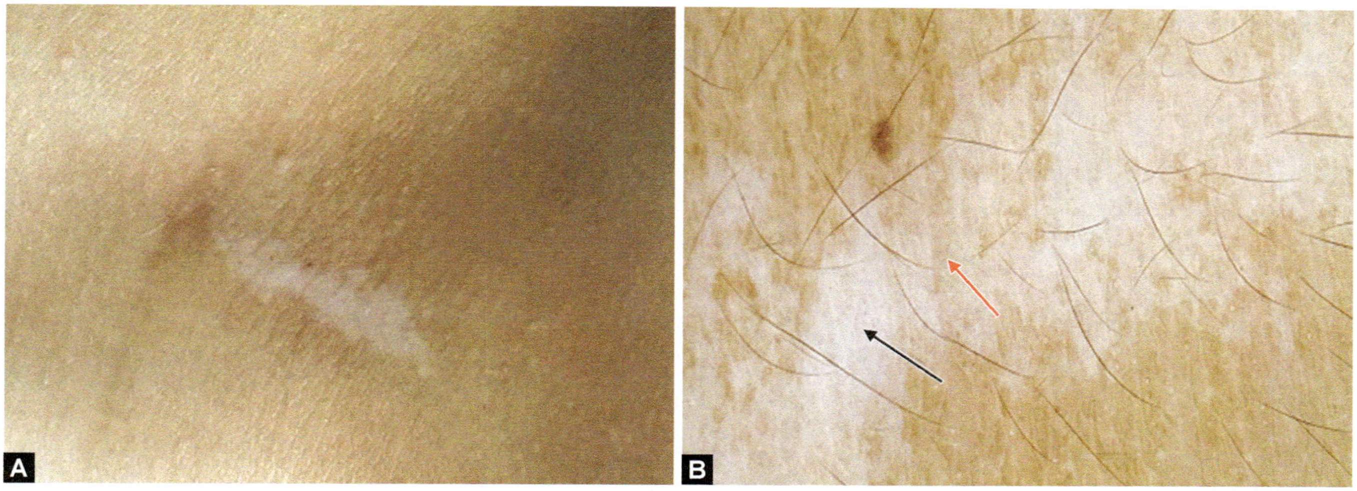

Figs. 1A and B: (A) Depigmented macule on the anterior part of the neck; (B) Dermoscopy of ash leaf macule shows white areas with zones of total loss pigment network (black arrow) among the zones of faint pigment network (red arrow).

REFERENCES

1. Paller A, Mancini A. Disorders of Pigmentation. In: Paller A, Mancini A (Eds). Hurwitz clinical pediatric dermatology: A textbook of skin disorders of childhood and adolescence. Philadelphia: Elsevier Saunders; 2005: pp. 255.
2. Malakar S, Mukharjee S. Differentiation of nevus depigmentosus, ash leaf macule and nevus anemicus. In: Chatarjee M, Neema S, Malakar S (Eds). Dermoscopy in Darker Skin, 1st edition. New Delhi: Jaypee Brothers Medical Publishers (P) Ltd.; 2017. pp. 39-41.

HYPOMELANOSIS OF ITO

INTRODUCTION

Now included in the group of disorders of "pigmentary mosaicism", hypomelanosis of Ito is characterized by patterned streaks of hypopigmentation.[1] The linear streaks and whorls tend to follow lines of mosaicism (lines of Blaschko) or a phylloid pattern of mosaic distribution.

Around 30% of pediatric patients may have associated abnormalities of the eyes, bones or CNS, but they occur in those with widespread skin involvement.[1]

Hypomelanosis of Ito needs to be differentiated from incontinentia pigmenti, nevus depigmentosus, and epidermal nevi, where dermoscopy is of immense value.[2]

KEY DERMOSCOPIC FEATURES

- Uniform faint pigment network with pigment blotches
- Irregular and cloudy border is very characteristic.

DISCUSSION

Diagnosis of hypomelanosis of Ito needs to be made with caution owing to its remarkable similarities with nevus depigmentosus.

The pathophysiological difference between the two conditions is as follows:

1. *Nevus depigmentosus*: Transfer defect of melanosomes
2. *Hypomelanosis of Ito*: Significant reduction of melanosomes and melanocytes in a patchy distribution, with no transfer defect.

The significant reduction of melanocytes in hypomelanosis of Ito is reflected in the incomplete, faint reticular pigment pattern, whereas a reduction in melanin results in blotchy type of pigmentation in the remaining areas.

KEYNOTE

The dermoscopic clue to the diagnosis of hypomelanosis of Ito is its cloudy border.

Dermoscopy allows in rapid distinction between otherwise similar entities, thus proving to be indispensable in pediatric patients. To appreciate these subtle distinguishing features require some training to the naïve eye **(Figs. 2 to 5)**.

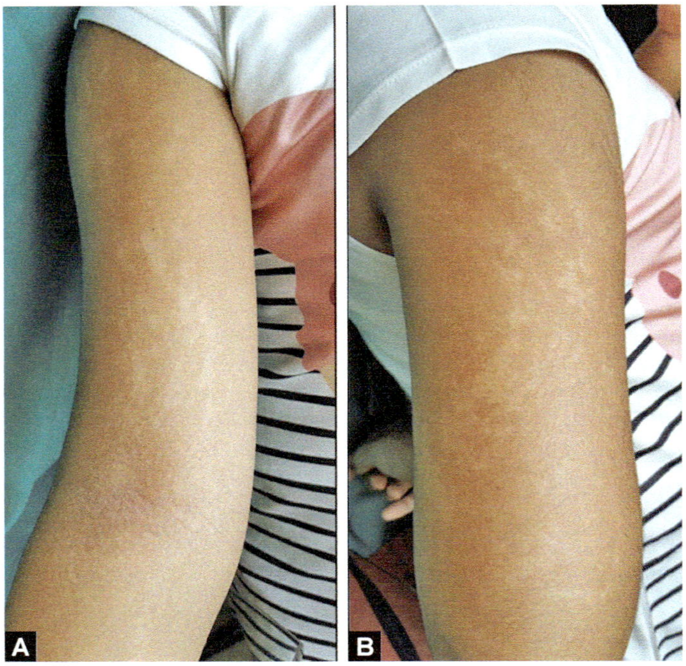

Figs. 2A and B: Linear hypopigmented streaks in a case of hypomelanosis of Ito.

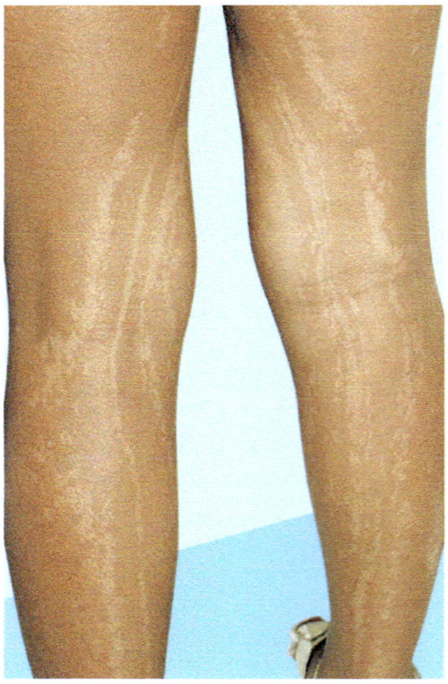

Fig. 3: Hypomelanosis of Ito: Lesions are seen along Blaschko's lines.

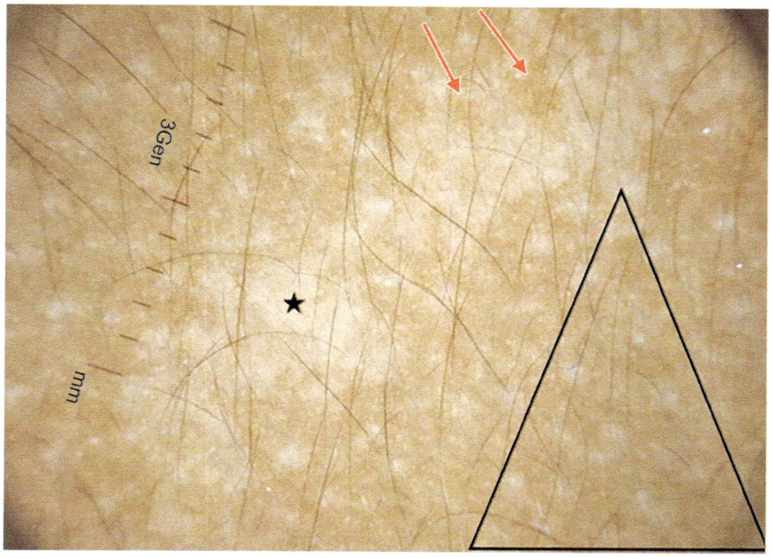

Fig. 4: Dermoscopic features of hypomelanosis of Ito include a diffuse light brown background (black star). In addition, there is also presence of blotchy pigmentation (red arrows). Irregular and cloudy border is a distinguishing feature here (black triangle).

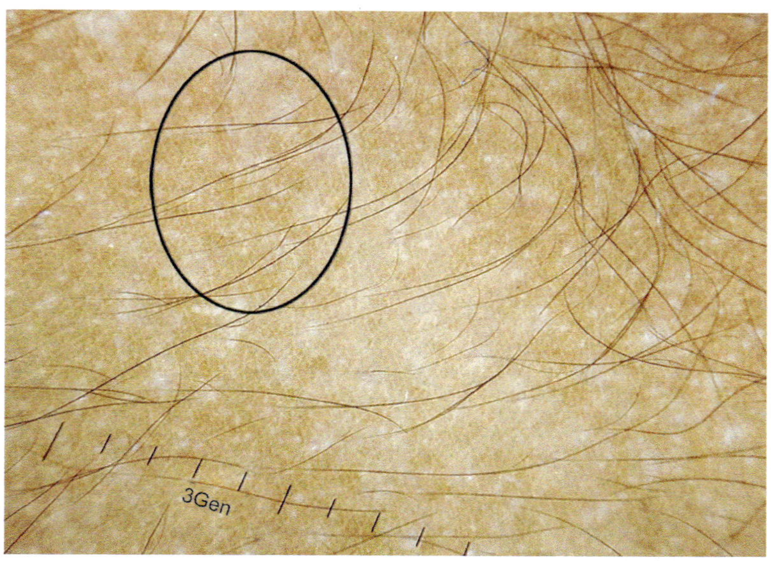

Fig. 5: Presence of blotchy pigmentation along with a cloudy border can be noted.

REFERENCES

1. Paller A, Mancini A. Disorders of Pigmentation. In: Paller A, Mancini A (Eds). Hurwitz clinical pediatric dermatology: A textbook of skin disorders of childhood and adolescence. Philadelphia: Elsevier Saunders; 2005. pp. 263-4.
2. Kumar HY, Jayaprasad S. Hypomelanosis of Ito: a rare cutaneous syndrome. Int J Health Allied Sci. 2013;2:203-5.

NEVUS DEPIGMENTOSUS

INTRODUCTION

Nevus depigmentosus (ND) is a common nevoid hypopigmentary condition characterized by white patches appearing on the skin at birth or may become apparent during infancy.[1]

Clinically, ND shows well-defined depigmented patches with serrated borders. Vitiligo, ash leaf macules, and nevus anemicus are clinical differentials. Dermoscopy can be utilized in this scenario to differentiate ND from these conditions.[2]

KEY DERMOSCOPIC FEATURES[3]

- Faint pigment network presents uniformly throughout the lesion
- Perifollicular pigmentation
- Pseudopods at periphery representing serrated borders.

DISCUSSION

Peripheral extensions of white areas appear as pseudopods. Here, presence of faint or subtle pigmentation in lesion indicates that melanin is definitely present in the epidermis. This feature of ND gives affirmation to the fact that melanosomes are not transferred to the keratinocytes in ND even though the number of melanocytes is normal. The number of melanocytes is normal whereas the amount of melanin is reduced.[4]

Perifollicular pigment is also a prominent feature of ND, so is an absence of leucotrichia.

Vitiligo reveals whites' structureless areas which are dense and glowing. Notably, pseudopods are not observed in vitiligo. Instead, perilesional and reverse pigmentation is frequently seen in vitiligo.[5]

KEYNOTE

Nevus depigmentosus is characterized by depigmented patches which do not change in color or texture throughout life. It has to be differentiated from other treatable diseases like vitiligo. Dermoscopy aids in the diagnosis of ND and also curtails the psychological impact of depigmented skin lesions **(Figs. 6 to 10)**.

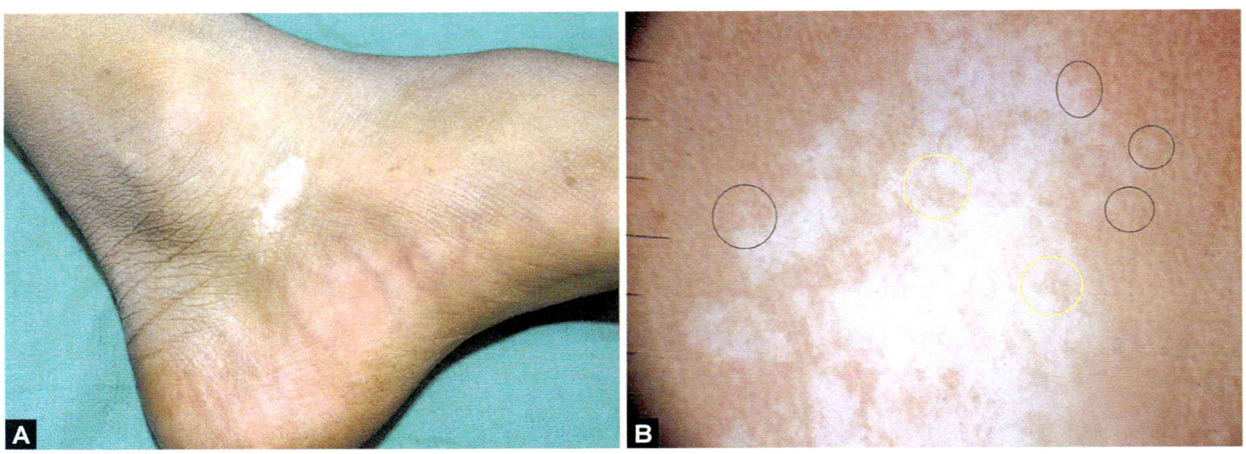

Figs. 6A and B: (A) Well-defined white patch of nevus depigmentosus with serrated borders on the ankle. (B) Dermoscopy shows white structureless areas with subtle pigment network (yellow circles) in white areas. Note the pseudopods at the periphery (black circles).

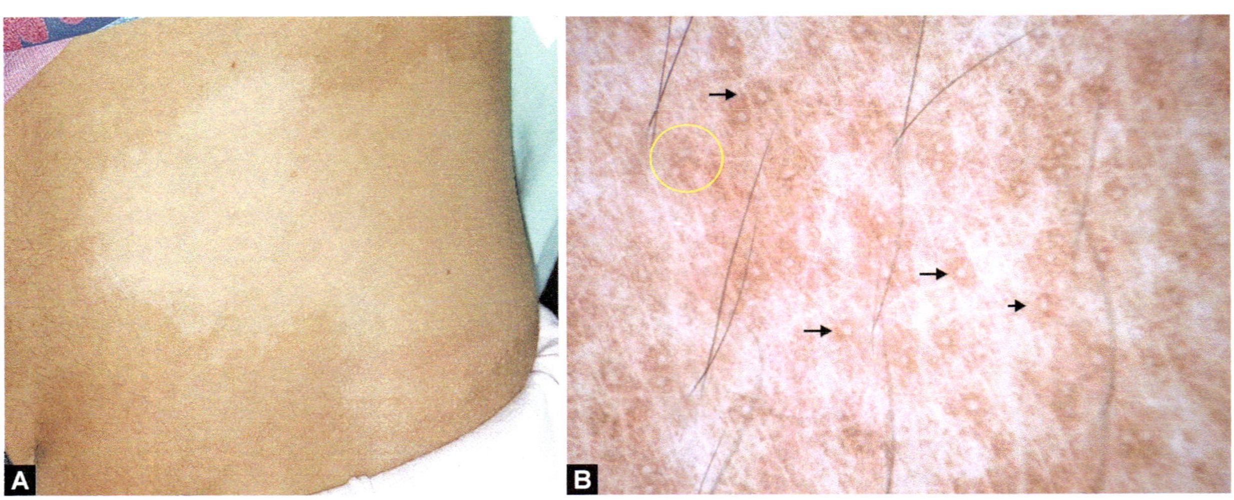

Figs. 7A and B: (A) A lesion of nevus depigmentosus on the trunk. (B) Dermoscopy reveals white areas, faint pigment network (yellow circle), and normal black colored hairs. White dots (eccrine openings) show peripheral pigmentation (black arrows).

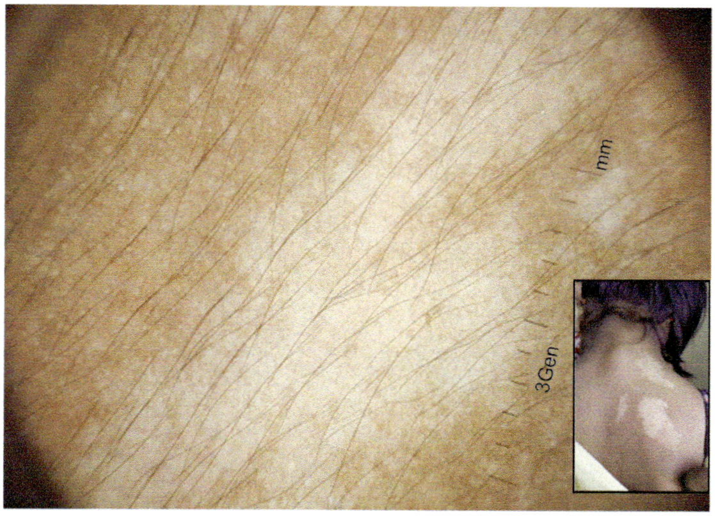

Fig. 8: Characteristic dermoscopic features of ND noted here are faint pigment network present uniformly throughout the lesion, along with retention of perifollicular pigment.

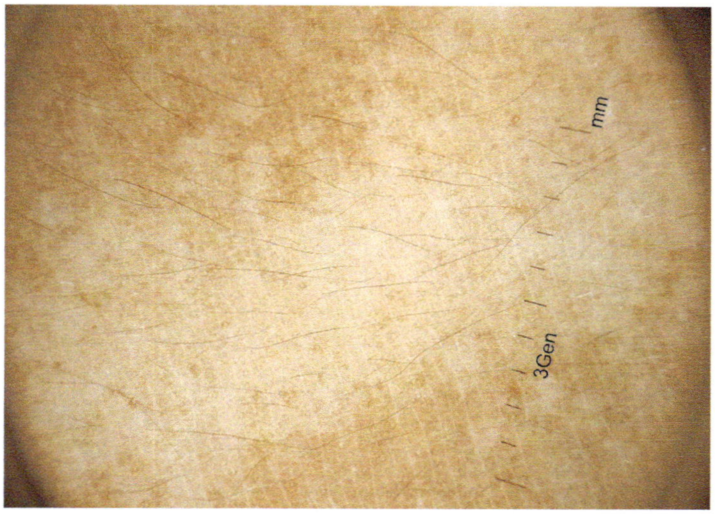

Fig. 9: Another case showing the typical serrated margin of ND. Note the absence of leucotrichia.

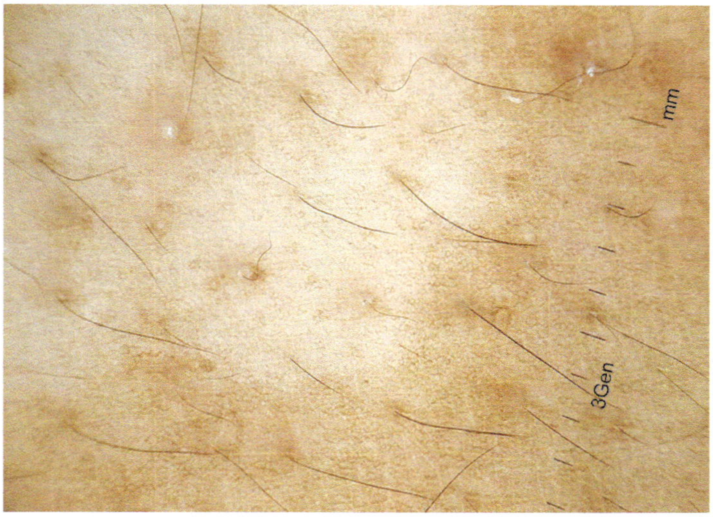

Fig. 10: Here, prominent perifollicular pigmentation can be seen.

REFERENCES

1. Deb S, Sarkar R, Samanta AB. A brief review of nevus depigmentosus. Pigment Int. 2014;1:56-8.
2. Oiso N, Kawada A. The diagnostic usefulness of dermoscopy for nevus depigmentosus. Eur J Dermatol. 2011;21(4):639-40.
3. Sarma N, Ankad BS. Dermoscopy in nevoid disorders. In: Chatarjee M, Neema S, Malakar S (Eds). Dermoscopy in darker skin, 1st edition. New Delhi: Jaypee Brothers Medical Publishers (P) Ltd.; 2017. pp. 127-33.
4. Lee HS, Chun YS, Hann SK. Nevus depigmentosus: clinical and histopathologic characteristics in 67 patients. J Am Acad Dermatol. 1999;40:21-6.
5. Thatte SS, Khopkar US. The utility of dermoscopy in the diagnosis of evolving lesions of vitiligo. Indian J Dermatol Venereol Leprol. 2014;80:505-8.

PIEBALDISM

INTRODUCTION

It is characterized by congenital patterned areas of depigmentation that may or may not include a white lock of hair above the forehead (white forelock) in affected individuals. It results from defective migration of melanoblasts from the neural crest to the ventral midline and a defect in the differentiation of melanoblasts to melanocytes.[1]

In piebaldism, there are depigmented patches interspersed with islands of normal or increased pigmentation. In contrast to vitiligo, piebaldism presents at birth, with lesions lacking convex borders, and being present mainly on the ventral surfaces.[2]

KEY DERMOSCOPIC FEATURES

- Vast areas of depigmentation, giving a white background
- Distorted melanocytic network
- Absence of perifollicular pigment
- Islands of normal or hyperpigmented skin
- Irregular margins
- Leucotrichia may or may not be present (we have rarely encountered leucotrichia either clinically or dermoscopically, as we have examined mostly cases of piebaldism over the other parts of the body except the scalp and eyebrows, where white forelock is an integral part of the condition).

DISCUSSION

Piebaldism results from defective migration of melanoblasts from the neural crest to the ventral midline thus manifesting dermoscopically as vast areas of depigmentation and islands of normal or hyperpigmentation.

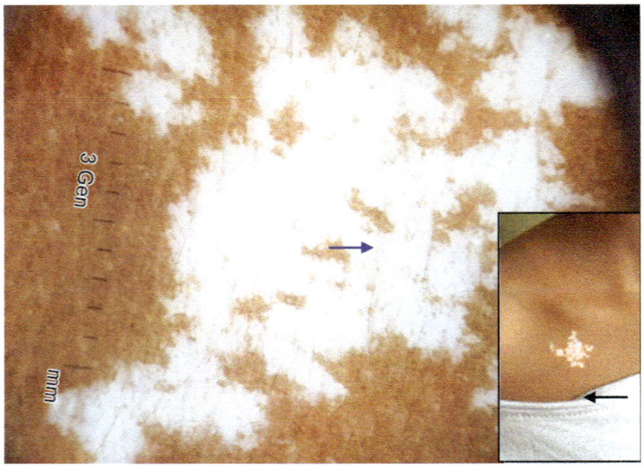

Fig. 11: Dermoscopy of piebaldism reveals distorted pigment network (black arrow), absence of perifollicular pigment (blue arrow), and vast areas of depigmentation (inset shows the clinical picture: depigmented patch with irregular margins, present over the anterior chest).

The distorted melanocytic network with reduced intensity of pigmentation results from a defect in the differentiation of melanoblasts to melanocytes.

We hypothesize that the absence of perifollicular pigment may be due to defect in transfer of melanosomes from the melanocytes in the hair bud to the surrounding keratinocytes, however, further studies may be necessary to substantiate this.

KEYNOTE

The clue to dermoscopic feature of piebaldism is distorted melanocytic network. Another distinguishing diagnostic feature of piebaldism is presence of islands of normal or hyperpigmented skin **(Figs. 11 to 14)**.

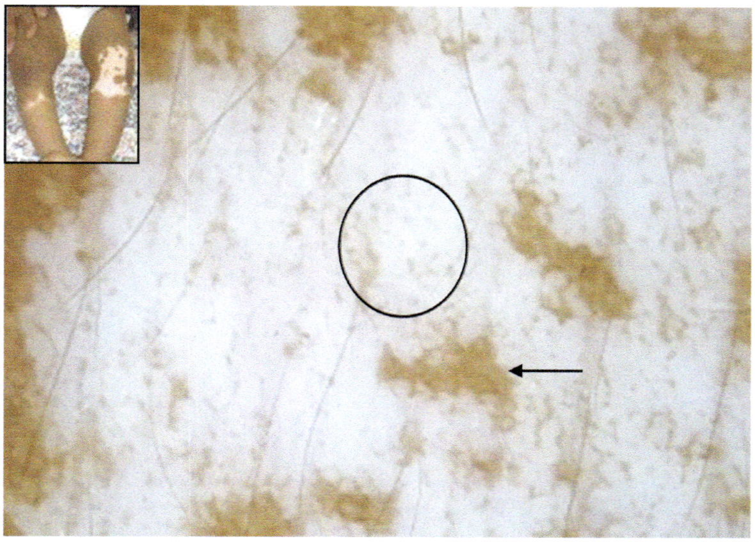

Fig. 12: Magnified dermoscopic image showing areas of distorted pigment network (black circle) and islands of normal pigmentation (black arrow), on a white background (inset shows patches of piebaldism present over both the knees. Note the depigmented patches with interspersed islands of pigmentation).

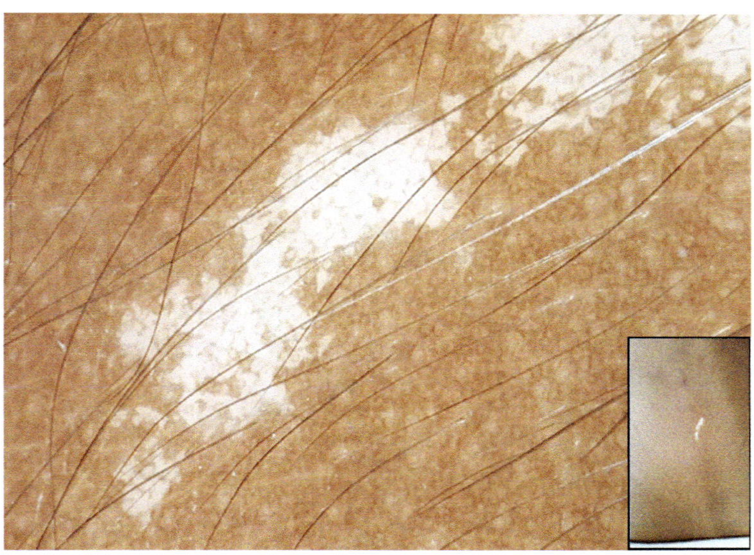

Fig. 13: The clinical picture shows a linear, hypopigmented lesion over the back over a 4-year-old boy, resembling an ash leaf macule. But dermoscopy of the lesion showed the distorted pigment network, which hints toward the diagnosis of piebaldism.

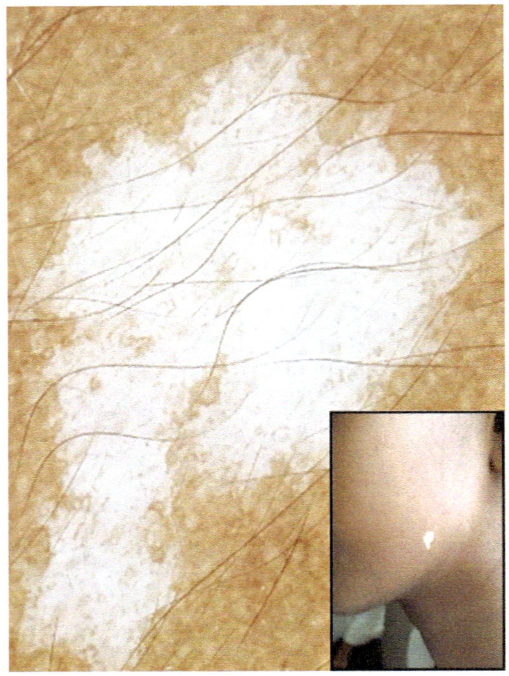

Fig. 14: Tiny, hypopigmented patch over the left mandibular area, mimicking vitiligo. However, dermoscopic examination reveals the most striking feature of piebaldism—distorted pigment network.

REFERENCES

1. Paller A, Mancini A. Disorders of Pigmentation. In: Paller A, Mancini A (Eds). Hurwitz clinical pediatric dermatology: A textbook of skin disorders of childhood and adolescence. Philadelphia: Elsevier Saunders; 2005. pp. 253-4.
2. Malakar S, Mukherjee SS, Malakar S. Looking through the dermoscope in a case of piebaldism. Our Dermatol Online. 2019;10(3): 312-3.

CHAPTER 12

Vascular Lesions

Subrata Malakar, Surit Malakar

INTRODUCTION

Vascular lesions can be divided into two categories—tumors and malformations. Neoplasms of the vasculature, resulting from endothelial cell proliferation, and cause vascular tumors such as infantile hemangioma and pyogenic granuloma.[1]

On the other hand, vascular malformations represent developmental anomalies without any endothelial proliferation that can further be categorized into capillary malformations (such as port-wine stain), venous, and lymphatic malformations. In contrast to infantile hemangiomas, vascular malformations are present at birth, persistent lifelong and show no spontaneous resolution.

REFERENCE

1. Paller A, Mancini A. Vascular disorders of infancy and childhood. In: Paller A, Mancini A (Eds). Hurwitz clinical pediatric dermatology: A textbook of skin disorders of childhood and adolescence. Philadelphia: Elsevier Saunders; 2005; pp. 307-44.

INFANTILE HEMANGIOMA PRECURSORS

INTRODUCTION

About 30–50% of hemangiomas present as precursor lesions. These are termed as "infantile hemangioma precursors (IHP)". Clinically, they appear in various forms: an area of pallor along with fine thread-like telangiectasias or a macular erythematous stain or a violaceous bruise-like area or a tiny scratch/ulcer.[1] They can be a source of diagnostic confusion, especially in infants, where anxious parents are concerned.

Most of the IHPs eventually proliferate into fully formed hemangiomas, but occasionally they may do so only in part of the lesion, or not at all. The later type is known as abortive or minimal growth hemangiomas. These hemangiomas without a proliferative phase are Glut-1 positive on immunohistochemistry.[2]

KEY DERMOSCOPIC FEATURES[3]

- Red linear vessels **(Fig. 1)**
- Red round globular vessels **(Fig. 2)**
- Red, comma-like vessels **(Fig. 3)**.

DISCUSSION

Dermoscopic features of IHP are polymorphous, showing red round globular vessels, comma vessels, and red linear vessels.

Histopathological correlates of dermoscopic findings are given in **Table 1**.

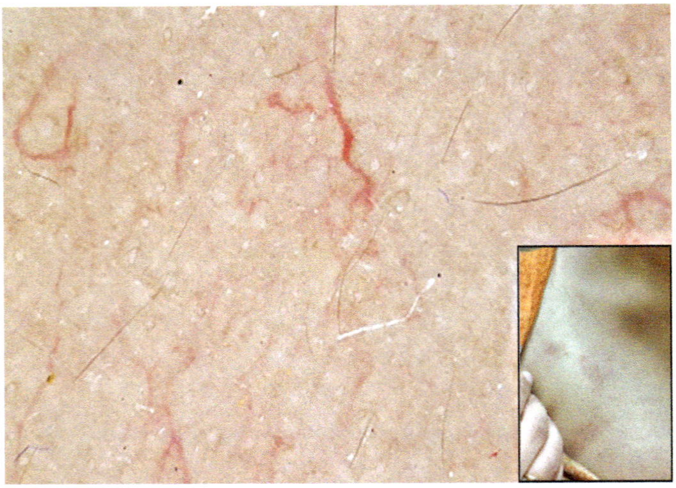

Fig. 1: Inset shows clinical picture of infantile hemangioma precursor showing macular erythematous stain on the upper chest present since infancy. Dermoscopy shows linear dilated vessels which correspond to vessels in the subpapillary and upper reticular dermis.

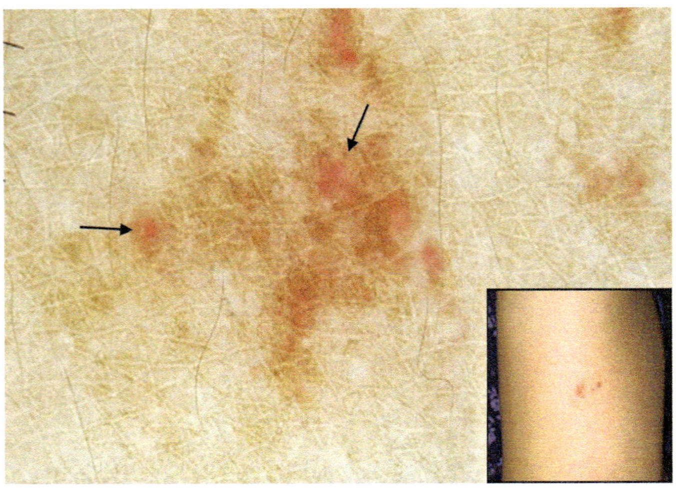

Fig. 2: An inconspicuous macular, erythematous stain present since birth in a young girl. Dermoscopy of the lesion shows red round large globular vessels (arrows) which denote their location in the superficial dermis.

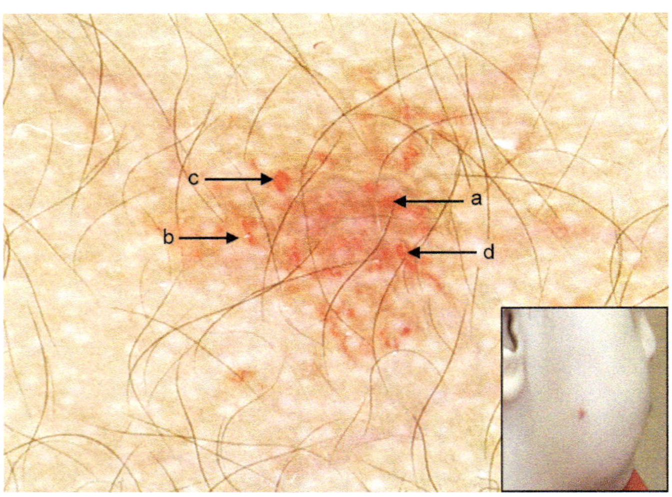

Fig. 3: A solitary, tiny erythematous papule present on the right cheek of an infant. Dermoscopy of the lesion revealing polymorphous appearance of vessels showing: (a) red round globular vessels; (b) red comma shaped vessels; (c) twisted red capillaries; and (d) red linear vessels; on an erythematous background.

Table 1: Dermoscopic findings of infantile hemangioma precursors.

Dermoscopic feature	*Histopathological correlation*
Red round globular vessels	Dilated capillaries in the papillary dermis
Red, comma-like vessels	Superficially dilated vasculature changing direction and transitioning to deep dilated horizontal subpapillary capillaries
Red linear vessels	Dilated linear vascular structures in the subpapillary and upper reticular dermis

The significance of IHP lies in their evolution. Following an accurate diagnosis from dermoscopy of IHP, parents can be counseled about the course of the condition.

KEYNOTE

Based on the depth of the vessels, a variety of vascular patterns ranging from dots to linear vessels can be seen in IHP.

REFERENCES

1. Hidano A, Nakajima S. Earliest features of the strawberry mark in the newborn. Br J Dermatol. 1972;87:138-44.
2. Corella F, Garcia-Navarro X, Ribe A, et al. Abortive or minimal-growth hemangiomas: immunohistochemical evidence that they represent true infantile hemangiomas. J Am Acad Dermatol. 2008;58:685-90.
3. Oiso N, Kimura M, Kawara S, et al. Clinical, dermoscopic, and histopathological features in a case of infantile hemangioma without proliferation. Pediatr Dermatol. 2011;28(1):66-8.

PYOGENIC GRANULOMA

INTRODUCTION

The term pyogenic granuloma (PG) is a misnomer as the lesions of PGs are neither pyogenic nor granulomatous. It is better termed as "lobular capillary hemangioma". Its pathogenesis is mainly reactive.

Pyogenic granuloma presents as a solitary, rapidly growing papulonodule, with a tendency to bleed on minor trauma. Thus, diagnosis is fairly straight forward but, occasionally, common benign and malignant tumors may be confused with PG.[1,2]

KEY DERMOSCOPIC FEATURES[3,4]

- Homogeneous reddish or reddish-white areas
- A whitish collarette which surrounds the reddish white area
- White rail lines
- Various vascular patterns such as hairpin, dotted, linear irregular, and polymorphous vessels
- Hemorrhagic crusts.

DISCUSSION

- The most common dermoscopic pattern of PG is a *homogeneous reddish or reddish white area* surrounded by a white collarette (in 85% of cases).[5] The reddish/reddish-white areas correspond histologically to proliferating capillaries and veins. It is the most common dermoscopic sign associated with PG.[6]
- The *white collarette* located at the periphery of the lesion is a ring-shaped squamous structure. It represents hyperplastic epithelium that partially or totally embraces the proliferating blood vessels in PG. It has also been observed in clear cell acanthoma.

- Homogeneous reddish areas are often intersected by *white rail lines* which appear dermoscopically as whitish streaks or bands. Histologically these rail lines correlate with the fibrous septae that surround the capillary tufts or lobules in advanced forms of PG. These structures have a good specificity but low sensitivity. Similar feature has been observed in dermatofibroma.
- Additional criteria are various *vascular patterns* such as hairpin, dotted, linear irregular, polymorphous vessels, and hemorrhagic crusts.

The four main dermoscopic features of PG in various combination give rise to seven dermoscopic patterns, which have been described by Zaballos et al. **(Table 2)**.[6]

After comparing all dermoscopic structures in PG, red homogeneous area is found to be present in all patterns. Zaballos et al. stated that P1, P4, and P5 are the most common patterns of PG.

KEYNOTE

Pyogenic granuloma is a common condition in pediatric patients. Dermoscopy can help to exclude other close differentials such as nodular amelanotic melanoma **(Figs. 4 to 10)**.

Table 2: Dermoscopic features of PG.

Patterns	*Red homogeneous area*	*White collarette*	*White rail lines*	*Vascular structures*
P1	+	+		
P2	+		+	
P3	+			+
P4	+	+	+	
P5	+	+		+
P6	+		+	+
P7	+	+	+	+

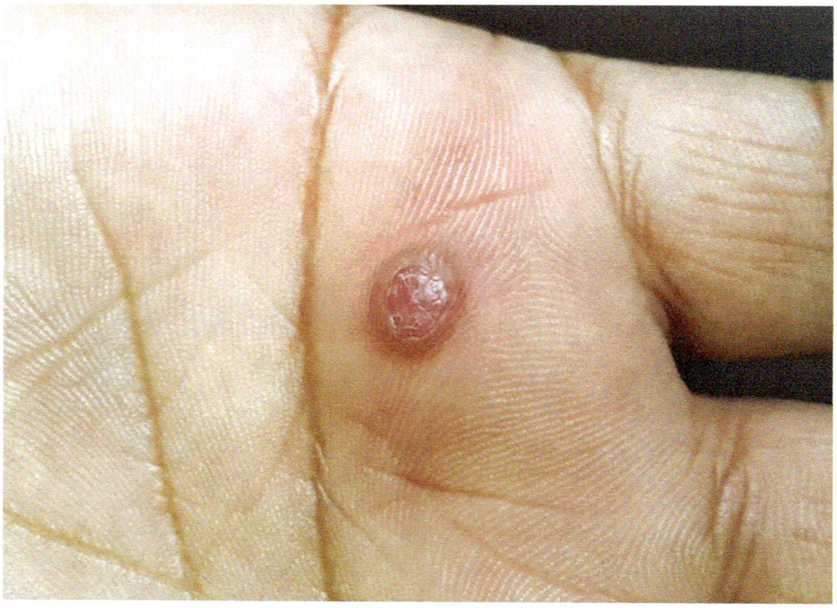

Fig. 4: Pyogenic granuloma over palm presenting as a solitary, red-brown, raised, and sessile nodule for 3 months. The base reveals a peripheral collarette of scale.

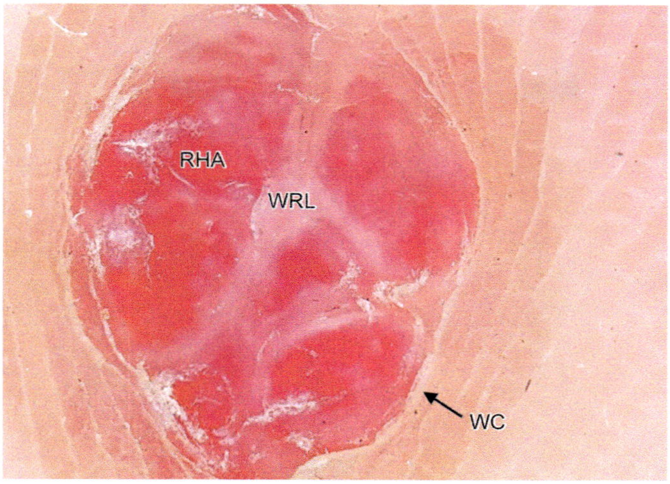

Fig. 5: P4 pattern of pyogenic granuloma (PG)—dermoscopy shows white collarette (WC), red homogeneous area (RHA), and white rail lines (WRL). This pattern composed of WC, RHA, and WRL has been demonstrated to be 100% specific for pyogenic granuloma.

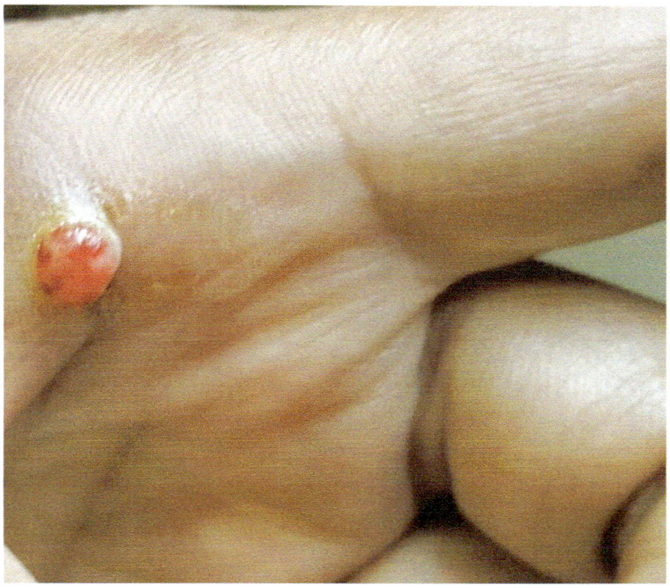

Fig. 6: Lesion of pyogenic granuloma: Painless, glistening red nodule over palm that bleed spontaneously.

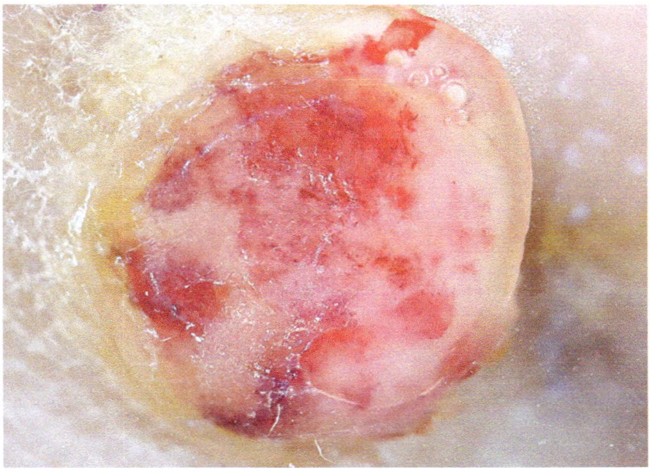

Fig. 7: P5 pattern of pyogenic granuloma (PG) in which there are white collarette (WC), red homogeneous area (RHA), and vascular structures. Vascular patterns seen in this picture are dotted, atypical, and hairpin vessels.

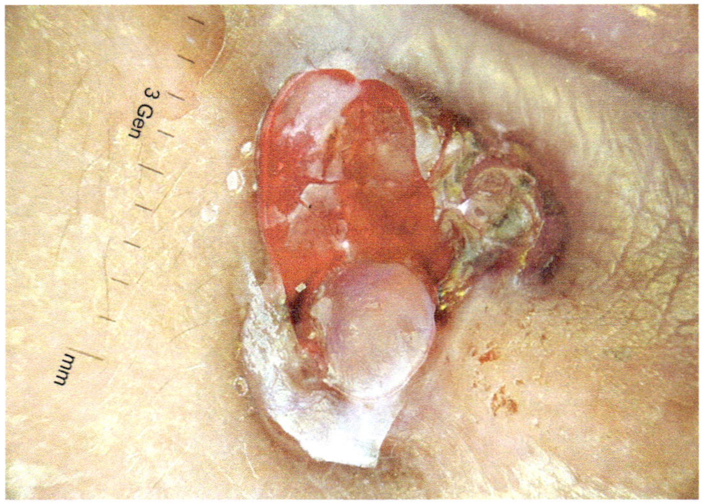

Fig. 8: P1—pyogenic granulomas are frequently eroded and crusted. This feature may explain the dermoscopic finding of ulceration and crusts.

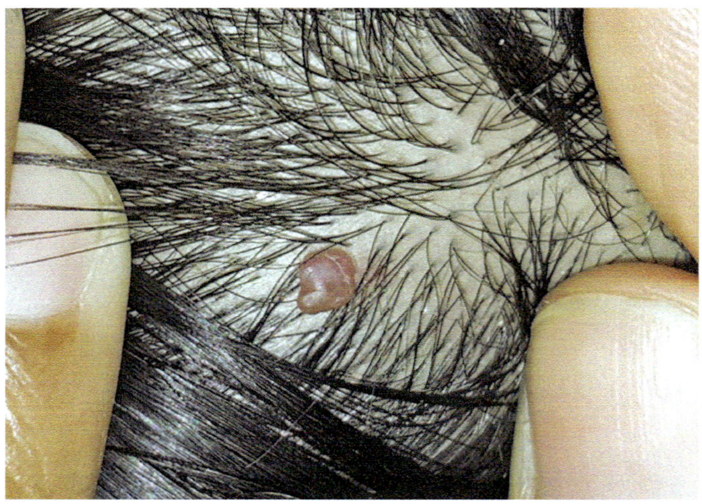

Fig. 9: A shiny red nodule of pyogenic granuloma (PG) on the scalp for 4 months.

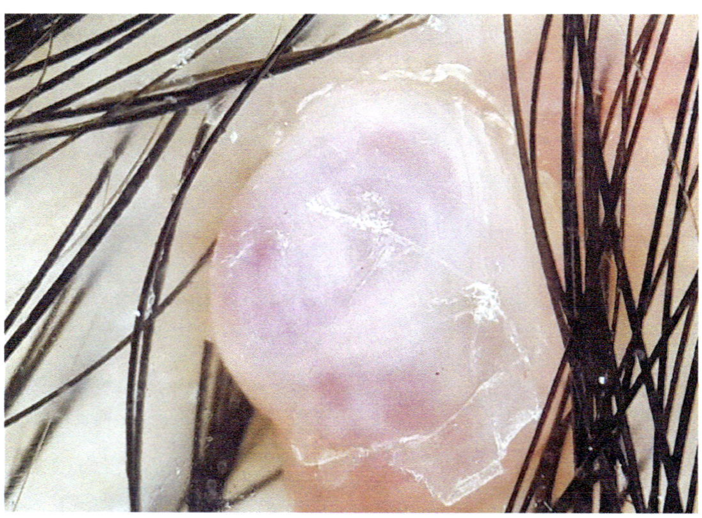

Fig. 10: P4 pattern of pyogenic granuloma (PG)—white collarette (WC), red homogeneous area (RHA), and white rail lines (WRL).

REFERENCES

1. Pagliai KA, Cohen BA. Pyogenic granuloma in children. Paediatr Dermatol. 2004;21:10-3.
2. Requena L, Sangueza OP. Cutaneous vascular proliferation. Part II. Hyperplasias and benign neoplasms. J Am Acad Dermatol. 1997;37:887-919.
3. Zaballos P, Llambrich A, Cuellar F, et al. Dermoscopic findings in pyogenic granuloma. Br J Dermatol. 2006;154:1108-11.
4. Zaballos P, Salsench E, Puig S, et al. Dermoscopy of pyogenic granulomas. Arch Dermatol. 2007;143:824.
5. Martin JM, Bella-Navarro R, Jorda E. Vascular patterns in dermoscopy. Actas Dermosifiliogr. 2012;103(5):357-75.
6. Zaballos P, Carulla M, Ozdemir F, et al. Dermoscopy of pyogenic granuloma: a morphological study. Br J Dermatol. 2010;163: 1229-37.

CAPILLARY MALFORMATIONS

PORT-WINE STAIN (FIGS. 11 TO 14)

Introduction

Port-wine stain (PWS) presents as a macular area, the color of which varies from pink to dark red. It is composed of dilated capillaries in the superficial and deep dermis. If the vessels are superficially placed the lesion looks bright red. It appears pink in case of deep and small vessels but purple in case of deep and larger vessels.[1]

Key Dermoscopic Features

- Red globules and dots
- Prominent red lines.

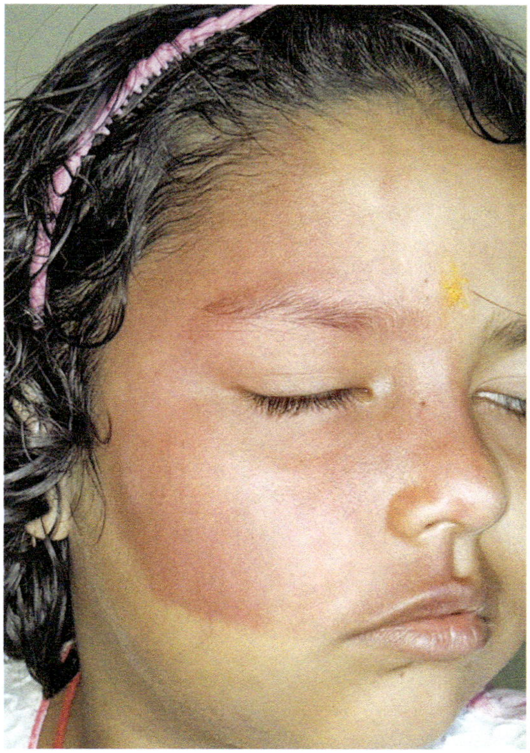

Fig. 11: Clinical picture of port-wine stain.

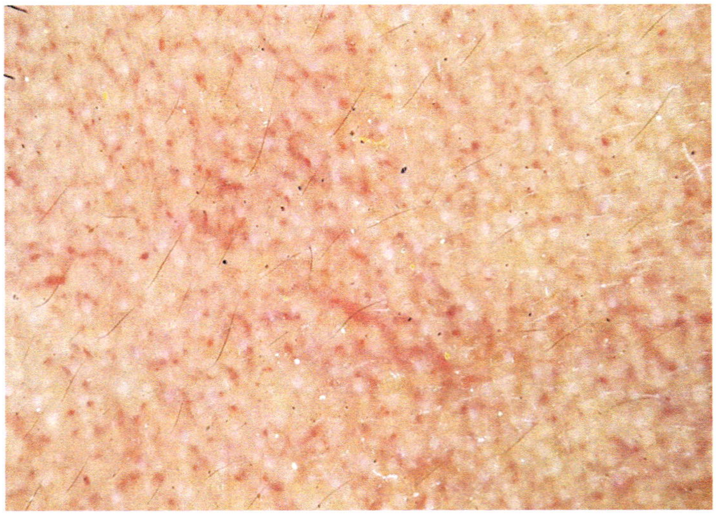

Fig. 12: Dermoscopy shows red globules and dots along with prominent red lines. Horizontal capillaries on dermoscopy signify that the location of the vessels is in the subpapillary plexus.

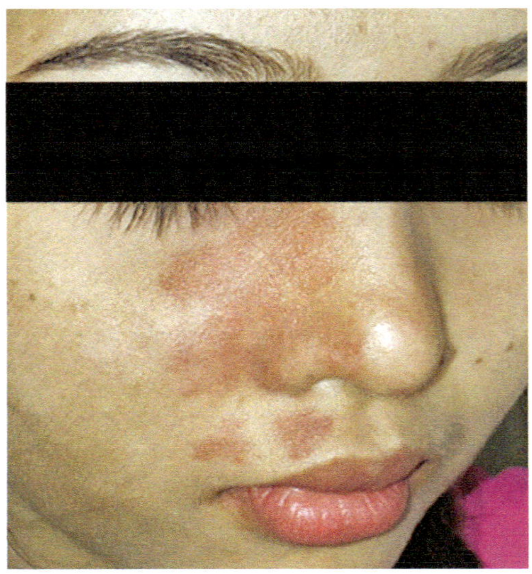

Fig. 13: PWS in a young girl.

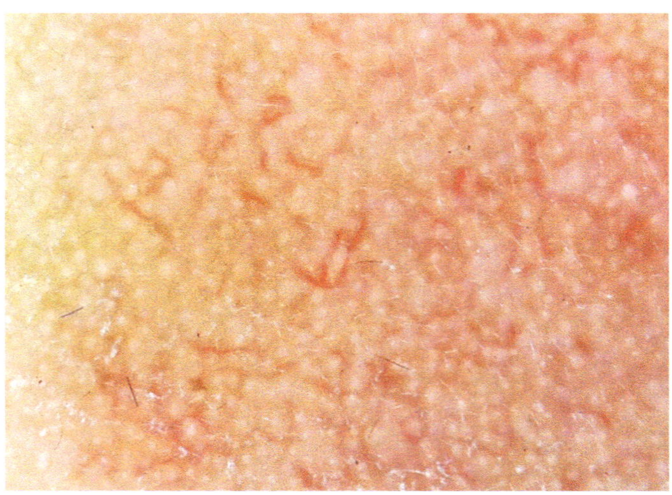

Fig. 14: Dermoscopy reveals mostly the prominent linear vessels. As the vessels are in a comparatively deeper plane, treatment with pulse dye laser here might lead to scarring. Thus, dermoscopy can aid in better management plan as well, on a case-to-case basis.

Discussion

Red globules and dots correspond to perpendicular vessels in the papillary dermis. On the other hand, prominent red lines correlate with thicker, horizontal capillaries present in the subpapillary plexus.

Knowledge regarding the location of vessels in the dermis dermoscopically is essential with regard to the treatment outcome, as laser treatment of deeper vessels often lead to scarring. The lesions revealing a superficial pattern consisting of red globules and dots on dermoscopy have the best response to pulsed dye laser.[2]

Keynote

Dermoscope is not only a useful tool for the selection of lesions for treatment; it also serves as a monitoring tool to record effectiveness of laser treatment on PWS.

References

1. Sevila A, Nagore E, Botella-Estrada R, et al. Videomicroscopy of venular malformations (port wine stain type): prediction of response to pulsed dye laser. Pediatr Dermatol. 2004;21:589-96.
2. Motley RJ, Lanigan SW, Katugampola GA. Videomicroscopy predicts outcome in treatment of port-wine stains. Arch Dermatol. 1997;133:921-2.

NEVUS SIMPLEX (FIGS. 15A AND B)

Introduction

Nevus simplex, more commonly known as salmon patch, is the most common capillary malformation of infancy which usually fades away in 1–2 years of age. Lesions on the posterior neck or scalp may fade, although some of these persist indefinitely. It appears as a flat, dull pink macular rash over the posterior neck and scalp, glabella, forehead, upper eyelid and occasionally the nose, or nasolabial folds.[1]

Key Dermoscopic Feature

Prominent linear vessels.

Discussion

The prominent linear vessels seen on dermoscopy are due to the ectatic dermal vessels (subpapillary plexus). Absence of red dots and globules helps in differentiating it from port-wine stain while the absence of polymorphous vessels helps in differentiating it from infantile hemangioma precursor.

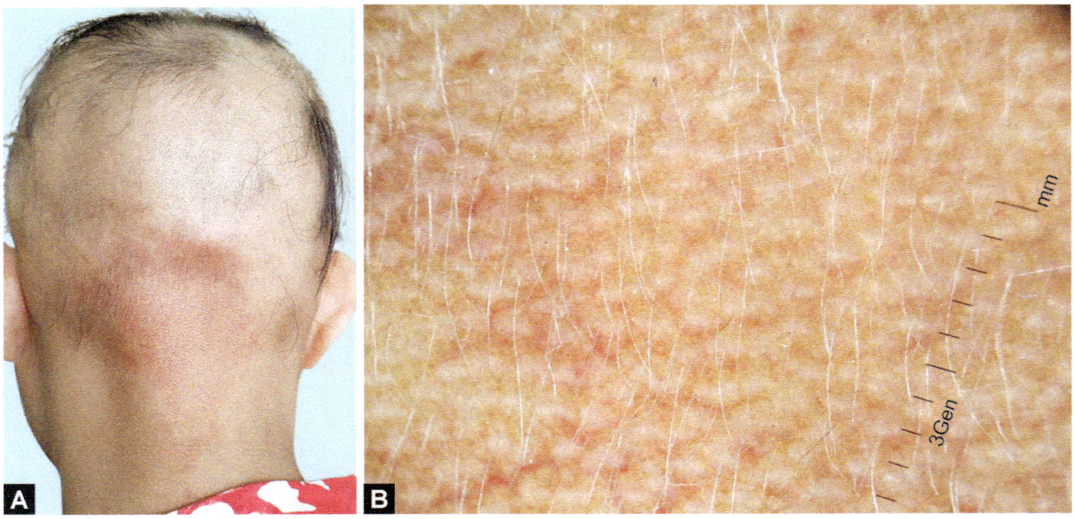

Figs. 15A and B: (A) Salmon patch over the posterior part of neck and scalp in a 3-year-old girl. (B) Dermoscopy of salmon patch showing some in-focused but mostly out-focused multiple linear vessels (dilated subpapillary plexus).

Reference

1. Amy PS, Mancini AJ. Vascular Disorders of Infancy and Childhood. Hurwitz Clinical Pediatric Dermatology: A Textbook of Skin Disorders of Childhood and Adolescence. 5th edition. Elsevier; 2016. pp. 295-6.

LYMPHANGIOMA CIRCUMSCRIPTUM

INTRODUCTION

Lymphangiomas are congenital lymphatic malformations, accounting for 4% of all vascular tumors. They originate from the lymphatic endothelial cells. They are classified into cutaneous lymphangioma circumscriptum (LC), cavernous lymphangiomas, and cystic hygromas.

Of these, cutaneous LC is the most common. It presents clinically as clusters of translucent vesicles; occasionally containing varying amounts of blood.[1] When cutaneous LC has a marked content of blood, it may be confused with hemangioma.[2] Histology of cutaneous LC shows thin-walled lymphatic vessels in the papillary and reticular dermis.

KEY DERMOSCOPIC FEATURES[2,3]

- Yellow/brown lacunae surrounded by pale septa; thin linear vessels may or may not be visible
- Reddish to bluish lacunae
- Hypopyon-like lesions.

DISCUSSION

Lesions containing clear lymphatic fluid appear as yellow/brown lacunae surrounded by pale septa on dermoscopy.

Varying amount of blood within the vesicle displays varied dermoscopic features which range from focal red to diffuse pink to violaceous-colored lacunae. The most plausible explanation to the presence of blood inside the lymphatic dilatation is the presence of microshunts between the lymphatic channels and small blood vessels.[4,5]

The development of hypopyon-like structures in LC is an interesting phenomenon. Over a period of time, red blood cells (RBCs) and white blood cells (WBCs) sediment at the bottom while the serum is suspended in the upper part. This leads to a color transition from light to dark as one progressively examines the top and bottom in some lacunae, creating an effect known as hypopyon.[2]

KEYNOTE

Cutaneous LC may sometimes contain marked amount of blood that mimics hemangioma. Consequently, it may be difficult to differentiate both conditions clinically and even dermoscopically. Hence, hypopyon-like feature can be a very useful dermoscopic pattern to differentiate between cutaneous LC from hemangioma, where such hypopyon formation is not seen **(Figs. 16 to 21)**.

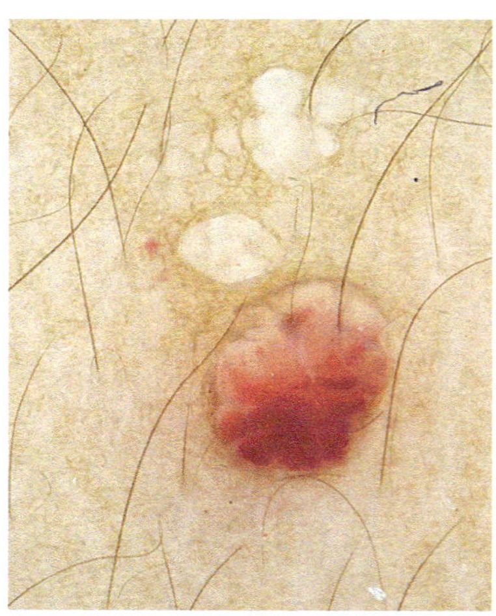

Fig. 16: Dermoscopy of a classic case of lymphangioma circumscriptum shows yellowish-white lacunae surrounded by pale septa. One of the lacunae contains blood that has accumulated in its lowest part producing "hypopyon".

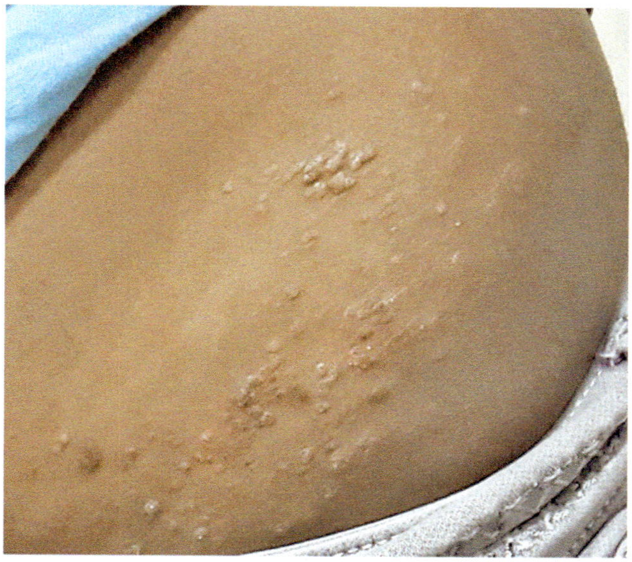

Fig. 17: Lymphangioma circumscriptum: Frogspawn appearance of the lesions.

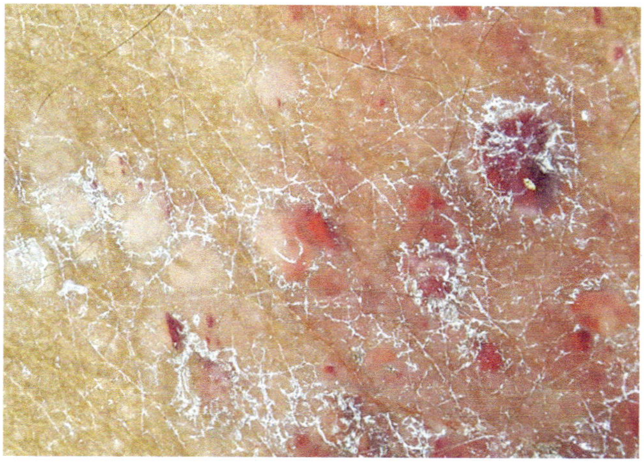

Fig. 18: Dermoscopy of the above lesion reveals yellow-white lacunae, red lacunae, and hypopyon-like structures.

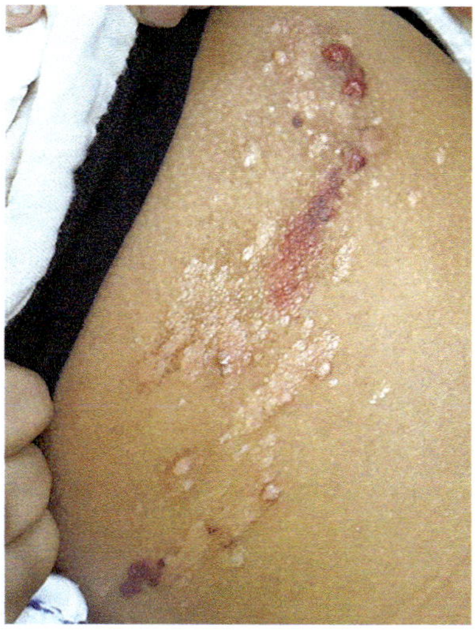

Fig. 19: Usually microcystic LMs are asymptomatic, but at times there is drainage of clear fluid from ruptured vesicles or even spontaneous bleeding.

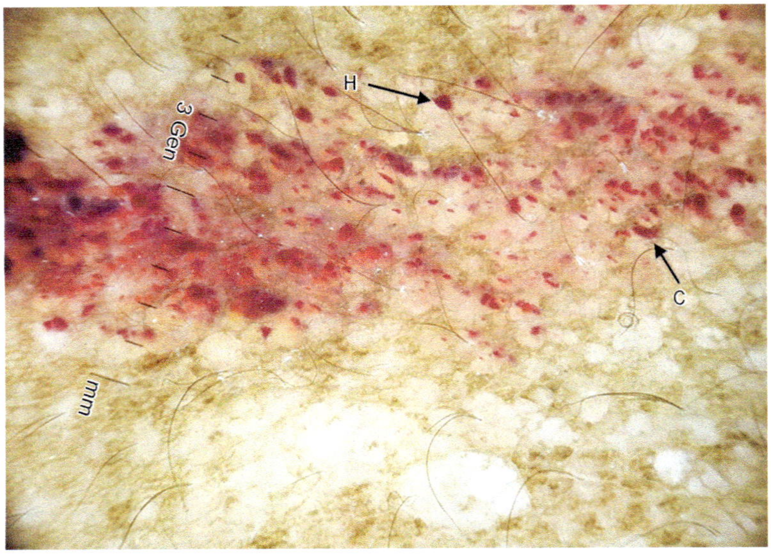

Fig. 20: Red lacunae are arranged in a linear fashion where multiple hypopyon-like structures are observed. Hypopyon-like structures may have different shapes like crescent (C) and half (H).

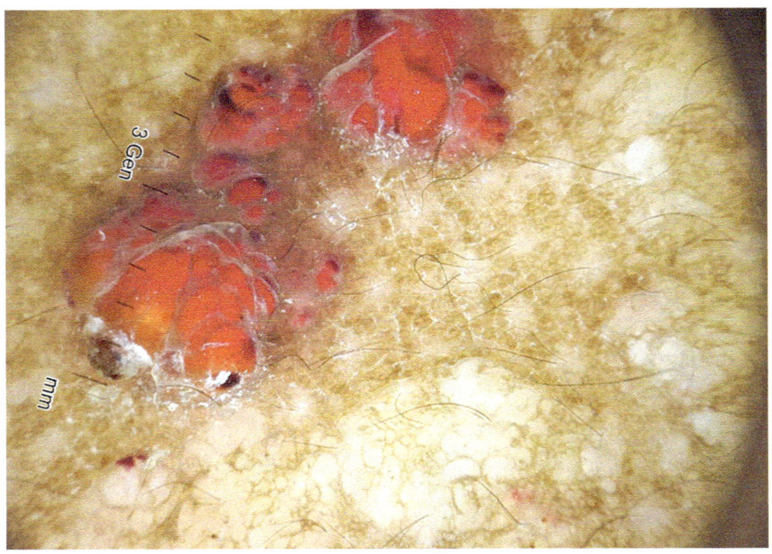

Fig. 21: Red lacunae on magnification which are in turn surrounded by plenty of yellow-white lacunae with septa.

REFERENCES

1. Patel GA, Schwartz RA. Cutaneous lymphangioma circumscriptum: frog spawn on the skin. Int J Dermatol. 2009;48:1290-5.
2. Gencoglan G, Inanir I, Ermertcan AT. Hypopyon-like features: new dermoscopic criteria in the differential diagnosis of cutaneous lymphangioma circumscriptum and hemangiomas? J Eur Acad Dermatol Venereol. 2012;26:1023-5.
3. Massa AF, Moreira AI, Menezes N, et al. Cutaneous lymphangioma circumscriptum: dermoscopic features. An Bras Dermatol. 2015;90(2):262-4.
4. Franke FE, Steger K, Marks A, et al. Hobnail hemangiomas (targetoid hemosiderotic hemangiomas) are true lymphangiomas. J Cutan Pathol. 2004;31:362-7.
5. Paller A, Miancini A. Vascular Disorders of Infancy and Childhood. In: Paller A, Miancini A (Eds). Hurwitz Clinical Paediatric Dermatology: A Textbook of Skin Disorders of Childhood and Adolescence. London: Elsevier; 2016. p. 304.

ANGIOKERATOMA

INTRODUCTION

Angiokeratomas are vascular malformations of the upper dermis which present clinically as blue-black papules.

The clinical forms of angiokeratomas are:

- Solitary and multiple angiokeratomas
- Angiokeratoma circumscriptum
- Angiokeratoma of Mibelli
- Angiokeratoma of Fordyce
- Angiokeratoma corporis diffusum (Fabry's disease).[1]

KEY DERMOSCOPIC FEATURES[1,2]

- Dark lacunae and red lacunae
- Whitish veil
- Peripheral erythema
- Hemorrhagic crusts.

DISCUSSION

Dark lacunae are the hallmark dermoscopic feature of solitary angiokeratoma and correspond histopathologically to partially or completely thrombosed dilated vessels.[2,3]

On the other hand, red lacunae denote presence of dilated vascular spaces in the upper dermis but which do not have thrombosis.

The whitish veil represents hyperkeratosis and acanthosis. Additional dermoscopic features include erythema and hemorrhagic crusts.

Zaballos et al. described three patterns of angiokeratoma on dermoscopy:[2]

1. Red lacunae, dark lacunae, and whitish veil (most common pattern).
2. Peripheral erythema along with the features of pattern 1.
3. Hemorrhagic crusts in addition to features of pattern 1.

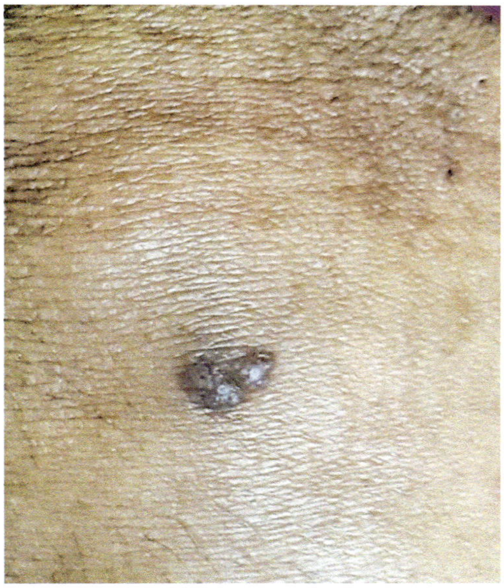

Fig. 22: Blue-red papulonodule over the knee with slight scaling on the surface. On histology, there are dilated thin-walled vessels in the upper dermis and the epidermis is hyperplastic.

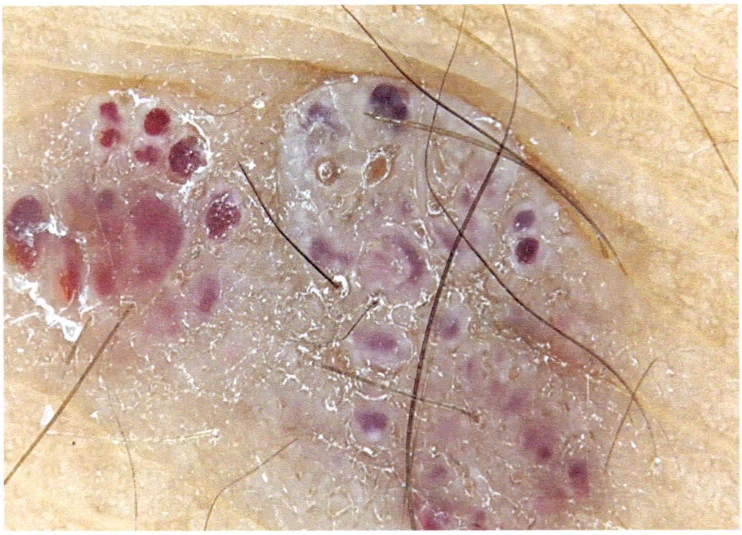

Fig. 23: Dermoscopically red and blue lacunae can easily be recognized. Red lacunae correspond to dilated vascular spaces without thrombosis whereas blue lacunae represent dilated blood vessels with thrombosis. The blue white veil denotes hyperkeratosis and acanthosis.

KEYNOTE

Angiokeratomas are sometimes confused clinically with pigmented lesions such as melanomas and spitz nevi, nonpigmented lesions such as dermatofibromas, and vascular lesions such as angiomas and pyogenic granulomas.

Dermoscopic patterns such as red and blue lacunae and white veils of angiokeratomas easily distinguish them from other vascular and nonvascular lesions **(Figs. 22 and 23)**.

REFERENCES

1. Wolf IH. Dermoscopic diagnosis of vascular lesions. Clin Dermatol. 2002;20:273-5.
2. Zaballos P, Daufi C, Puig S, et al. Dermoscopy of solitary angiokeratoma: a morphological study. Arch Dermatol. 2007;143:318-25.
3. Campos-do-Carmo G, Ramos-e-Silva M. Dermoscopy: basic concepts. Int J Dermatol. 2008;47:712-9.

CHAPTER 13

Connective Tissue Disorders

Subrata Malakar, Rashmi Agarwal, Seujee Das

JUVENILE DERMATOMYOSITIS

INTRODUCTION

Juvenile dermatomyositis (JDM) is an uncommon autoimmune condition of childhood affecting mostly the skin and striated muscles. The mean age of onset is 7 years of age. Characteristic clinical findings include heliotrope rash, Gottron's papules, malar rash, poikiloderma, arthritis, proximal muscle weakness, periungual telangiectasia, calcinosis, and lipodystrophy.

In contrast to adult dermatomyositis, JDM is more frequently associated with small vessel vasculopathy, periungual and gingival telangiectasia, ulceration, calcinosis, and lipodystrophy.[1]

Periungual telangiectasia, a characteristic feature of JDM and a marker of cutaneous disease activity, can be easily viewed with the help of a dermoscope.

KEY DERMOSCOPIC FEATURES

- *Gottron's papules*: Numerous rosettes on discrete whitish structures along with background erythema.
- *Nailfold capillaroscopy (NFC)*: Tortuous and enlarged capillaries, areas of capillary loss, ramified capillaries, and microhemorrhages.
- *Scalp*: Thin, sparse hair along with interfollicular pigmented dots and globules.

DISCUSSION

Dermoscopy of Gottron's papule has rarely been described in literature. Namiki et al. described the dermoscopic feature of Gottron's papules in an adult male as "surface scales with dotted vessels in a homogeneous pink background".[2]

Each individual Gottron's papule is denoted by the discrete whitish structures. The presence of numerous rosettes on a background of erythema overlying these discrete whitish structures is the striking dermoscopic feature of Gottron's papule. Whitish areas may correspond histopathologically to acanthosis and erythema to the dilated deeper vessels.

Nailfold capillaroscopy findings in JDM show a scleroderma like pattern with tortuous and enlarged capillaries, areas of capillary loss, ramified/bushy capillaries, and microhemorrhages. NFC changes in JDM are a potential marker of disease activity and severity and hence play an important role in taking treatment decisions, even in the absence of obvious clinical signs like muscle weakness or JDM rash.[3]

Trichoscopy of scalp in DM of adults have shown vascular findings similar to those seen on NFC like elongated and tortuous vessels and arborizing vessels with extravasation.[4] Julio et al. described the presence of peripilar casts, tufting, and interfollicular scales on scalp trichoscopy of adults with DM.[5] But no such characteristic trichoscopic changes were noted in the scalp in case of JDM.

Sparse and thin hair with interfollicular pigmented dots and globules may be observed probably due to pigmentary incontinence with dermal melanophages (personal observation).

KEYNOTE

Nailfold capillaroscopy findings in JDM show a scleroderma like pattern, which is an important marker of disease severity and activity **(Figs. 1 to 8)**.

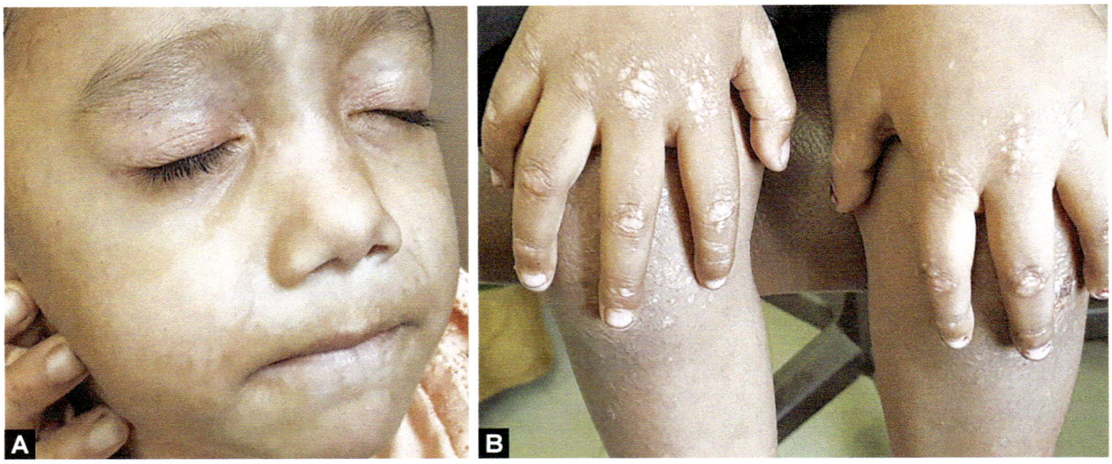

Figs. 1A and B: Dermatomyositis in a 2-year-old child with (A) heliotrope rash and (B) Gottron's papules.

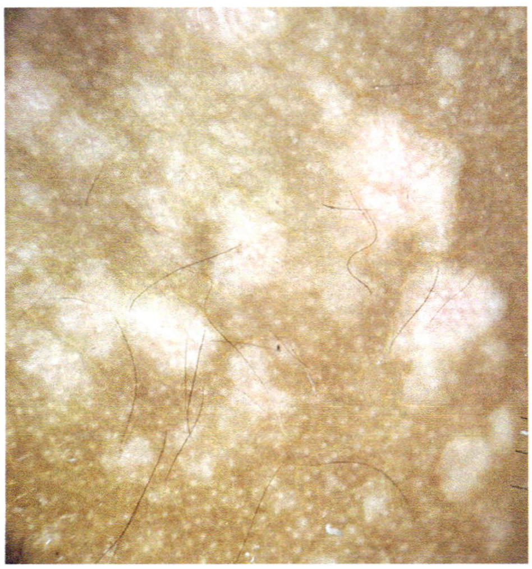

Fig. 2: Dermoscopy of Gottron's papules showing discrete whitish structures with irregular borders and background erythema. Numerous rosettes and few out-focused linear vessels are noted.

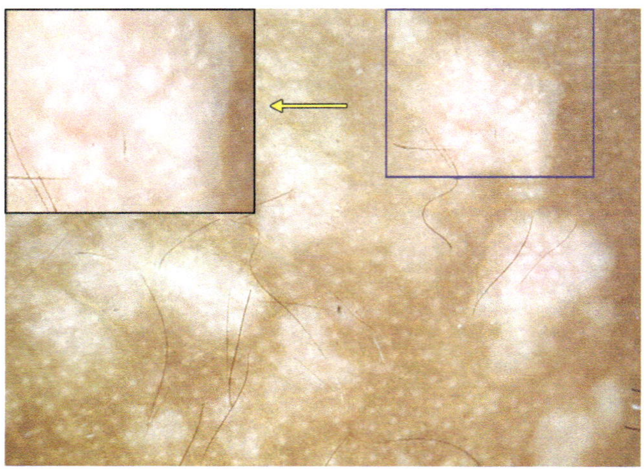

Fig. 3: Offset showing zoomed in view of the marked field. Note the numerous rosettes and linear vessels.

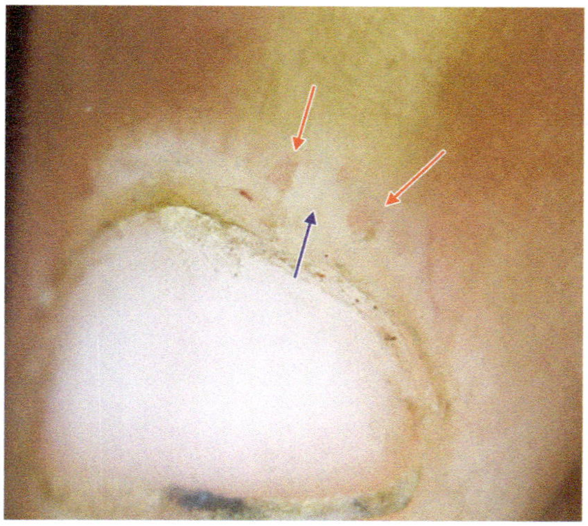

Fig. 4: Nailfold capillaroscopy showing ramified capillaries (red arrows) and avascular areas (blue arrow).

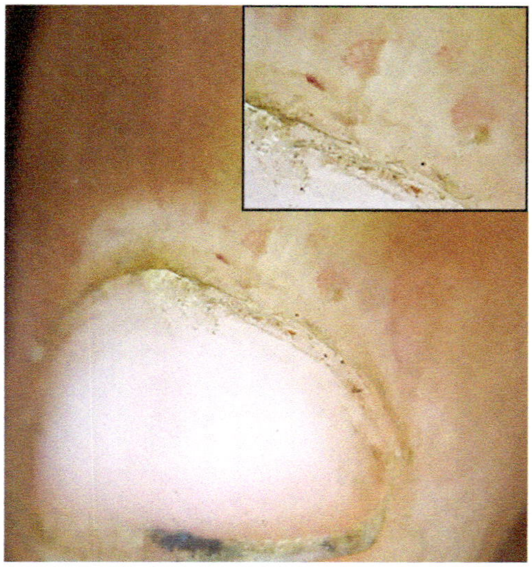

Fig. 5: Note the ramified capillaries in the zoomed-in image.

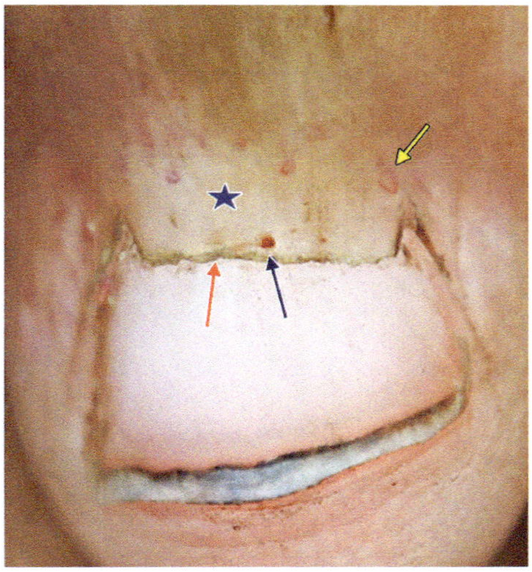

Fig. 6: Nailfold capillaroscopy showing ragged cuticle (red arrow), microhemorrhages (blue arrow), enlarged capillaries (yellow arrow), and large areas of capillary loss (blue star).

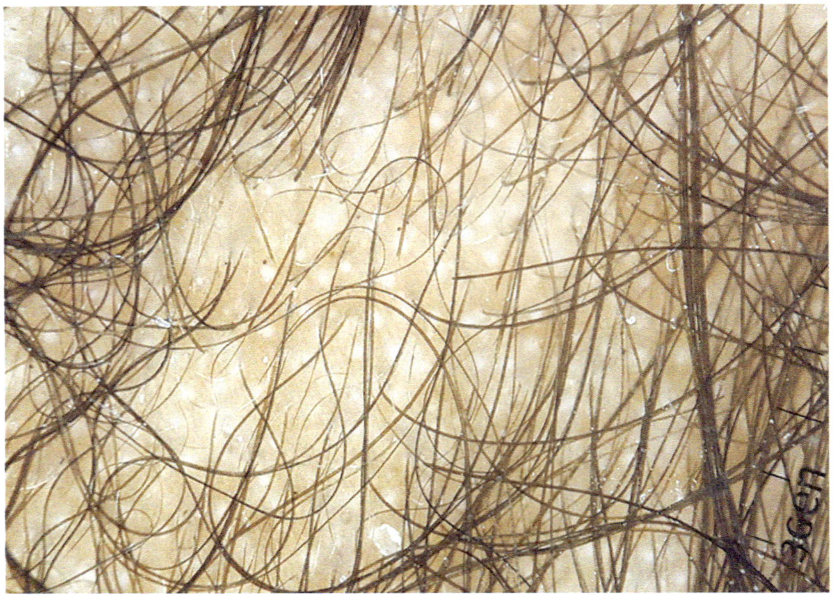

Fig. 7: Trichoscopy of scalp of the same child shows nonspecific features like sparse and thin hairs, decreased number of hairs per follicular unit.

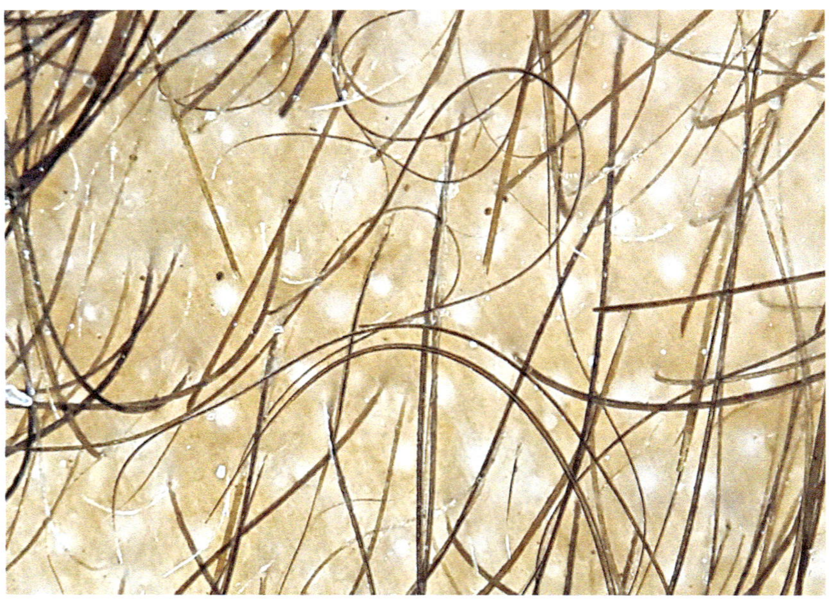

Fig. 8: Close-up view of the previous trichoscopic image shows the pigmented dots and globules mostly in the interfollicular area.

REFERENCES

1. Paller AS, Mancini AJ. Collagen vascular disorders. In: Paller AS, Mancini AJ (Eds). Hurwitz Clinical Pediatric Dermatology. China: Elsevier Inc; 2016. pp. 521-7.
2. Namiki T, Hashimoto T, Hanafusa T, et al. Case of dermatomyositis with Gottron papules and mechanic's hand: Dermoscopic features. J Dermatol. 2017;45(1):e19-e20.
3. Schmeling H, Stephens S, Goia C, et al. Nailfold capillary density is importantly associated over time with muscle and skin disease activity in juvenile dermatomyositis. Rheumatology. 2011;50(5):885-93.
4. Miteva M, Tosti A. Hair and scalp dermatoscopy. J Am Acad Dermatol. 2012;67:1040-8.
5. Jasso-Olivares J, Tosti A, Miteva M, et al. Clinical and dermoscopic features of the scalp in 31 patients with dermatomyositis. Skin Appendage Disorders. 2017;3(3):119-24.

LICHEN SCLEROSUS ET ATROPHICUS

INTRODUCTION

Lichen sclerosus et atrophicus (LSA) is an autoimmune, inflammatory disorder. It may occur in genital or extragenital sites. It has a bimodal age distribution, being seen in preadolescence as well.[1] It is clinically characterized by well-defined, ivory white, and atrophic papules that coalesce into plaques. Extragenital LSA is often confused with morphea and vitiligo (especially in its early stages).[2]

KEY DERMOSCOPIC FEATURES

- Comedo-like openings
- White structureless areas
- Chrysalis structures
- Linear branching vessels
- *Other vascular patterns*: Dotted, comma, and hairpin.

DISCUSSION

The earliest dermoscopic hallmark of LSA is presence of comedo-like openings. They correspond histopathologically to follicular plugging.[3,4]

White structureless areas are another major finding. These are seen due to both the epidermal atrophy and upper dermal fibrosis. Chrysalis structures are seen more frequently than they are reported (personal observation).

Linear branching vessels are the main vascular pattern of LSA. These represent the deep horizontal, subpapillary plexus, being easily visualized through the atrophic epidermis.

KEYNOTE

In early stages of the disease, diagnosis of LSA may be difficult on the basis of clinical examination alone. Here, dermoscopy proves to be an invaluable tool, by demonstrating the hallmark feature of comedo-like openings in LSA **(Figs. 9 and 10)**.

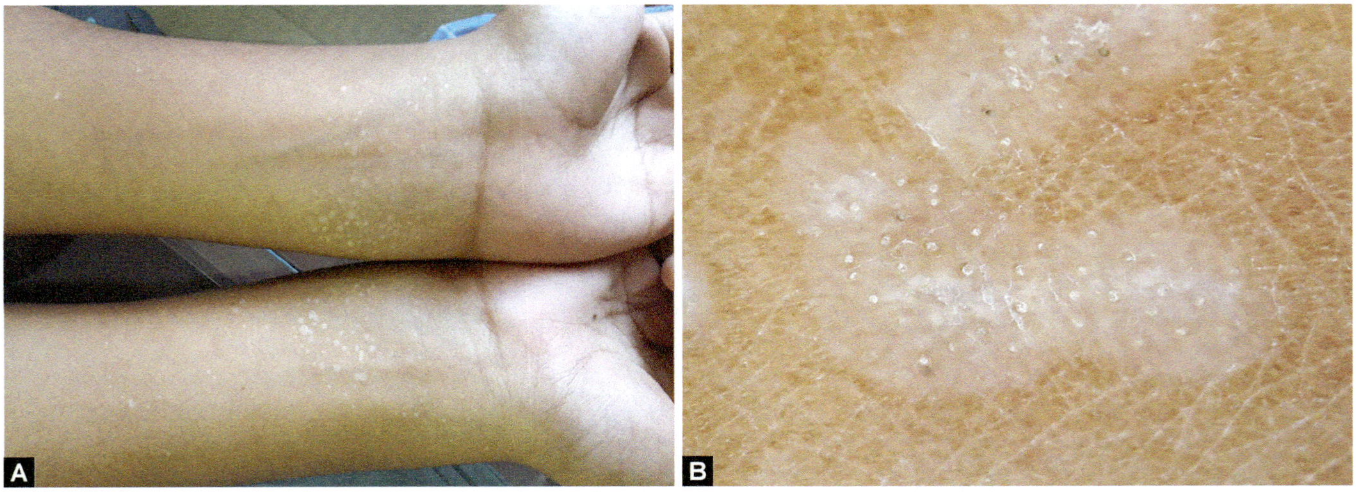

Figs. 9A and B: (A) An 11-year-old girl presented with shiny, atrophic papules over both the forearms. A clinical differential diagnosis of lichen nitidus and guttate lichen sclerosus et atrophicus was considered; (B) Dermoscopic evaluation revealed numerous comedo-like openings and a few white, structureless areas. Thus, a diagnosis of extragenital lichen sclerosus et atrophicus was made.

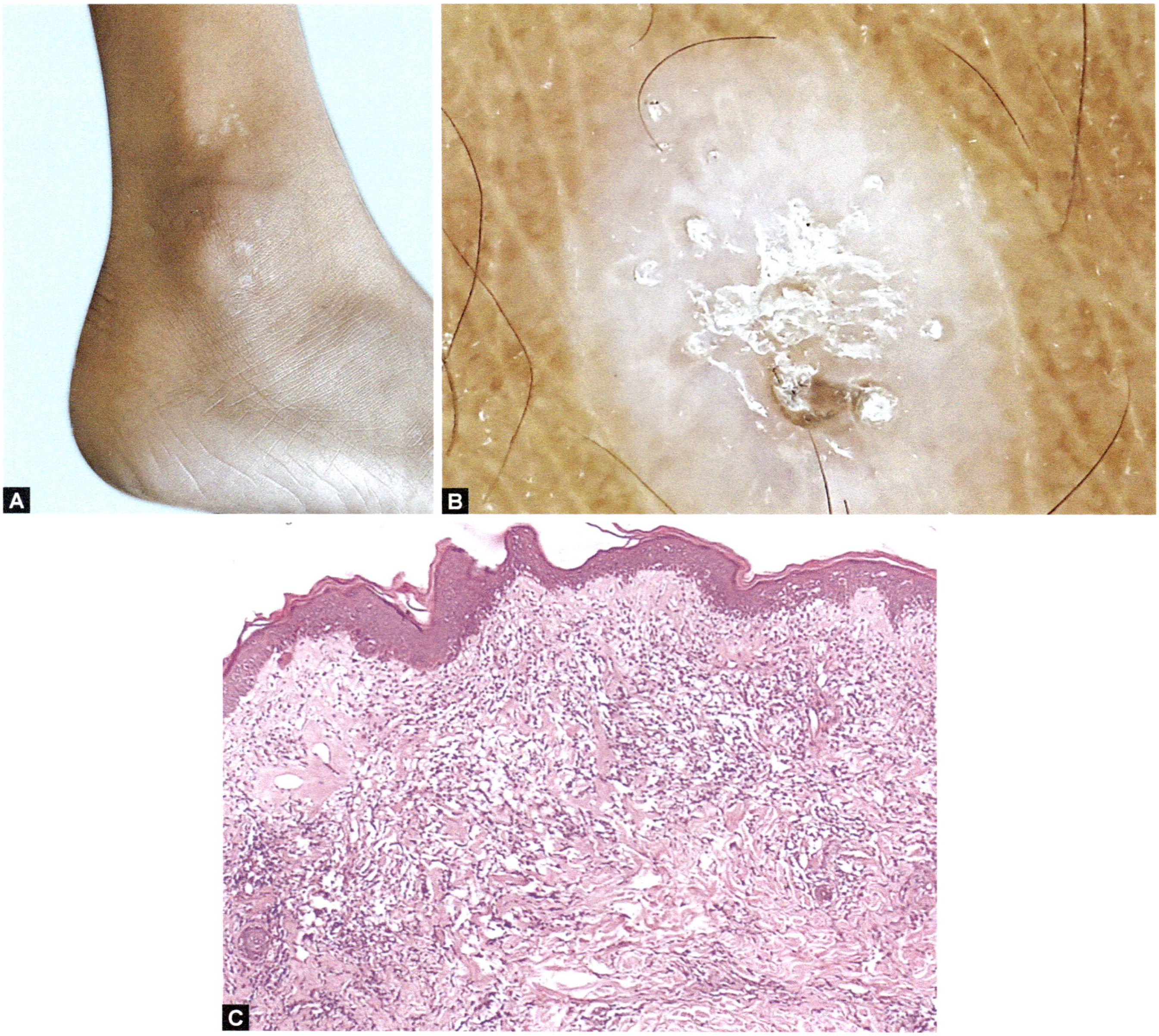

Figs. 10A to C: (A) A 10-year-old boy presenting with multiple, shiny, white, and flat-topped papules over the legs. These resembled lichen nitidus clinically. Koebnerization was noted; (B) Comedo-like openings, which are the hallmark of LSA, were seen on dermoscopy. White structureless areas were noted in the periphery of the lesion; (C) Histopathology of LSA shows interface vacuolar dermatitis along with epidermal atrophy. There is compact orthokeratosis and follicular plugging. In the dermis, there is dense lichenoid infiltrate with subepidermal hyalinization.

REFERENCES

1. Paller AS, Mancini AJ. Collagen vascular disorders. In: Paller AS, Mancini AJ (Eds). Hurwitz Clinical Pediatric Dermatology. China: Elsevier Inc; 2016. pp. 534-36.
2. Larre Borges A, Tiodorovic-Zivkovic D, Lallas A, et al. Clinical, dermoscopic and histopathologic features of genital and extragenital lichen sclerosus. J Eur Acad Dermatol Venereol. 2013;27(11):1433-9.
3. Garrido-Ríos AA, Álvarez-Garrido H, Sanz-Muñoz C, et al. Dermoscopy of extragenital lichen sclerosus. Arch Dermatol. 2009;145(12):1468.
4. Ankad BS, Beergouder SL. Dermoscopic patterns in lichen sclerosus: A report of three cases. Indian Dermatol Online J. 2015;6: 237-40.

MORPHEA

INTRODUCTION

Morphea is an autoimmune disorder clinically characterized by localized skin plaques of skin sclerosis.[1] Superficial, plaque-type morphea begins as skin-colored, erythematous patches, which evolve into firm, hyperpigmented or ivory-colored plaques. These plaques have a surrounding lilac inflammatory zone; however, in darker skin, this may not be readily perceptible.

The ivory plaques may sometimes resemble lichen sclerosus. Dermoscopy helps in differentiating between the two.

KEY DERMOSCOPIC FEATURES

***Superficial morphea*:**
- White fibrotic beam
- Linear branching vessels
- White shiny structures (personal observation).

***Deep morphea (personal observations)*:**
- Fibrotic beams
- Pigment patterns include pigmentation around hair follicles, spoke and wheel pattern, and dots and globules
- Linear vessels.

DISCUSSION

The hallmark dermoscopic feature of morphea is presence of white fibrotic beams. The fibrotic beams indicate dermal sclerosis on histopathology.[2] In some lesions, white shiny structures also corresponding to sclerosis, are observed.

Linear branching vessels may be seen crossing the white fibrotic beams.

KEYNOTE

Sometimes, differentiation of morphea and extragenital lichen sclerosus is a diagnostic dilemma. Each of them has distinct dermoscopic findings as follows: morphea is characterized by fibrotic beams and crossing linear vessels while LS reveals comedo-like openings and white patches. Hence, dermoscopic analysis can be very useful in case of doubt **(Figs. 11 and 12)**.

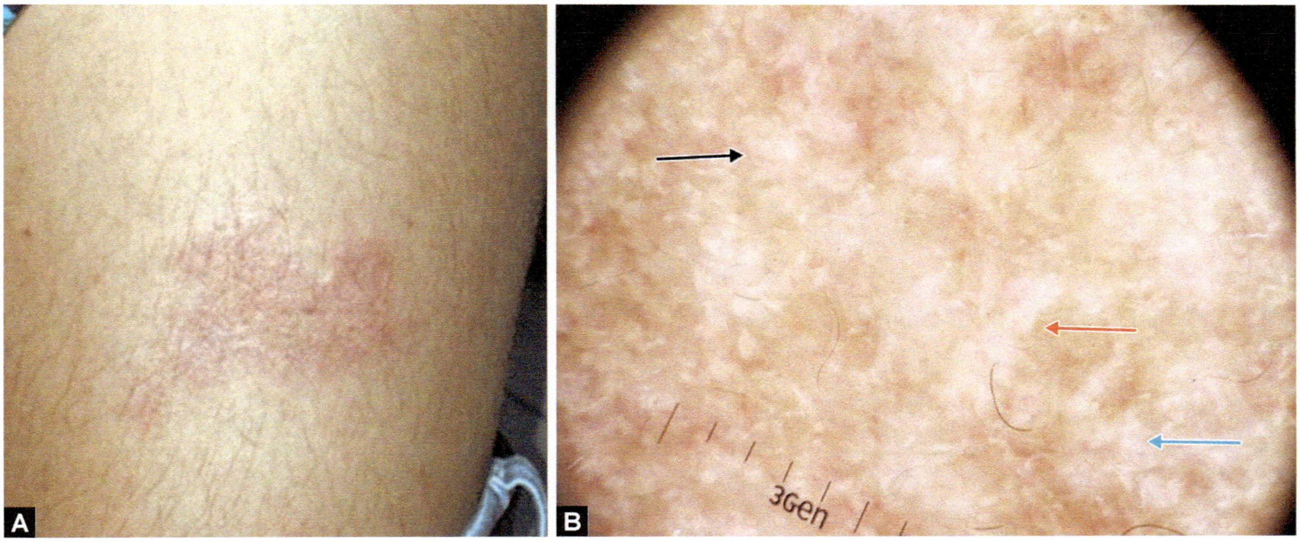

Figs. 11A and B: (A) A young female presented with an asymptomatic erythematous patch over the left thigh of 4 months duration; (B) Dermoscopy reveals fibrotic beams (red arrow). Linear vessels are also seen in the upper and extreme right side of the field. Some of the vessels are seen crossing the fibrotic beams (black arrow). White shiny structures (blue arrow) are also present.

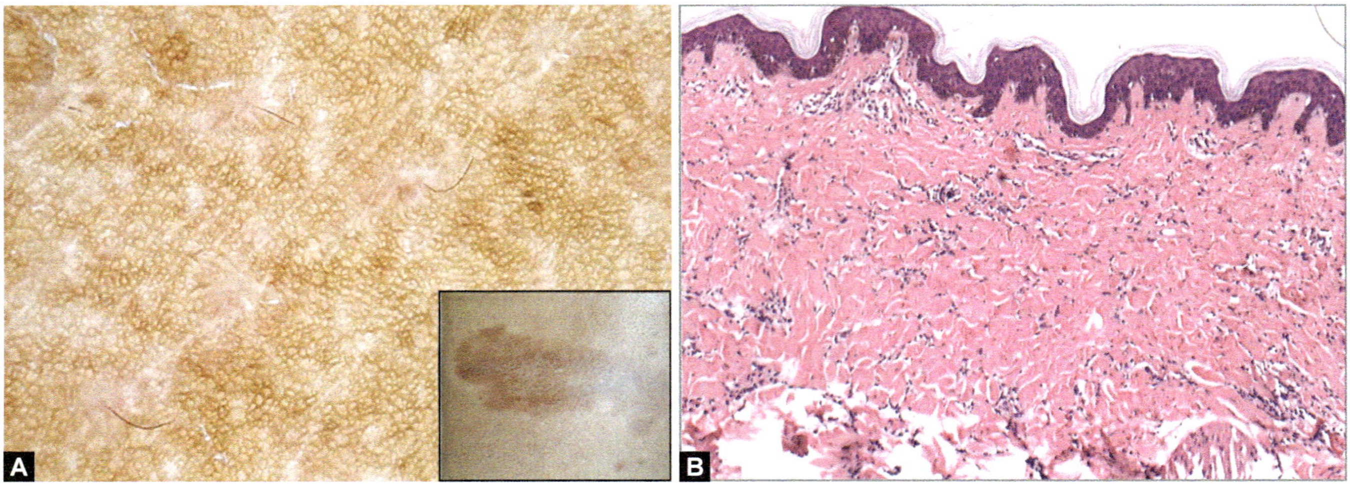

Figs. 12A and B: Localized, plaque-type morphea. Multiple fibrotic beams are visible dermoscopically; (B) Histopathology of the above lesion showed marked thickening and hyalinization of the collagen in the papillary and reticular dermis. There is also presence of a sparse superficial and deep lymphohistiocytic infiltrate.

REFERENCES

1. Pope E, Laxer RM. Diagnosis and management of morphea and lichen sclerosus and atrophicus in children. Pediatr Clin North Am. 2014;61(2):309-19.
2. Shim WH, Jwa SW, Song M, et al. Diagnostic usefulness of dermatoscopy in differentiating lichen sclerous et atrophicus from morphea. JAAD. 2012;66:690-1.

SYSTEMIC LUPUS ERYTHEMATOSUS

INTRODUCTION

Cutaneous lupus erythematosus (CLE) may occur as an isolated finding, or in the setting of underlying systemic lupus erythematosus (SLE). Cutaneous manifestations of SLE include malar rash, photosensitivity, and discoid lesions. Discoid lesions can develop in 25% of patients with SLE. 80% of pediatric SLE patients have cutaneous involvement.

Lupus specific subsets of CLE include:

- *Acute CLE*: Malar rash, generalized photodistributed morbilliform eruption
- Subacute CLE (rare in children)
- Chronic CLE (discoid LE).

Hair loss is a typical complaint in patients with SLE. Presentations may be acute telogen effluvium (TE), patchy nonscarring alopecia, or patchy scarring alopecia (discoid LE).

KEY DERMOSCOPIC FEATURES[1]

- ***Acute CLE***
  - White scales
  - Multicomponent vascular pattern
  - Red starburst pattern
  - Red pink background
- ***Discoid LE:*** It depends on the stage of progression **(Box 1)**.
- ***Scalp:*** Enlarged branching vessels, red dots, keratotic plugs, speckled pigmentation, upright regrowing hairs.
- ***Nail:*** Dilated tortuous vessels, microhemorrhages.

Box 1: Stage of progression of discoid lupus erythematosus.

Early lesions:
- Perifollicular whitish halo
- Follicular plugging
- Whitish scales

Long-standing lesions:
- Telangiectatic structures
- Pigmentation structures
- White structureless areas

Unclassified:
- Follicular red dots

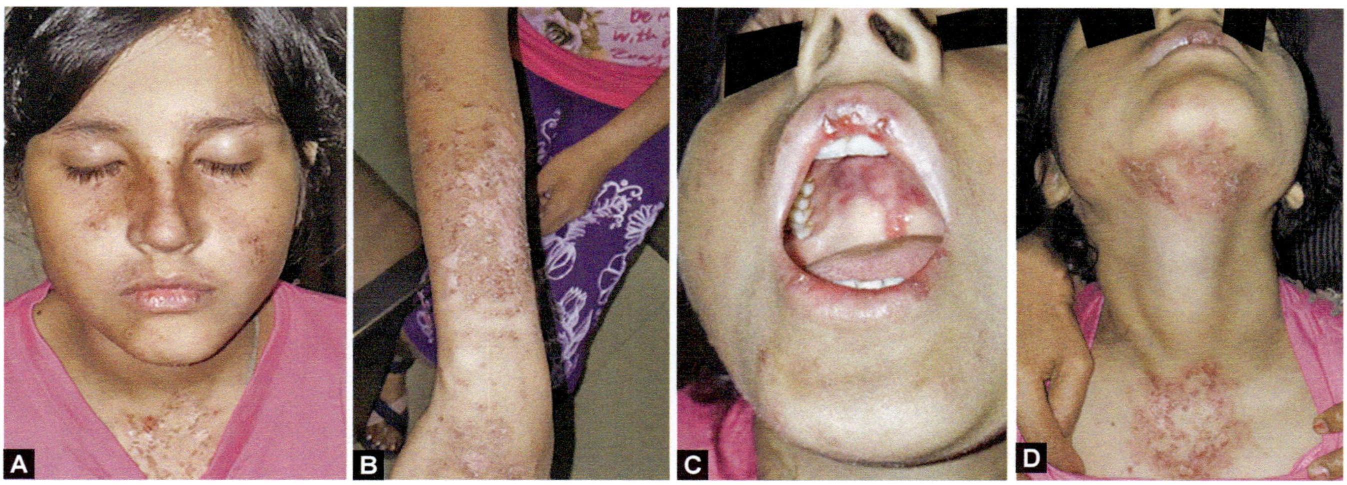

Figs. 13A to D: (A and B) A 12-year-old girl with SLE having malar rash and a photosensitivity rash; (C) Same patient showing palatal ulcers; (D) Lesions of acute cutaneous lupus erythematosus (CLE) over the neck and upper chest.

DISCUSSION

Dermoscopy of specific acute LE lesions has not been described in the literature. The photosensitivity rash in acute CLE (ACLE) shows presence of whitish scales in a pinkish red background with multicomponent vessels (linear, linear-irregular, branching, and dotted vessels). Histopathologically, the scales represent hyperkeratosis while the pinkish red background is because of vasodilatation. The targetoid areas within the ACLE lesions (personal observation) are probably due to cutaneous vasculitic process in the acute stages.

In contrast, dermoscopy of DLE lesions mainly displays pigmentation structures and follicular findings, i.e. keratotic plugs, dilated follicles, and perifollicular whitish halos, and the vascular pattern is typically monomorphic.[2]

Nailfold capillaroscopic changes in SLE is usually nonspecific (tortuous capillaries, microhemorrhages, and abnormal morphology) and is usually seen during the active stage.[3]

Trichoscopy of the scaly plaque over scalp showed numerous rosettes (personal observation) with multicomponent vascular pattern and a violaceous hue probably due to lichenoid dermatitis. Other features of scalp trichoscopy in cases of SLE are enlarged branching vessels, red dots, keratotic plugs, speckled pigmentation, and upright regrowing hairs **(Figs. 13 to 20)**.[1]

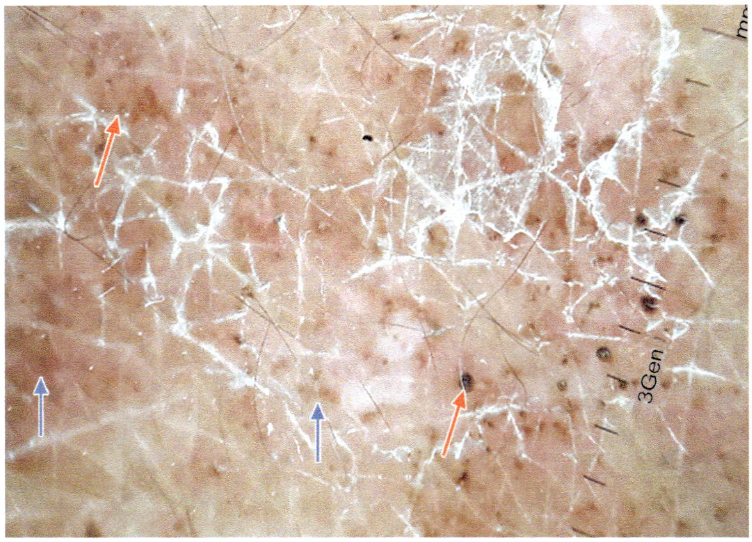

Fig. 14: Dermoscopy of acute cutaneous lupus erythematosus (CLE) rash showing white scales, on a red pink background with pigmented dots and globules. Multiple scattered small targetoid lesions (red arrows) can be seen. Blue arrows mark the pigmented dots and globules.

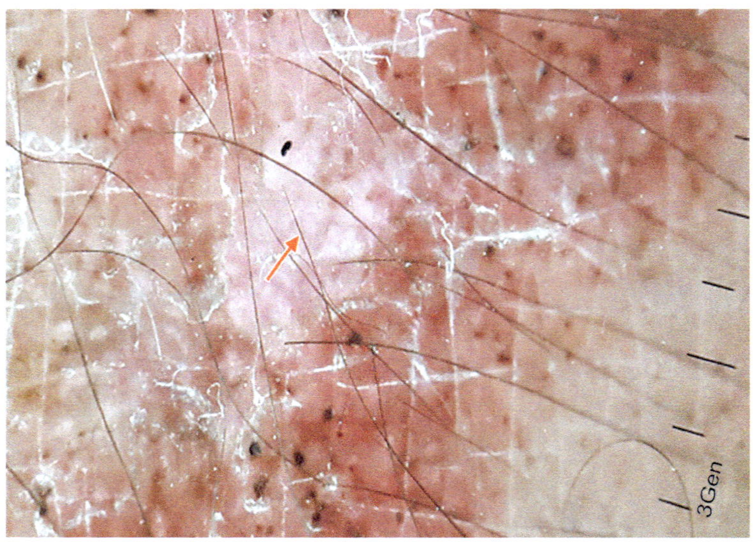

Fig. 15: Dermoscopy showing whitish scales on a pinkish red background with peripheral erythema along with multicomponent vessels. Some amorphous globular structures (red arrow) are also seen.

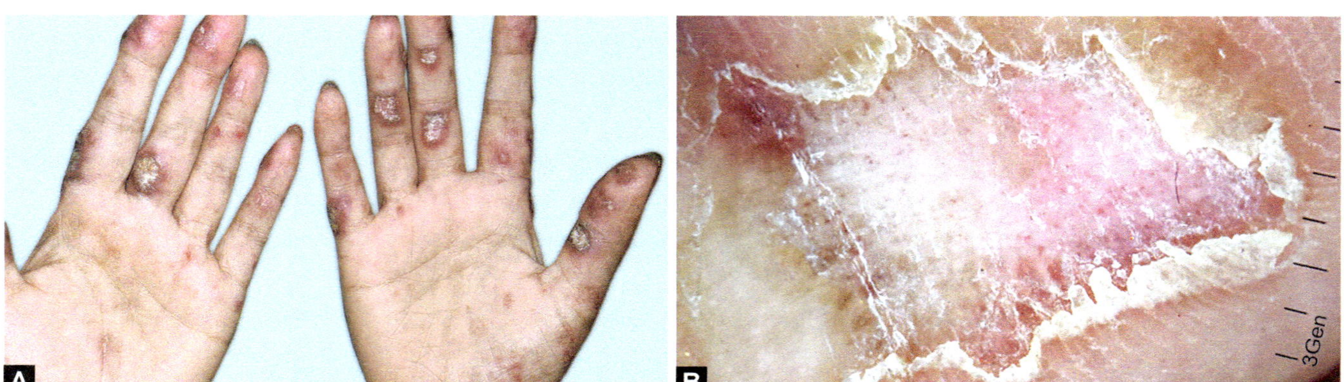

Figs. 16A and B: (A) Erythematous papulosquamous lesions on the palms of the above patient; (B) Dermoscopy of the palmar lesions showing multicomponent vascular pattern.

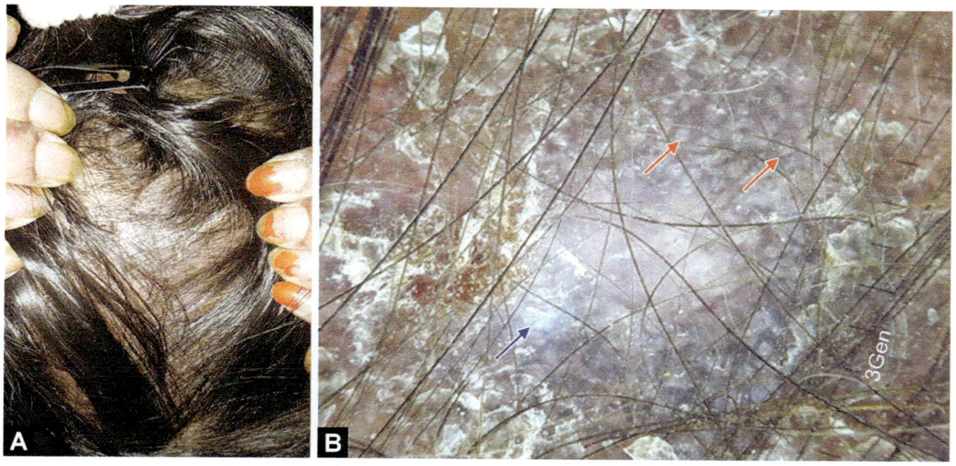

Figs. 17A and B: (A) Scaly plaques over the scalp with sparse hair of the same girl with systemic lupus erythematosus (SLE). (B) Trichoscopy of scalp lesions showing multiple rosettes (red arrows), white amorphous globular structures (blue arrow), multicomponent vascular pattern in the periphery masked by the overlying scales. Note the violaceous hue of the lesion (probably due to lichenoid dermatitis).

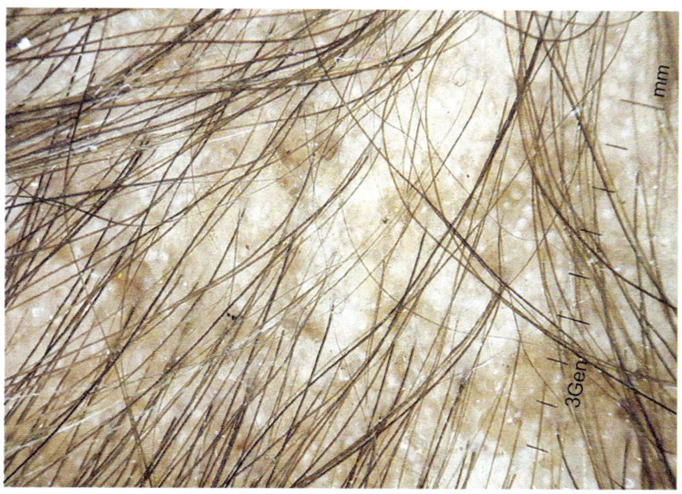

Fig. 18: Trichoscopy showing thin and sparse hair with grayish brown pigmentary changes around the follicle and in the interfollicular areas. The pigmentary changes represent the interface dermatitis leading to incontinence of pigment.

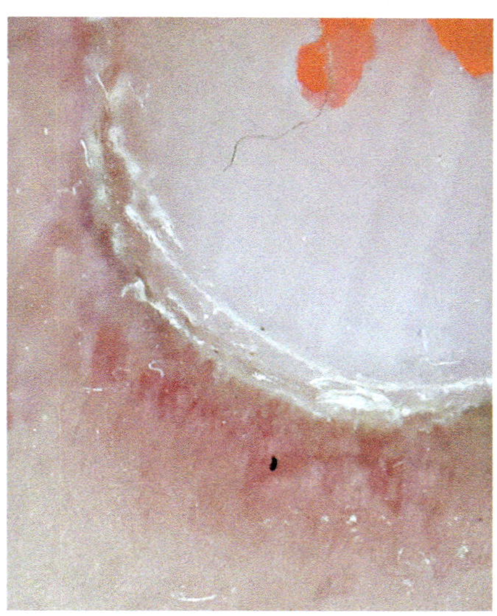

Fig. 19: Nailfold capillaroscopy showing ragged cuticle with dilated and disorganized capillary loops.

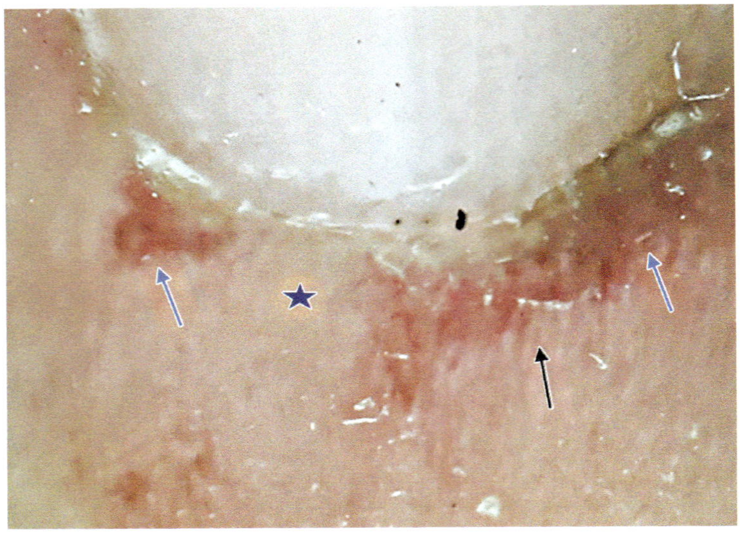

Fig. 20: Note the presence of avascular areas (star) alongside increased capillary density (black arrow). Blue arrows indicate areas of sludging of blood.

REFERENCES

1. Souvik S, Malakar S. Trichoscopy in autoimmune connective tissue diseases. In: Malakar S (Ed). Trichoscopy: A Text and Atlas. New Delhi: Jaypee Brothers Medical Publishers; 2017. p. 300.
2. Errichetti E, Piccirillo A, Viola L, et al. Dermoscopy of subacute cutaneous lupus erythematosus. Int J Dermatol. 2016;55(11): e605-7.
3. Cutolo M, Melsens K, Wijnant S, et al. Nailfold capillaroscopy in systemic lupus erythematosus: A systematic review and critical appraisal. Autoimmun Rev. 2018;17(4):344-52.

CHAPTER 14

Miscellaneous

Subrata Malakar, Surit Malakar

ENDOCRINE DISORDERS AND THE SKIN

ACANTHOSIS NIGRICANS

Introduction

Acanthosis nigricans presents as dark brown, velvety thickening of the skin involving the intertriginous areas, such as the axillae, neck, genital, and submammary regions. The initial change is hyperpigmentation followed by eventual thickening with intensification of skin markings.[1]

Key Dermoscopic Features

- Linear crista cutis
- Sulcus cutis
- Focal hyperpigmented dots.

Discussion

The dermoscopic features of linear crista cutis would correspond to papillomatous projections of the dermis. The origin of the hyperpigmented dots is not confirmed yet. The proposed hypotheses include increased melanin granules per melanocytes, an increased number of melanin contents containing keratinocytes, or some other nonmelanin associated pigmentation.[2]

Keynote

Hyperpigmented dot is a characteristic dermoscopic feature of acanthosis nigricans that is not apparent on naked eye examination **(Figs. 1A to D)**.

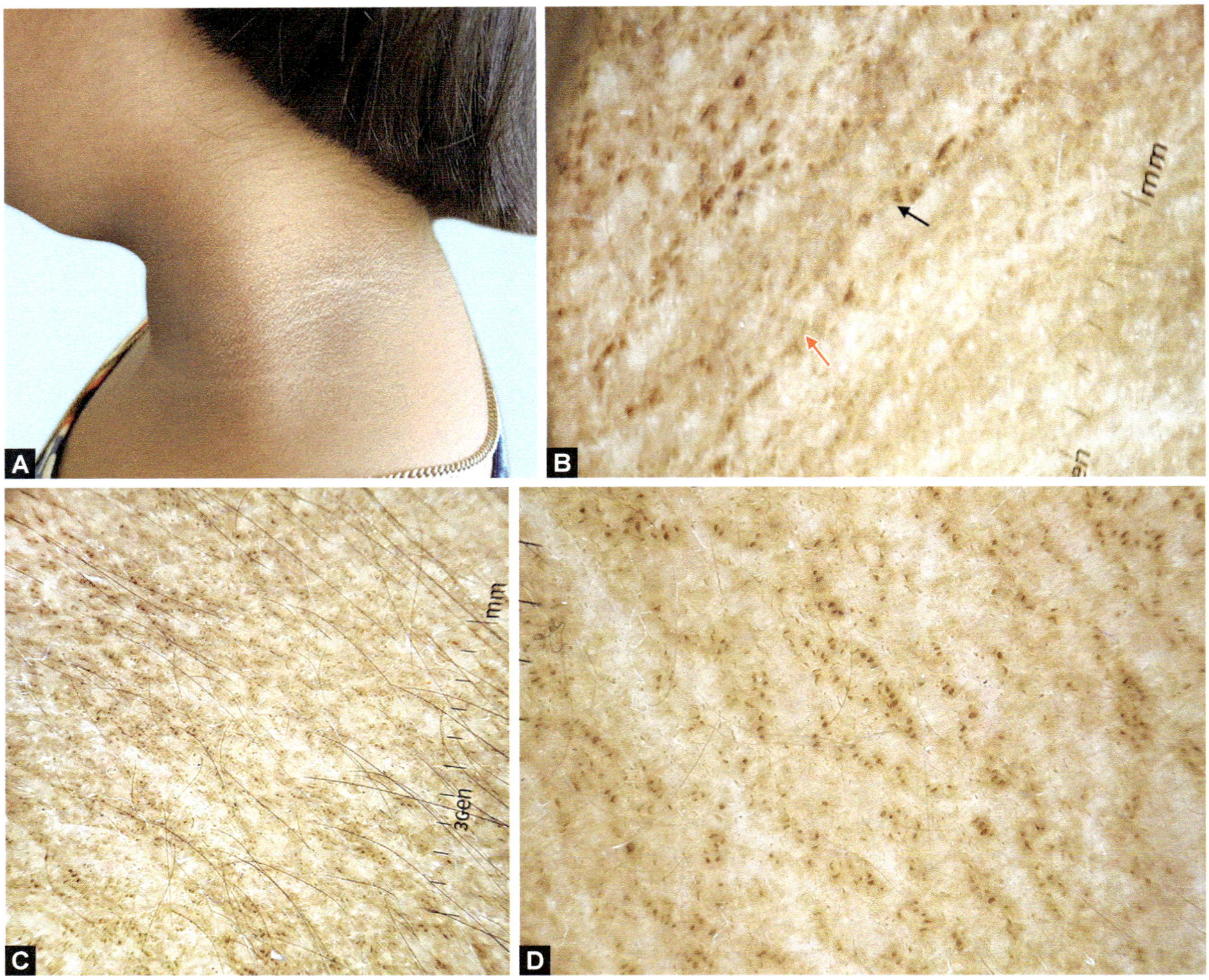

Figs. 1A to D: (A) Velvety hyperpigmentation involving the neck; (B) Dermoscopy shows linear crista cutis (black arrow), sulcus cutis (red arrow); (C) Presence of hyperpigmented dots throughout the lesional skin. These are appreciated in the polarized mode; (D) Magnified view of the above image showing numerous hyperpigmented dots and streaks.

References

1. Paller S Amy, Anthony J Mancini, et al. Hereditary disorders of cornification. Hurwitz Clinical Pediatric Dermatology: A Textbook of Skin Disorders of Childhood and Adolescence. 5th edition. Elsevier: 2016. pp. 554-5.
2. Uchida S, Oiso N, Suzuki T, et al. Dermoscopic features of hyperpigmented dots in crista cutis in two siblings in a Japanese family with inherited acanthosis nigricans. Journal of Cosmetics, Dermatological Sciences and Applications. 2012;2:252-3.

STRIAE DISTENSAE

Introduction

Striae distensae are characterized by linear, smooth, and atrophic bands over the skin. They reflect breaks in the connective tissue and occur at the areas of dermal damage. They may be the end result of various physiological conditions like pregnancy, adrenocortical excess, and change in the body habitus or can be the marker of excessive topical steroid use.[1]

Key Dermoscopic Features

- Linear atrophic bands
- Telangiectasia.

Discussion

The misuse of steroid on the face can be picked up easily by the signs like erythema, telangiectasia, acneiform eruptions, striae, and eventually atrophy and scarring. However, these signs can be easily missed on scalp due to the presence of hair. So trichoscopy is important in identifying the signs of steroid misuse on scalp at an early stage.[2]

Keynote

Periodic monitoring of patients on topical corticosteroid treatment on scalp via trichoscopy is important in order not to miss the signs of steroid misuse. Trichoscopy is not only a diagnostic tool but also a monitoring tool wherein it can reveal the tell-tale signs of inadvertent topical therapy **(Figs. 2 and 3)**.

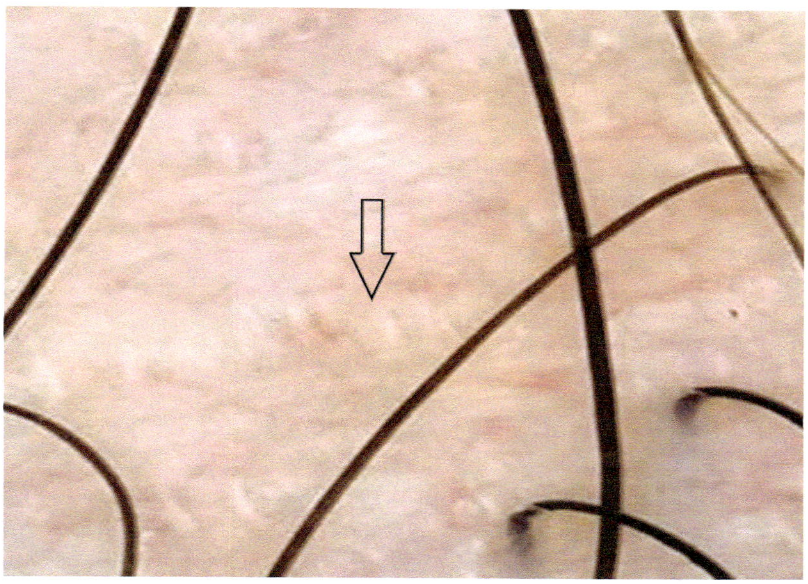

Fig. 2: Linear atrophic bands (striae distensae) and telangiectasia over scalp on a patient with alopecia areata.

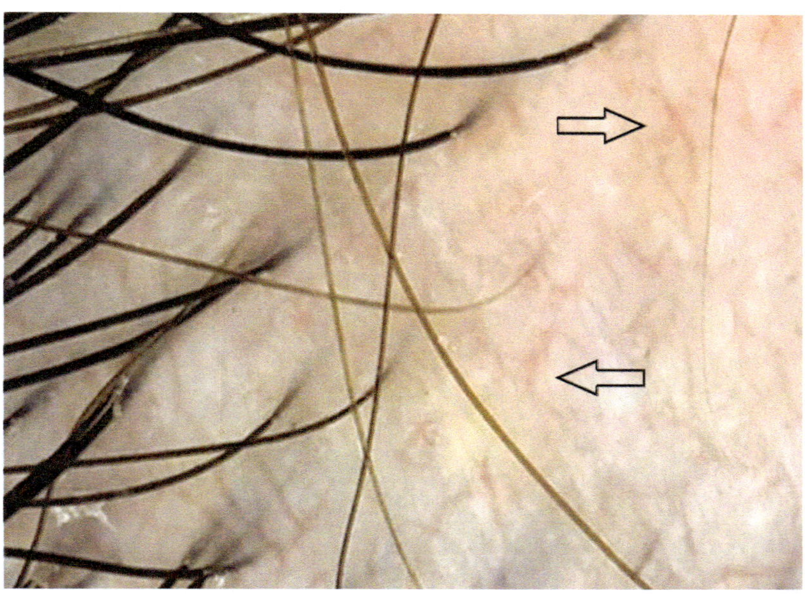

Fig. 3: Telangiectasia over the scalp seen after steroid misuse.

References

1. Awley TJ, Yancey KB. Skin changes and diseases in pregnancy. In: Freedberg IM, Eisen AZ, Wolff K, Austen KF, Goldsmith LA, Katz SI (Eds). Fitzpatrick's Dermatology in General Medicine, 6th edition. New York: McGraw-Hill; 2003. pp. 1362.
2. Malakar S, Diwaker P. Striae distensae over scalp: A trichoscopic revelation. Our Dermatol Online. 2018;9(2):227-8.

GRANULOMA ANNULARE

INTRODUCTION

Granuloma annulare (GA) was first described in 1895 by Colcott-Fox who reported an 11-year-old girl with a "ring eruption of the fingers". GA usually presents clinically with an annular plaque without scales, the border of which consists of numerous small papules. Several clinical variants of GA have been recognized such as localized, generalized, subcutaneous, perforating, and arcuate dermal erythema. Type IV cell-mediated immunity, immune complex vasculitis, and abnormality of tissue monocytes are proposed mechanism of pathogenesis.

KEY DERMOSCOPIC FEATURES[1-3]

- Peripheral structureless orange-reddish borders
- Unfocused vessel. However, in pediatric age group, we tend to get in-focus vessels owing to the physiologically thinner skin in children, as compared to adults.

DISCUSSION

Dermoscopy of GA is characterized by peripheral yellow-orange rim surrounding the structureless center. The yellow-orange rim corresponds to the "palisading granuloma" on histology.

The lesions usually lack vessels. When present, they are focused vessels, having variable patterns such as dotted, branching, and linear-irregular, on a reddish-pink background. In contrast, vessels in adult patients tend to be out-of-focus due to the dermal thickness.

KEYNOTE

Evaluation using dermoscopy often helps to narrow the clinical differentials. This is true for necrobiosis lipoidica (NL) and GA when investigating using dermoscopy; arborizing vessels are present in NL whereas in GA vessels are scant to absent **(Figs. 4 and 5)**.[4,5]

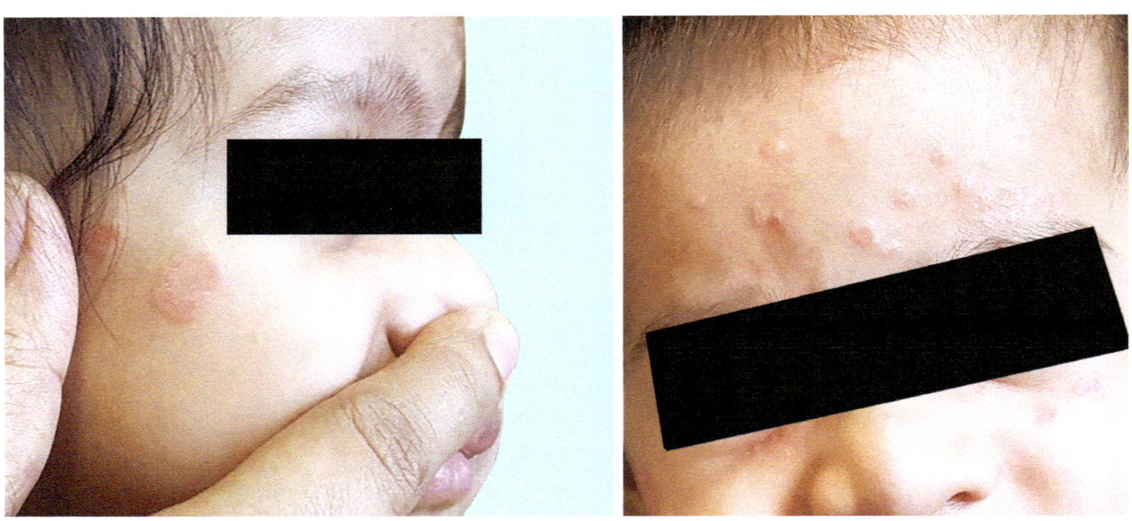

Fig. 4: A 10-month-old child presented with erythematous annular lesions with mild pruritus of 3 months duration.

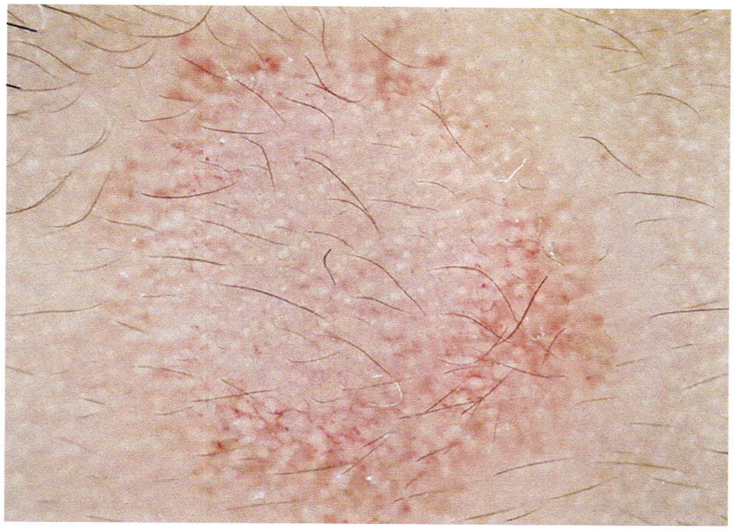

Fig. 5: Dermoscopy showing peripheral structureless orange reddish areas with mainly linear vessels, more so in the periphery than the center. This is in contrast to the unfocused vessels found in adult GA patients.

REFERENCES

1. Errichetti E, Lallas A, Apalla Z, et al. Dermoscopy of granuloma annulare: A clinical and histological correlation study. Dermatology. 2017;233(1):74-9.
2. Pellicano R, Caldarola G, Filabozzi P, et al. Dermoscopy of necrobiosis lipoidica and granuloma annulare. Dermatology. 2013;226(4):319-23.
3. Navarrete-Dechent C, Puerto Cd, Bajaj S, et al. Dermoscopy of elastosis perforans serpiginosa: A useful tool to distinguish it from granuloma annulare. J Am Acad Dermatol. 2015;73(1):e7-9.
4. Pellicano R, Caldarola G, Filabozzi P, et al. Dermoscopy of necrobiosis lipoidica and granuloma annulare. Dermatology. 2013;226:319-23.
5. Lallas A, Zaballos P, Zalaudek I, et al. Dermoscopic patterns of granuloma annulare and necrobiosis lipoidica. Clin Exp Dermatol. 2013;38:425-7.

JUVENILE XANTHOGRANULOMA

INTRODUCTION

Juvenile xanthogranuloma (JXG) is one of the common pediatric tumors. It usually presents as an erythematous papule or nodule which eventually turns bright yellow-orange in color. Resolving lesions form atrophic brown macules or patches.[1,2] They present with single or multiple lesions on the flexural areas or scalp, but can be found anywhere on the body.

Histopathologically, they consist of dense dermal infiltration of lipid-laden vacuolated cells, along with Touton cells, and lymphocytes and eosinophils in varying proportion.[3] The quality of infiltrate varies with the clinical evolution of the lesion.

KEY DERMOSCOPIC FEATURES[4,5]

- "Setting sun" appearance
- Clouds of pale yellow globules
- Whitish streak
- Linear and/or branched vessels.

DISCUSSION

Song et al. suggested a schematic overview of evolving clinical and dermoscopic presentation of JXG, in accordance with the histopathological changes in the lesion.

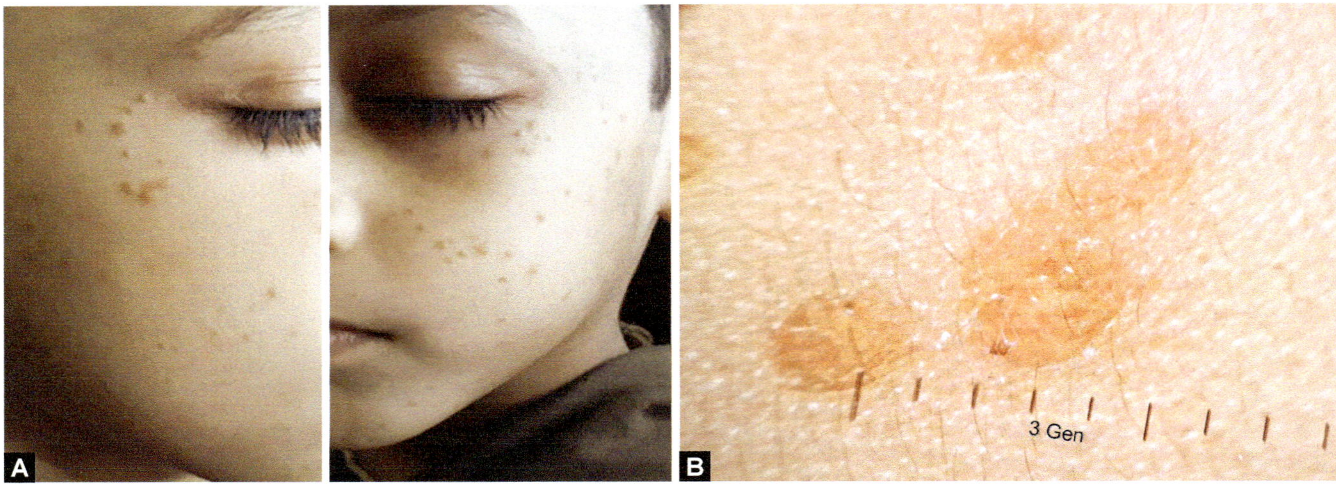

Figs. 6A and B: (A) A 6-year-old boy presented with asymptomatic yellow brown papules over the face of 8 months duration; (B) Clouds of pale yellow globules. In darker skin, "setting sun" appearance is rarely visible, rather clouds of pale yellow globules is the main dermoscopic feature (personal observation).

- *Early evolutionary*:
  - The setting sun appearance is the dermoscopic hallmark.
  - However, in darker skin, "setting sun" appearance is rarely visible probably due to the masking of the vessels and erythema by prominent melanocytic network and more melanin.
- *Fully developed stages*:
  - As the vacuolated cells of the early stage evolve to xanthomatized cells, yellow globular clouds manifest more. These yellow globular clouds are the consistent features of fully developed and late stages.
  - They are also the main dermoscopic feature in dark skin (personal observation).
- *Regressive phase*:
  - The surrounding erythema decreases in the late regressive phase, thus setting sun become less apparent or absent.
  - Whitish streaks become visible in the late regressive phase, which shows infiltration of spindle-shaped cells in variable amounts on histology.

In all the stages of JXG, linear and branched vessels are observed in high percentage of cases.

KEYNOTE

A thorough clinical examination along with a careful dermoscopy of the lesion avoids skin biopsy in JXG of the pediatric age group. Furthermore, follow-up dermoscopy allows a lot for the dermatologists who want to learn practical clues for the natural course of JXG.

Dermoscopy in darker skin rarely shows the setting sun appearance, rather clouds of pale yellow color are the most common dermoscopic feature in them **(Figs. 6A and B)**.

REFERENCES

1. Hernandez-Martin A, Baselga E, Drolet BA, et al. Juvenile xanthogranuloma. J Am Acad Dermatol. 1997;36(3 Pt 1): 355-67.
2. Janssen D, Harms D. Juvenile xanthogranuloma in childhood and adolescence: A clinicopathologic study of 129 patients from the Kiel pediatric tumor registry. Am J Surg Pathol. 2005;29:21-8.
3. Burgdorf WH, Gerami P, Yan AC. Benign and malignant tumors. In: Schachner L, Hansen RC (Eds). Pediatric Dermatology: New York: Elsevier; 2011. p. 1215.
4. Palmer A, Bowling J. Dermoscopic appearance of juvenile xanthogranuloma. Dermatology. 2007;215:256-9.
5. Rubegni P, Mandato F, Fimiani M. Juvenile xanthogranuloma: Dermoscopic pattern. Dermatology. 2009;218:380.

SECTION 3

Trichoscopy

CHAPTERS

CHAPTER 15

Trichoscopy in Pediatric Age Group

Purva Mehta, Subrata Malakar

INTRODUCTION

The diagnostic algorithm in pediatric trichology is based on the clinical acumen of the dermatologist and the investigative tools at hand. Invasive investigative techniques like scalp biopsies are cumbersome and nonfeasible in the pediatric age group. A trichoscope serves as an effective, noninvasive tool in the diagnostic armamentarium of pediatric trichology. It not only aids in the diagnosis but also acts as a prognostic and therapeutic marker. This section on pediatric trichoscopy elaborates the trichoscopic language explaining follicular, peri- and interfollicular, and hair shaft patterns. It throws light on key trichoscopic features of various common and uncommon trichological disorders, and hair shaft disorders encountered in the pediatric age group. Decoding of varied clinical trichological mimics is possible through trichoscopy, obviating the need for a scalp biopsy.

Pediatric trichoscopy is performed via nonpolarized mode or polarized mode (contact and noncontact).

Polarized trichoscopy has the advantage of cross-polarized filters, which eliminate light reflected off the skin surface and allow light reflected from the deeper structures to reach the physician's eye. A trichoscope is a dermoscope used to examine scalp and trichological disorders, providing a magnification of 10- to 100-fold. Trichoscopes can be digital or handheld. Digital trichoscopes have the added advantage of higher magnification and also enable photography and storage of trichoscopic images.

To conclude, trichoscopy goes hand in hand with pediatric trichology and is a must in day-to-day clinical practice.

CHAPTER 16

Step-by-Step Trichoscopy

Subrata Malakar, Purva Mehta, Surit Malakar

To understand pediatric trichoscopy, it is imperative to have a thorough knowledge of basic patterns concerning the hair follicle.[1]

FOLLICULAR PATTERNS

Follicular patterns on trichoscopy comprises of "DOTS" which are circular follicular openings.[2] It may be of various types as described here.

YELLOW DOTS

Dilated follicular openings inspissated with kerato-sebaceous material are called yellow dots. They are commonly seen in conditions like alopecia areata, discoid lupus erythematosus (DLE), etc. **(Fig. 1)**.

BLACK DOTS

When the hair shaft breaks at the level of the scalp, it forms a black dot. Black dots are not a sign of a healthy scalp. They are seen in tinea capitis, trichotillomania, alopecia areata, etc. **(Fig. 2)**.

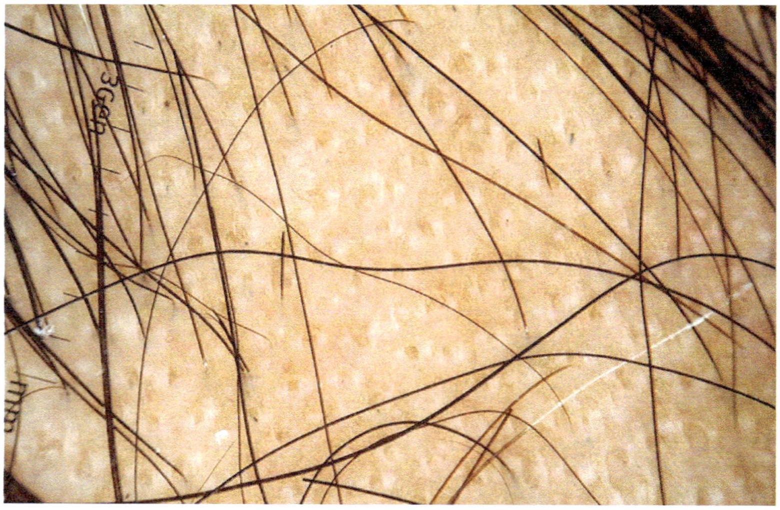

Fig. 1: Yellow dots are a characteristic trichoscopic feature of alopecia areata. They also occur in androgenetic alopecia, trichotillomania, etc.

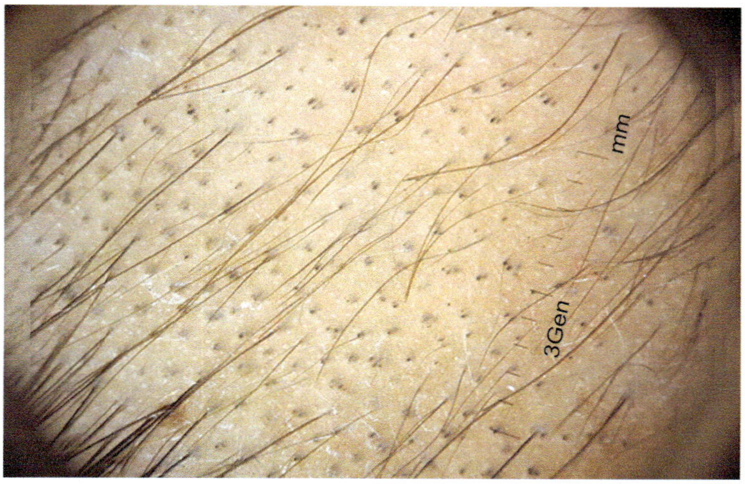

Fig. 2: Several black dots in this trichoscopic field denoting hair shafts broken at the surface of the scalp. Presence of numerous black dots is almost diagnostic of alopecia areata (AA) and they are a sign of disease activity.

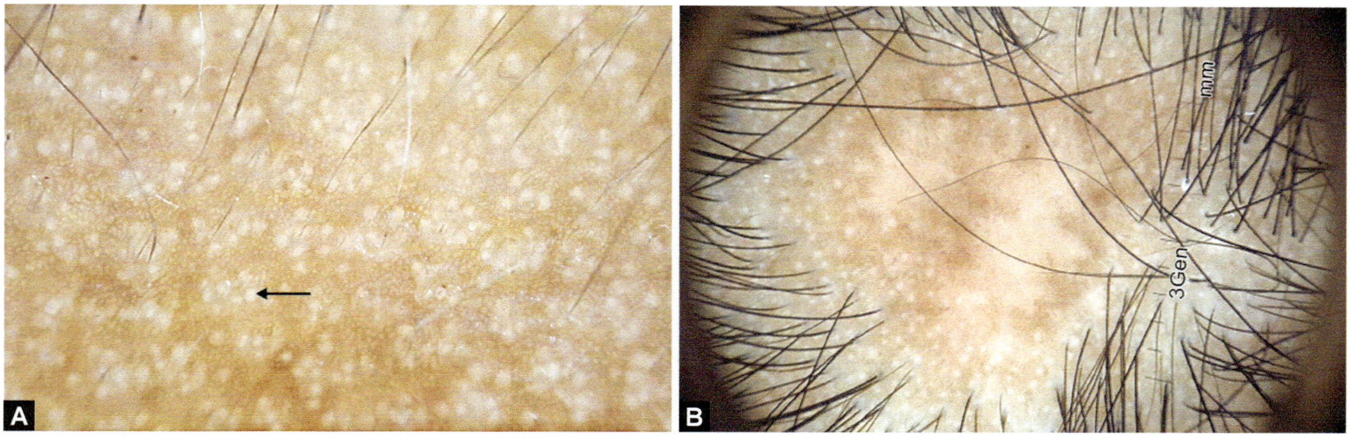

Figs. 3A and B: (A) Pinpoint white dots in a trichoscopic field of a normal scalp. They represent openings of either empty follicles or eccrine sweat glands and tend to be regular in distribution. They are also seen in nonscarring alopecias; (B) Fibrotic white dots implying cicatrization. They are irregularly placed in scarring alopecias. White dots coalesced in the center to form large white patches of fibrosis.

WHITE DOTS

White dots on trichoscopy are classified as pinpoint and fibrotic.

Pinpoint white dots are seen on normal scalp and in noncicatricial alopecias wherein they represent openings of empty follicles or eccrine sweat glands.

Fibrotic white dots are irregular in shape and are characteristically seen in cicatricial alopecias. They correspond to the underlying areas of fibrosis owing to cicatrization **(Figs. 3A and B)**.

BLUE-GRAY DOTS

They correspond to melanophages in the papillary dermis. Blue gray dots are characteristically seen in scarring alopecias such as DLE, where they are arranged in a speckled manner interfollicularly. This follicular pattern is more common in the darker phenotype **(Fig. 4)**.

RED DOTS

When a dilated follicular opening is surrounded by blood vessels, it forms a red dot on trichoscopy. Red dots are quite rare in the pediatric age group and are seen in DLE **(Fig. 5)**.[3,4]

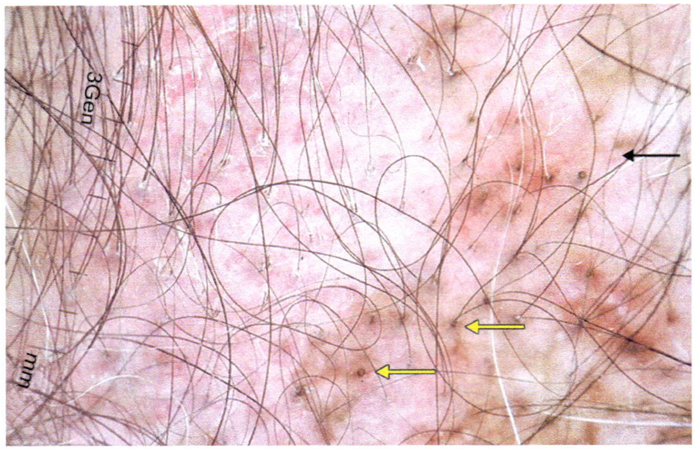

Fig. 4: Blue gray dots in a case of discoid lupus erythematosus, present both around the follicles (yellow arrows) and in between the hair follicles (black arrow).

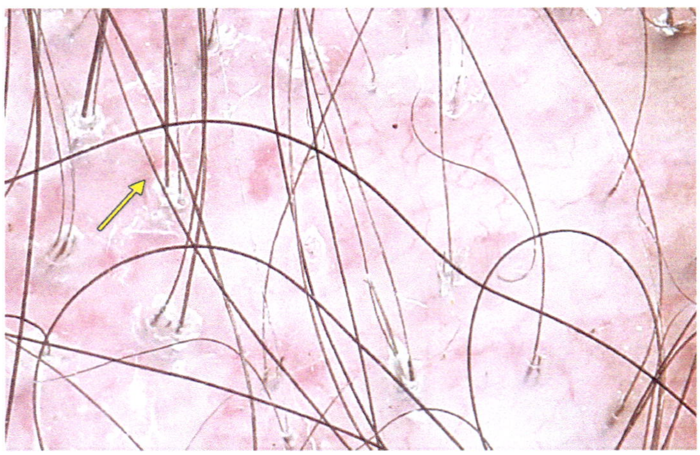

Fig. 5: Dilated blood vessel surrounding the dilated follicular opening forms the red dot, a trichoscopic feature of discoid lupus erythematosus.

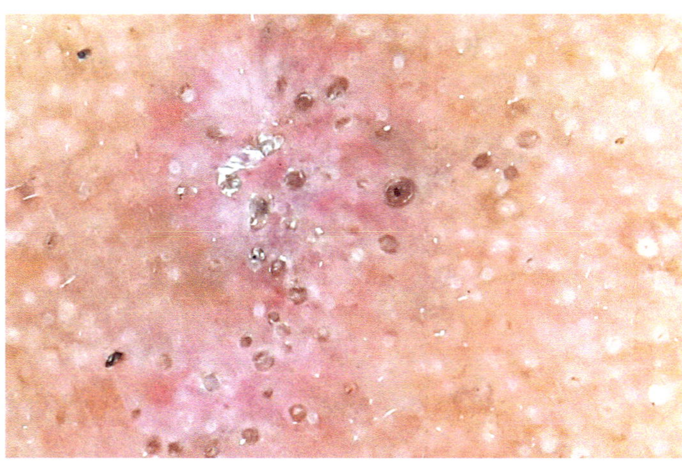

Fig. 6: In discoid lupus erythematosus, keratin occludes the dilated infundibular openings and protrudes out forming a keratotic plug.

KERATOTIC PLUGS

Dilated follicular openings occluded by keratotic material form keratotic plugs, a characteristic trichoscopic feature of DLE **(Fig. 6)**.

REFERENCES

1. Ross EK, Vincenzi C, Tosti A. Videodermoscopy in the evaluation of hair and scalp disorders. J Am Acad Dermatol. 2006;55(5): 799-806.
2. Kowalska-Oledzka E, Slowinska M, Rakowska A, et al. 'Black Dots' seen under trichoscopy are not specific for alopecia areata. Clin Exp Dermatol. 2012;37:615-9.
3. Malakar S, Mehta P. Follicular and perifollicular patterns. In: Malakar S, Chandrashekhar BS, Mukherjee S, Mehta P, Pradhan P (Eds). Trichoscopy: A Text and Atlas. New Delhi: Jaypee Brothers Medical Publishers (P) Ltd.; 2017. pp. 57-64.
4. Tosti A, Torres F, Misciali C, et al. Follicular red dots: a novel dermoscopic pattern observed in scalp discoid lupus erythematosus. Arch Dermatol. 2009;145(12):1406-9.

PERIFOLLICULAR PATTERNS

Perifollicular pattern deals with structures surrounding the hair follicle. Hair cast, perifollicular scales, and peripilar sign comprise the trichoscopic perifollicular pattern in the pediatric age group.[1,2]

HAIR CAST

It is a cylindrical whitish structure which not only surrounds the hair shaft but also extends beyond the surface of the scalp. Hair cast is a trichoscopic feature of tinea capitis, seborrheic dermatitis, and scalp psoriasis **(Fig. 7)**.

PERIFOLLICULAR SCALES

They surround the hair shaft at the proximal end and are seen in ichthyosis vulgaris, discoid lupus erythematosus, lichen planopilaris, etc. **(Fig. 8)**.

PERIPILAR SIGN

It is a trichoscopic feature of patterned alopecia which may be seen in late adolescence and denotes brown discoloration around the hair follicle. It corresponds to perifollicular inflammation **(Fig. 9)**.

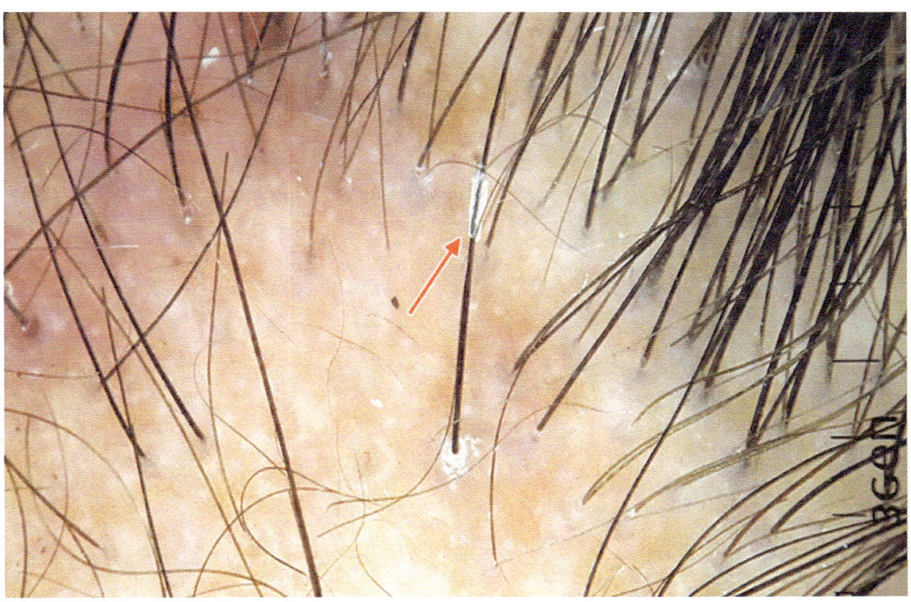

Fig. 7: Hair cast (red arrow).

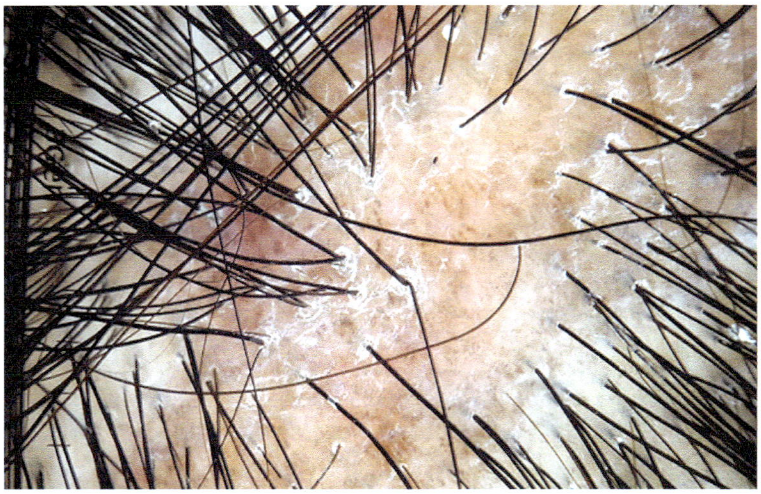

Fig. 8: Perifollicular scales.

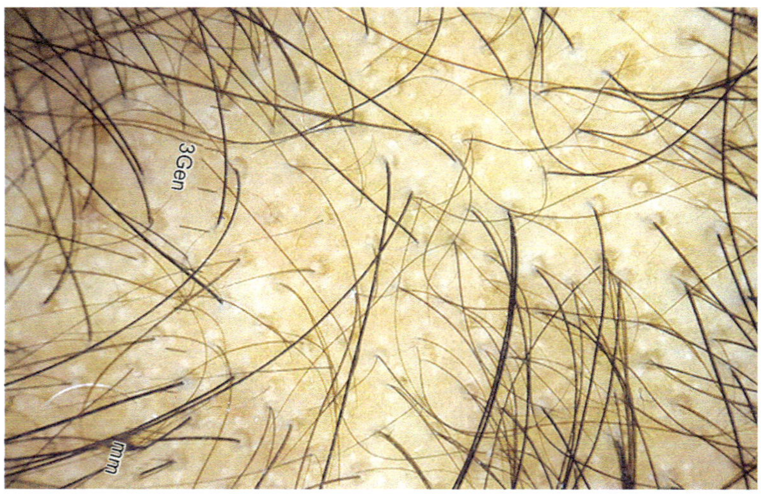

Fig. 9: Peripilar sign.

REFERENCES

1. Rudnicka L, Rakowska A, Olszewska M. Trichoscopy: how it may help the clinician. Dermatol Clin. 2013;31:29-41.
2. Rakowska A, Slowinska M, Kowalska-Oledzka E, et al. Trichoscopy of cicatricial alopecia. J Drugs Dermatol. 2012;11:753-8.

INTERFOLLICULAR PATTERNS

The space between hair follicles on trichoscopy consists of interfollicular scales, honeycomb pigment network, normal scalp vasculature, and white patches.[1]

INTERFOLLICULAR SCALES

Scalp psoriasis, seborrheic dermatitis, tinea capitis, ichthyosis vulgaris, etc., are some of the trichological disorders wherein interfollicular scales are a trichoscopic characteristic. They are placed in between the follicles. The color of the scale is a trichoscopic diagnostic marker as interfollicular scales are silvery white in scalp psoriasis and greasy yellow in seborrheic dermatitis **(Fig. 10)**.[2,3]

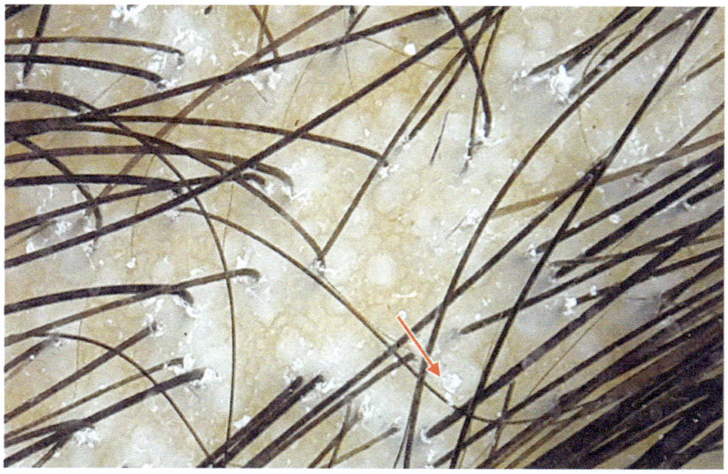

Fig. 10: Interfollicular scales are found in scalp psoriasis, seborrheic dermatitis, ichthyosis vulgaris, tinea capitis, discoid lupus erythematosus, etc.

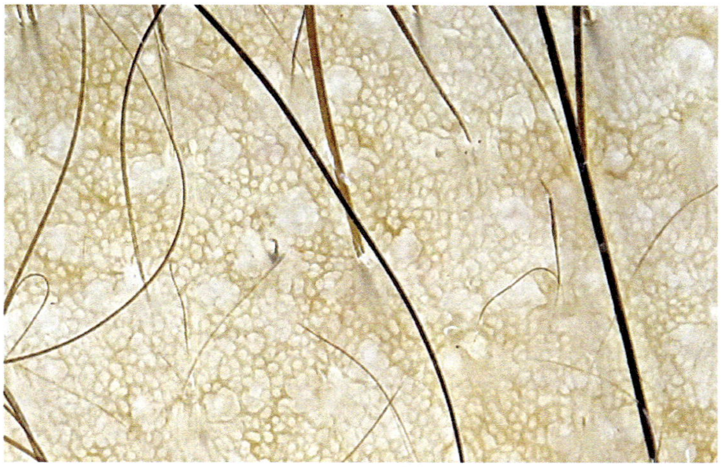

Fig. 11: Honeycomb pigment network on a normal scalp. It represents the melanocyte pigment network of the skin and scalp.

HONEYCOMB PIGMENT NETWORK

It is a homogeneous melanocytic network of contiguous brown rings. Honeycomb network is a nonspecific feature seen on the normal scalp, in scarring as well as nonscarring alopecias, barring discoid lupus erythematosus. The hyperchromic areas in the honeycomb pigment network correspond to rete ridges melanocytes while the hypochromic areas represent the melanocytes in the suprapapillary epidermis **(Fig. 11)**.

NORMAL SCALP VASCULATURE

Normal scalp vasculature includes superficial vessels such as interfollicular loops and deep vessels such as arborizing red lines. The interfollicular loops are hair pin-shaped capillaries placed in the dermal papillae, commonly seen in scalp psoriasis. On lower magnification, they will be seen as red dots on trichoscopy. Arborizing red lines are larger bore vessels placed in the subpapillary plexus. An exaggerated network of arborizing red lines is seen in seborrheic dermatitis **(Fig. 12)**.

WHITE PATCHES

White structureless areas corresponding to dermal areas of fibrosis are called as white patches. As they imply a cicatricial process, they are a trichoscopic hallmark of scarring alopecias. Numerous fibrotic white dots may progressively coalesce to form a white patch ultimately **(Fig. 13)**.[4]

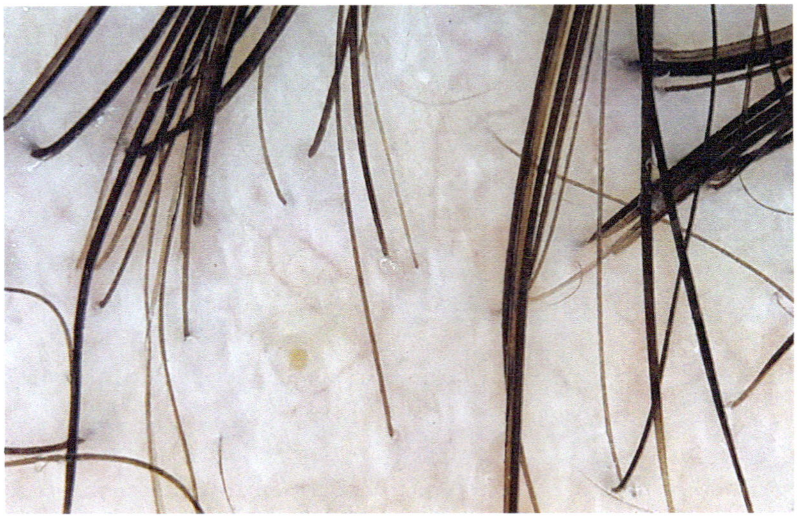

Fig. 12: Normal scalp vessels.

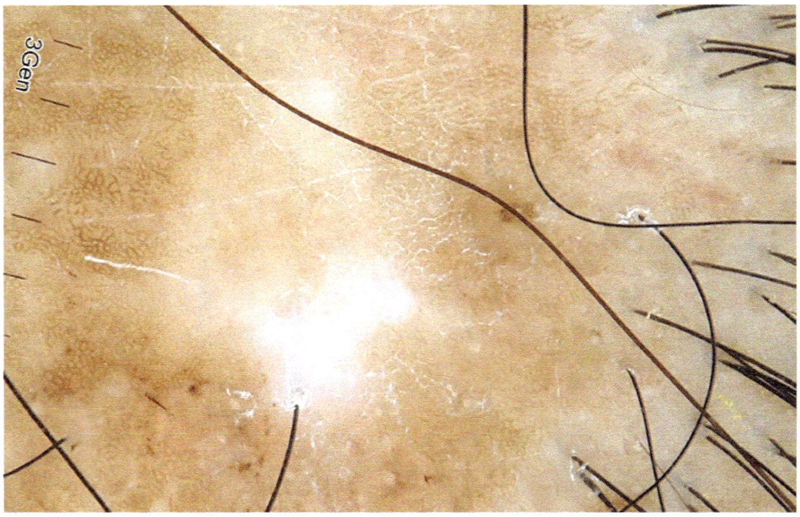

Fig. 13: White patch in the center of the trichoscopic field. It is a white, structureless area of fibrosis formed as a result of cicatrization.

REFERENCES

1. Braun RP, Rabinovitz HS, Oliviero M, et al. Dermatoscopy of pigmented skin lesions. J Am Acad Dermatol. 2005;52:109-21.
2. Rudnicka L, Olszewka M, Rakowska A, et al. Trichoscopy update 2011. J Dermatol Case Rep. 2011;5:82-8.
3. Kim GW, Jung HJ, Ko HC, et al. Dermatoscopy can be useful in differentiating scalp psoriasis from seborrheic dermatitis. Br J Dermatol. 2011;164:652-6.
4. Miteva M, Tosti A. Hair and scalp dermatoscopy. J Am Acad Dermatol. 2012;67:1040-8.

HAIR SHAFT PATTERNS

BLOCK HAIR

It is a very short hair and has a horizontal distal tip. Block hair is observed in tinea capitis trichoscopically. It can be seen rarely in other conditions **(Fig. 14)**.[1-3]

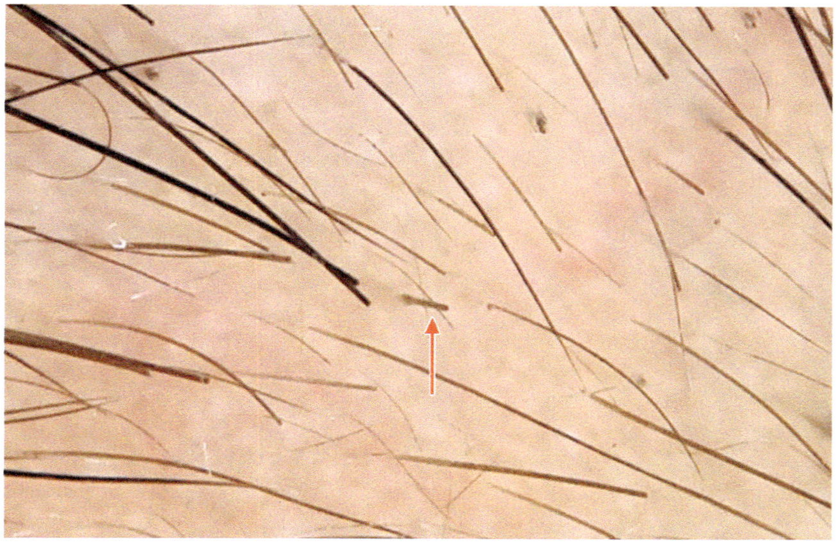

Fig. 14: Block hair is a very short hair with a horizontal distal end seen in the center of the field (red arrow). Block hair lacks the accentuated distal end of i hair thus differentiating it from i hair. Block hair is seen in tinea capitis, alopecia areata, etc.

BROKEN HAIR

Broken hairs are of varying lengths formed due to breakage of the hair shaft at different levels from the scalp surface. A chaotic trichoscopic field full of broken hairs is almost diagnostic of trichotillomania. However, broken hair is also seen in tinea capitis, alopecia areata, etc. **(Fig. 15)**.

CIRCLE HAIR

When a short and fine hair (vellus hair) coils up, it forms a circle hair. It is uniform in thickness and shape. Presence of numerous circle hair is a trichoscopic marker of alopecia areata **(Fig. 16)**.

COILED HAIR

Coiled hair is typically found in trichotillomania on trichoscopy. Due to a constant pulling force in this condition, the broken hair shaft contracts and ultimately curls back onto itself to form a coiled hair. Coiled hair is irregular in shape and thickness and thus can be differen-tiated from circle hair on trichoscopy.

A variant of the coiled hair is question mark hair. Partial coiling of the distal end gives rise to a hook-like appearance resulting in a question mark hair **(Fig. 17)**.

COMMA HAIR

It is a "c" shaped hair which is short and curved. Comma hair is a trichoscopic characteristic of both ectothrix and endothrix infections of tinea capitis in children **(Fig. 18)**.[4]

CORKSCREW HAIR

A short spirally arranged hair is a corkscrew hair. It resembles a corkscrew and is another trichoscopic feature of tinea capitis **(Fig. 19)**.[5]

FLAME HAIR

It is a trichoscopic characteristic of trichotillomania. Due to a constant pulling and twisting force, hair becomes wavy and cone shaped resulting in flame hair. On histopathology, flame hair correspond to pigmented casts **(Fig. 20)**.

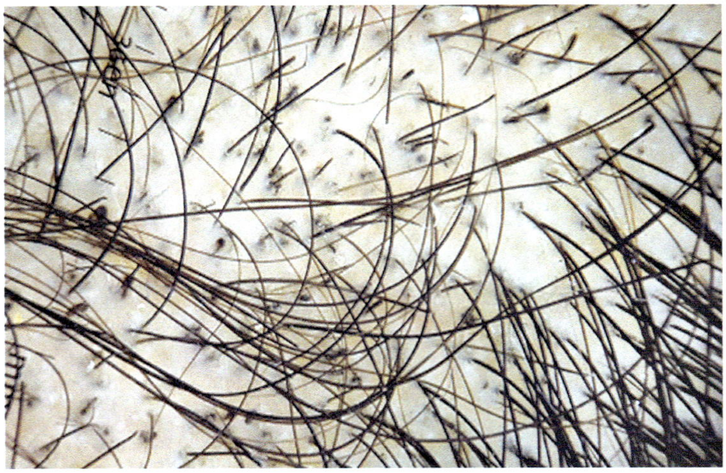

Fig. 15: Broken hairs at various lengths from the scalp surface. It is a trichoscopic feature of some disorders where hair breakage is very common such as trichotillomania, tinea capitis, alopecia areata, etc.

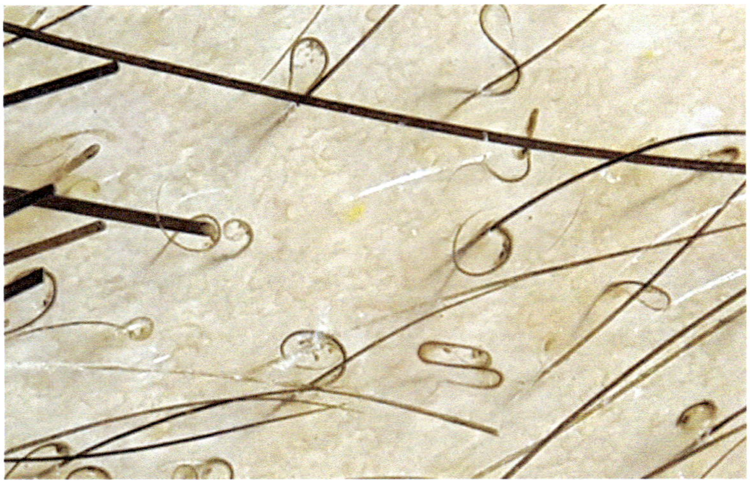

Fig. 16: Presence of numerous circle hair on trichoscopy is suggestive of alopecia areata. It is also seen in patterned alopecia.

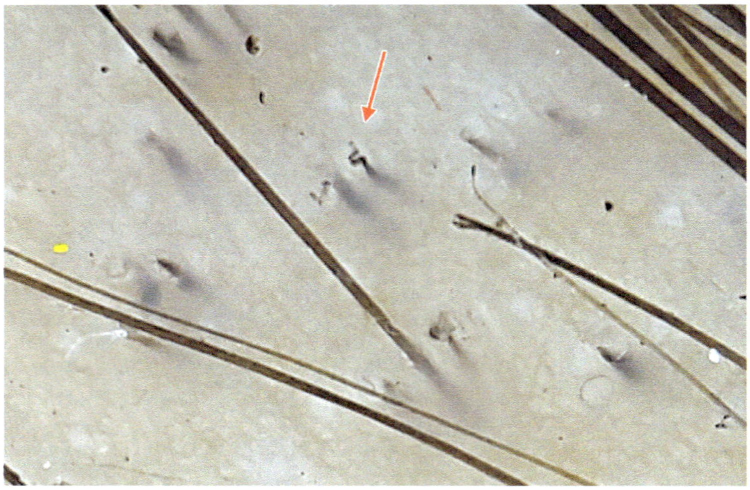

Fig. 17: Coiled hair (red arrow) is broken hair that curls back on itself irregularly.

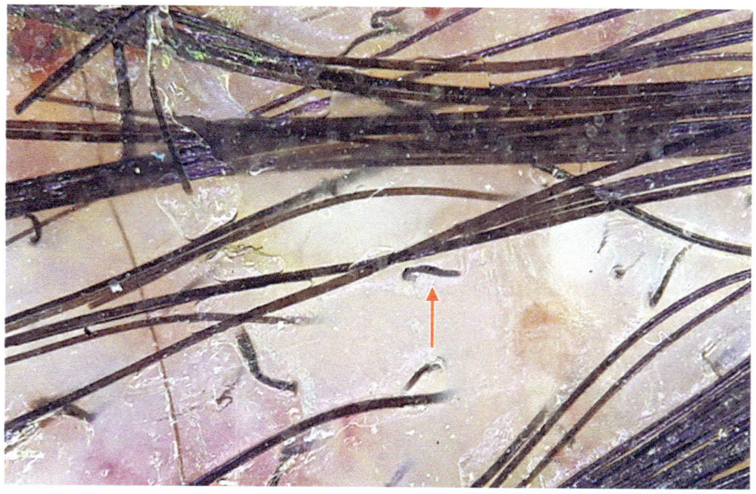

Fig. 18: Ectoparasites of the hair shaft by *Microsporum canis* species in tinea capitis causes the hair shaft to break. The short, broken hair shaft curls slightly to form a comma hair which resembles a "comma" and is a trichoscopic marker for tinea capitis in children.

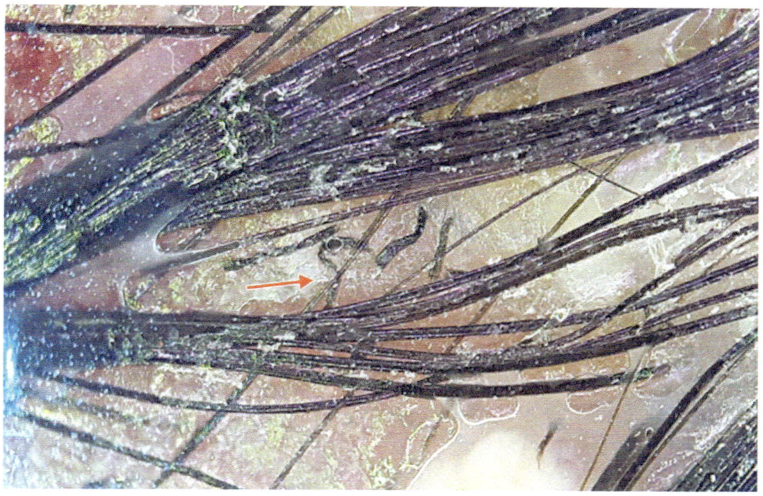

Fig. 19: Corkscrew hair is a short, broken hair which is spirally arranged, resembles a corkscrew (red arrow), and is a trichoscopic hallmark of tinea capitis. It has multiple twists and turns and hence can be differentiated from comma hair on trichoscopy.

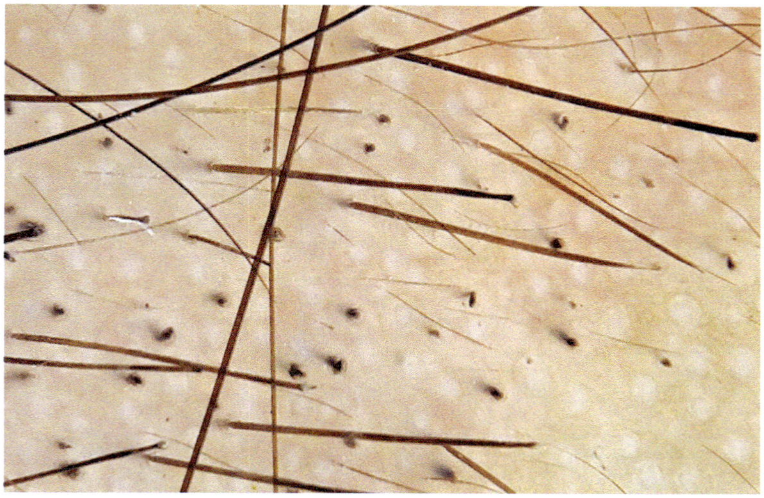

Fig. 20: Wavy, cone-shaped flame hair due to violent pulling in a chaotic trichoscopic picture of trichotillomania.

i HAIR

A short broken hair with an accentuated distal end is called i hair as it resembles the alphabet "i". A short broken hair without the accentuation forms a block hair. i hair is prevalent in conditions where breakage is common such as trichotillomania, tinea capitis, etc. **(Fig. 21)**.

POHL PINKUS CONSTRICTION

They are constrictions placed at irregular intervals on the hair shaft seen in conditions like alopecia areata, chemotherapy alopecia, etc. If these conditions respond to treatment, then the hair shaft regains its structure with a residual constriction. However, if the condition persists, then the hair shaft progressively weakens and ultimately breaks to form a broken hair or a black dot **(Fig. 22)**.

SHORT REGROWING HAIR

It is also called an upright regrowing hair. It is a short hair with a pointed distal tip and a thicker proximal end, the thickness being that of a normal shaft or less than that. Presence of several upright regrowing hair is a trichoscopic hallmark of telogen effluvium. However, they are also seen in the remission phase of alopecia areata, patterned alopecia, etc. **(Fig. 23)**.

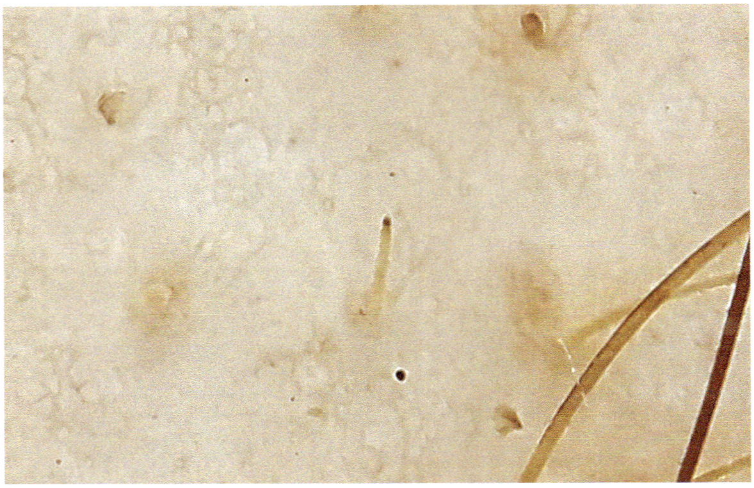

Fig. 21: Short broken hair with an accentuated distal end—i hair, prevalent in conditions like tinea capitis, trichotillomania, etc.

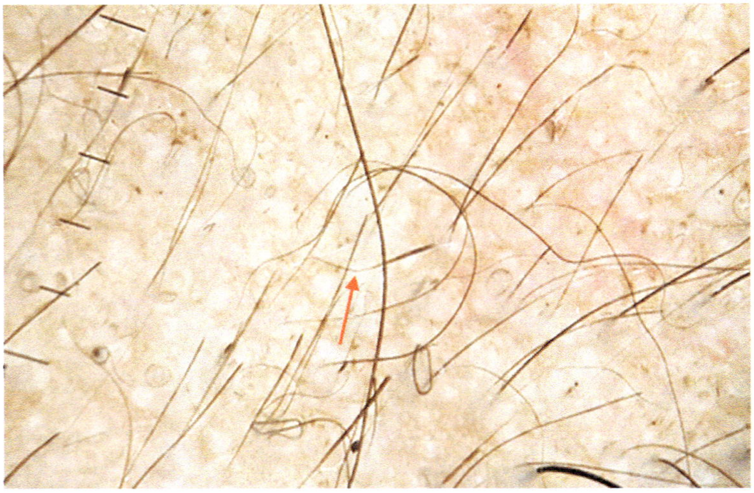

Fig. 22: Pohl Pinkus constriction (red arrow). It is a nonspecific feature seen in alopecia areata, chemotherapy alopecia, etc.

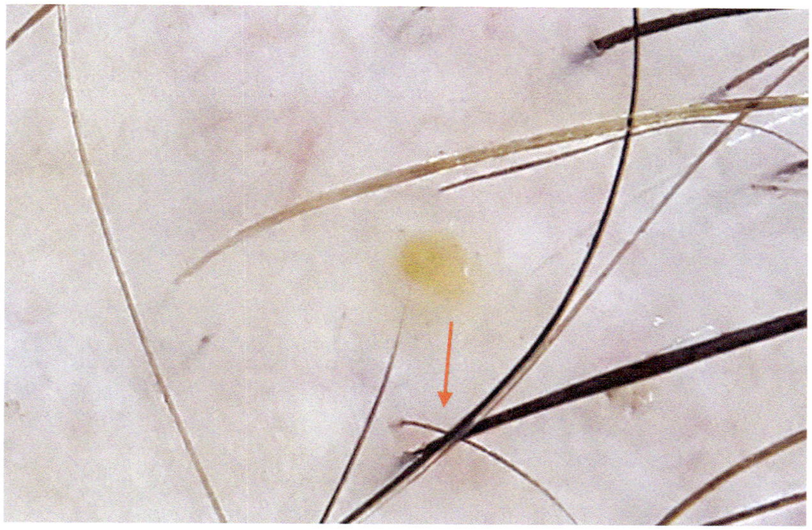

Fig. 23: Short regrowing hair is upright, uniformly pigmented and has a shaft tapering distally to end as a pointed tip and needs to be distinguished from a vellus hair which is short, hypopigmented (red arrow). Multiple upright regrowing hair on trichoscopy indicate telogen effluvium.

TAPERING HAIR

The term tapering hair encompasses exclamation mark hair and coudability hair, both of which are a trichoscopic feature of alopecia areata and also serve as a marker of disease activity.

Exclamation mark hair is a short broken hair with a hypopigmented, tapering proximal portion and a darker, thicker, frayed distal portion resembling an exclamation mark. It is generally present at the periphery of a patch of alopecia areata.

Coudability hair is a hair of normal length with a narrowed shaft toward the proximal end. It can be differentiated from normal hair as normal hair have a uniform thickness throughout the length of the shaft. Coudability hair on trichoscopy are located in the periphery of the alopecic patch **(Figs. 24A and B)**.[6,7]

TERMINAL HAIR

It is uniform in thickness and color along its entire length **(Fig. 25)**.

TUFTED HAIR

When a group of five or more hair emerges from a singular dilated hair orifice, it is called tufted hair. Tufted hair is a trichoscopic feature of scarring alopecias such as folliculitis decalvans, lichen planopilaris, discoid lupus erythematosus, etc. **(Fig. 26)**.

TULIP HAIR

A broken hair due to oblique fracture of the hair shaft, resembling a tulip flower is called "tulip hair". The presence of tulip hair is highly suggestive of trichotillomania but it is also seen in alopecia areata, traction alopecia, etc. **(Fig. 27)**.

VELLUS HAIR

It is a thin, hypopigmented, nonmedullated hair which is less than 3 mm long and less than 30 mm thick. Vellus hair in a clustered manner are seen in the remitting phase of alopecia areata. They are also present trichoscopically in congenital triangular alopecia, patterned alopecia, etc. Vellus hair needs to be differentiated from short regrowing hair on trichoscopy.

Vellus hair is short, thin, and hypopigmented while short regrowing hair is upright, uniformly pigmented, has a thicker proximal end and thins out distally to end with a pointed tip **(Fig. 28)**.

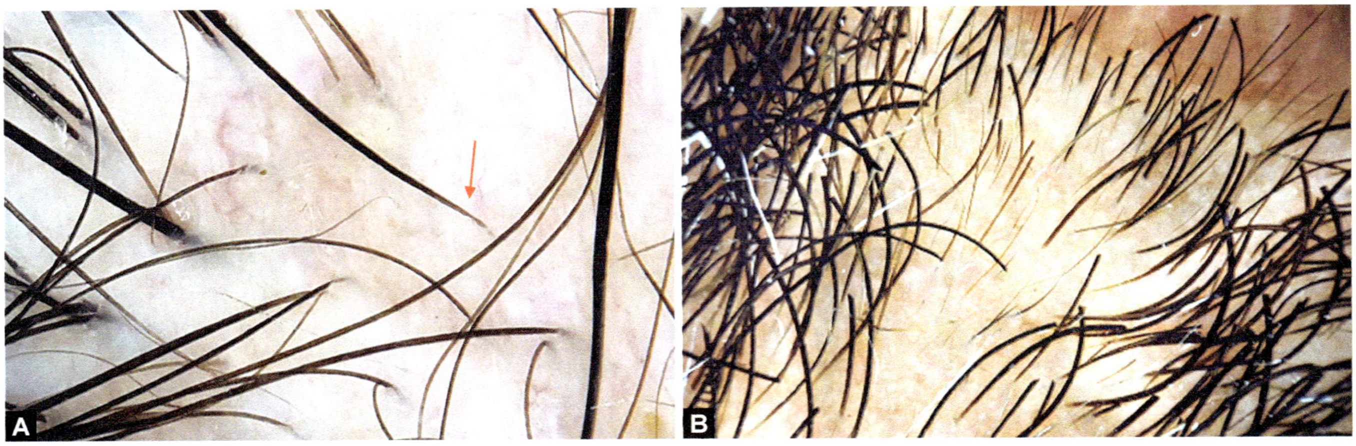

Figs. 24A and B: (A) Coudability hair is a type of tapering hair with a narrowed proximal shaft (red arrow) where as a normal hair shaft is uniform in thickness throughout. It is generally found in the periphery of patches of alopecia areata; (B) Exclamation mark hair—a trichoscopic hallmark of alopecia areata, generally present in the periphery of the alopecic patch. Note that exclamation mark tapers toward the distal end which is dark colored and frayed. Alopecia areata causes a rapid transition from the anagen to the catagen phase resulting in narrowing of the hair shaft and exclamation mark hair.

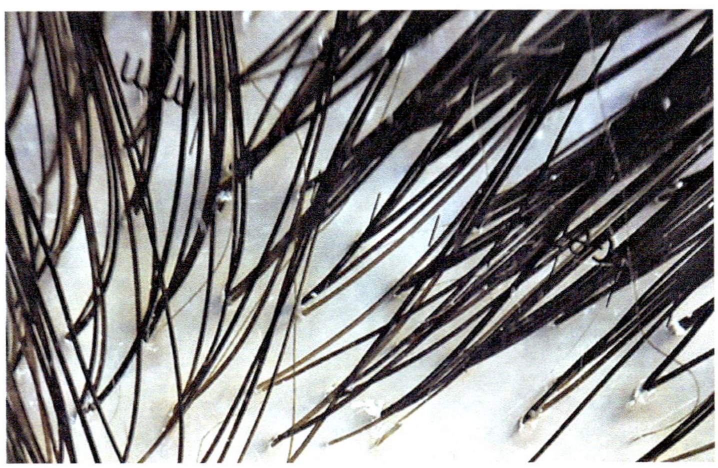

Fig. 25: Terminal hair.

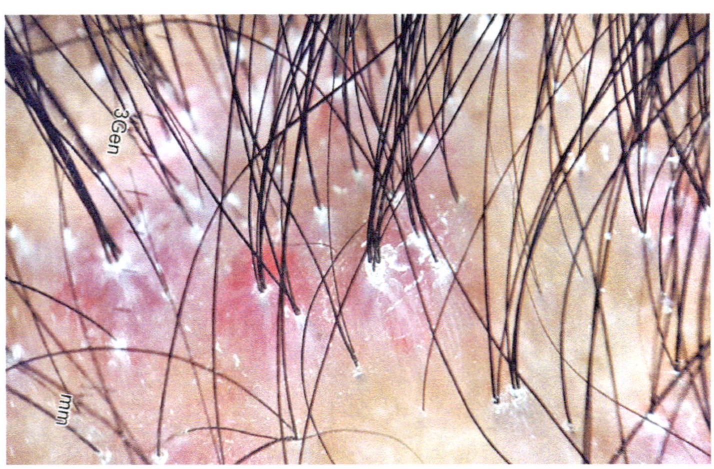

Fig. 26: Four to five hair shafts emerging from a dilated orifice forming tufts of hair, seen in scarring alopecias.

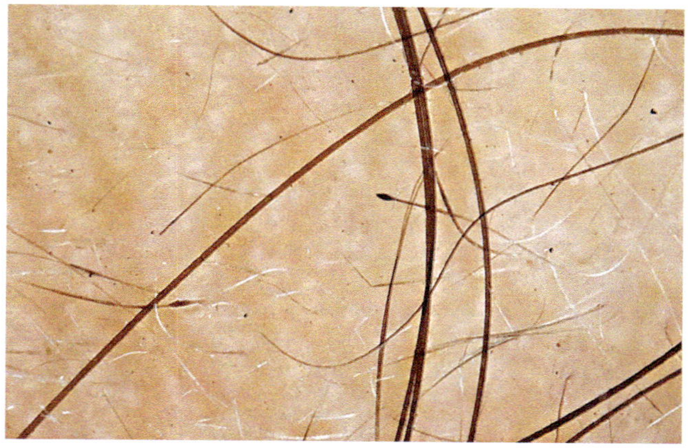

Fig. 27: Note the tulip hair at the center of the trichoscopic field. It is seen trichoscopically in conditions where breakage is common like trichotillomania, alopecia areata, traction alopecia, etc.

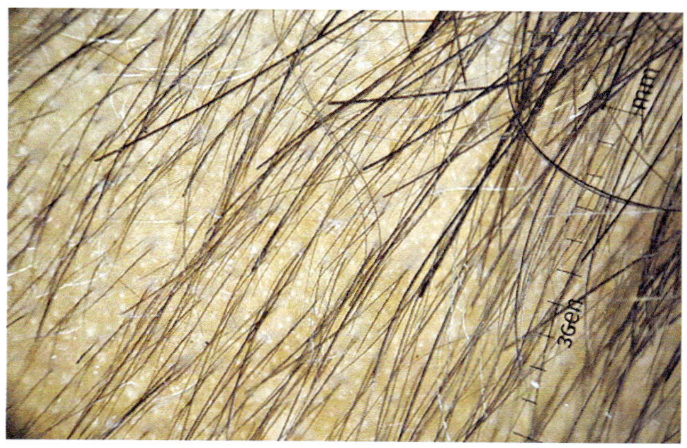

Fig. 28: Clustered vellus hair observed in this trichoscopic field, a common trichoscopic feature in the remission of alopecia areata.

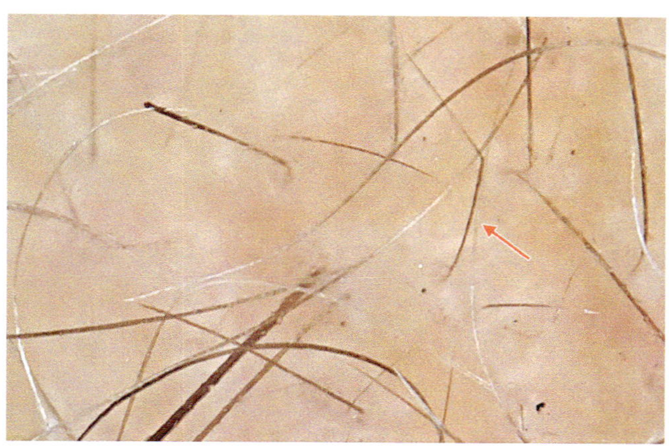

Fig. 29: Zigzag hair or Z hair is formed as a result of focal weakening of hair shafts at multiple points and a nonspecific feature found in many conditions (red arrow).

Z HAIR

In some trichological disorders, there is focal weakening of the hair shaft causing it to bend sharply at multiple points forming Z hair or zigzag hair resembling the letter "Z". It is observed in certain hair shaft disorders such as monilethrix, trichorrhexis nodosa and also in other common conditions such as tinea capitis, alopecia areata, etc. **(Fig. 29).**[8,9]

REFERENCES

1. Rakowsa A, Olszewska M, Rudnica L, et al. Hair shafts. In: Rudnica L, Olszewska M, Rakowsa A (Eds). Atlas of Trichoscopy. Springer; 2012. pp. 25-8.
2. Malakar S. Pattern of hair shafts. In: Malakar S, Chandrashekhar BS, Mukherjee S, Mehta P, Pradhan P (Eds). Trichoscopy: A Text and Atlas. New Delhi: Jaypee Brothers Medical Publishers (P) Ltd.; 2017. p. 72.
3. Rudnica L, Olszewska M, Rakowsa A. Trichotillomania and traction alopecia. In: Rudnica L, Olszewska M, Rakowsa A (Eds). Atlas of Trichoscopy. Springer; 2012. pp. 263-7.
4. Slowniska M, Rudnicka L, Schwartz RA, et al. Comma hairs: a dermatoscopic marker for tinea capitis: a rapid diagnostic method. J Am Acad Dermatol. 2008;59(5 Suppl):S77-9.
5. Hughes R, Chiaverini C, Bahadoran P, et al. Corkscrew hair: a new dermoscopic sign for diagnosis of tinea capitis in black children. Arch Dermatol. 2011;147(3):355-6.
6. Malakar S. Patterns of hair shaft. In: Malakar S, Chandrashekhar BS, Mukherjee S, Mehta P, Pradhan P (Eds). Trichoscopy: A Text and Atlas. Jaypee Brothers Medical Publishers (P) Ltd.; 2017. p. 84.
7. Inui S, NakajimaT, Itami S. Coudability hairs: a revisited sign of alopecia areata assessed by trichoscopy. Clin Exp Dermatol. 2010;35:361-5.
8. Mane M, Nath AK, Thappa DM. Utility of dermoscopy in alopecia areata. Indian J Dermatol. 2011;56(4):407-11.
9. Rudnicka L, Olszewska M, Rakowska A. Hair shaft. In: Rudnicka L, Olszewska M, Rakowska A (Eds). Atlas in Trichoscopy. Springer; 2012. p. 41.

CHAPTER 17

Non-scarring Alopecias

Subrata Malakar, Purva Mehta, Surit Malakar

ALOPECIA AREATA

INTRODUCTION

Alopecia areata (AA) presents as circumscribed bald patch on the scalp with a prevalence of 0.1–0.2% of the population. There has been a strong association between AA and atopic dermatitis, which is greatest among prepubertal children. Loss of function mutations in *FLG* that encodes filaggrin has been associated with a more severe course, and associated atopy but not a higher risk. The disorder has no sexual predilection.

The typical clinical picture of AA generally consists of a sudden appearance of one or more round or oval patches of hair loss.

KEY TRICHOSCOPIC FEATURES

- Yellow dots
- Black dots
- Tapered hairs (exclamation mark and coudability hairs)
- Broken hairs
- Vellus hairs
- Pohl-Pinkus constriction.

DISCUSSION

Disease activity can be monitored by trichoscopy as exclamation mark hairs, coudability hairs, black dots, and broken hairs are markers for disease activity. It is an excellent tool to record severity as the presence of yellow dots, and vellus hairs indicate the disease to be severe and in its late, inactive stage.[1,2]

Another trichoscopic marker for disease severity is "craters of the moon" sign in AA. This sign signifies extensive yellow dots which resemble the craters on the moon. In AA, sebum secreted by the sebaceous glands directly opens out onto the scalp surface as the alopecic patch is devoid of hair follicle to form a yellow dot, hence forming a depression resembling a crater on the moon.[3] Short regrowing hair and pigtail hair are trichoscopic indicators of hair regrowth.[4] Thus, trichoscopy should be used in the therapeutic assessment of AA in children **(Figs. 1 to 11)**.[5]

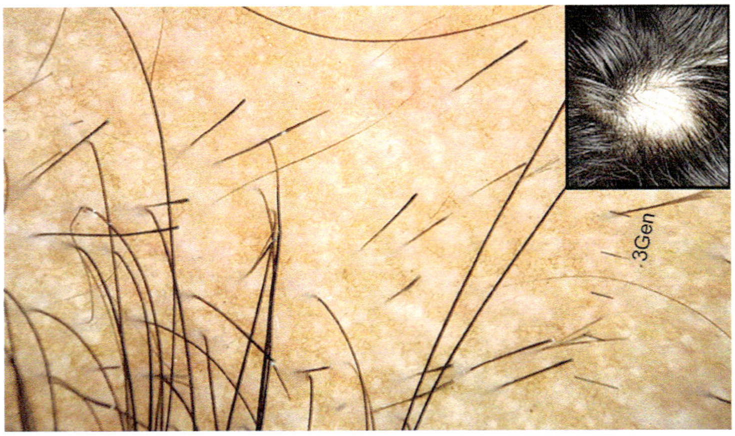

Fig. 1: Trichoscopy shows plenty of exclamation mark hairs in this field. Inset showing single circumscribed patch in an 11-year-old kid.

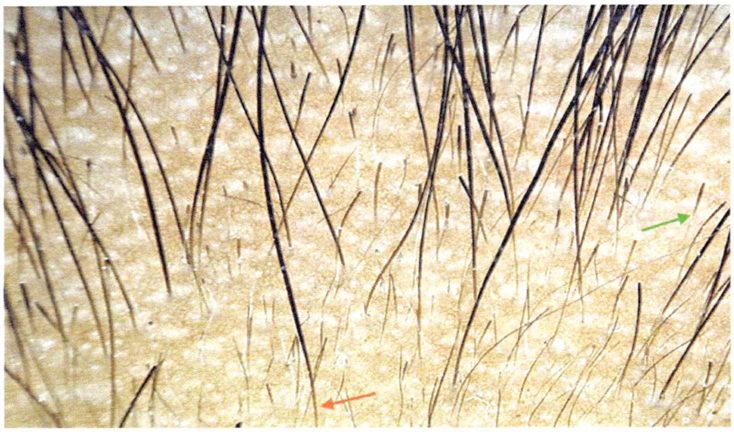

Fig. 2: The trichoscopic field is full of tapered hairs. Tapered hairs are of two types—exclamation mark hair (EMH) and coudability hairs (CH). EMH (green arrow) is a short hair while CH (red arrow) has normal length but the proximal part is narrow. Tapered hairs are indicative of activity of the disease.

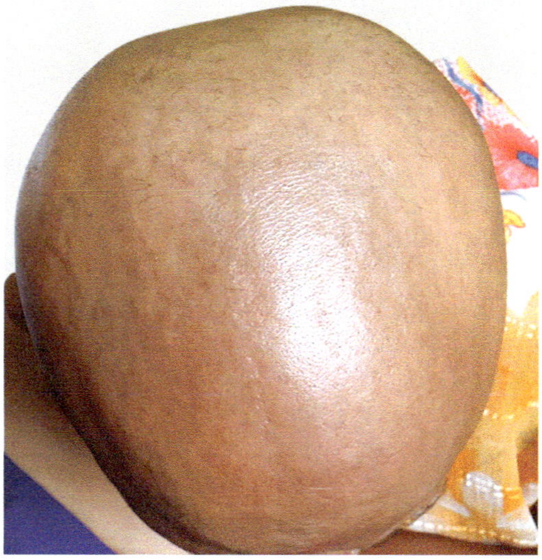

Fig. 3: Alopecia totalis may be difficult to diagnose by trichoscopy, though a clue may be provided by the regularly distributed yellow dots. In *very late cases* of alopecia areata, yellow dots may be absent. Sometimes, it may reappear after few months of topical corticosteroid therapy. So, it is a useful guide to repeat the trichoscopic examination in conditions of uncertain diagnosis.

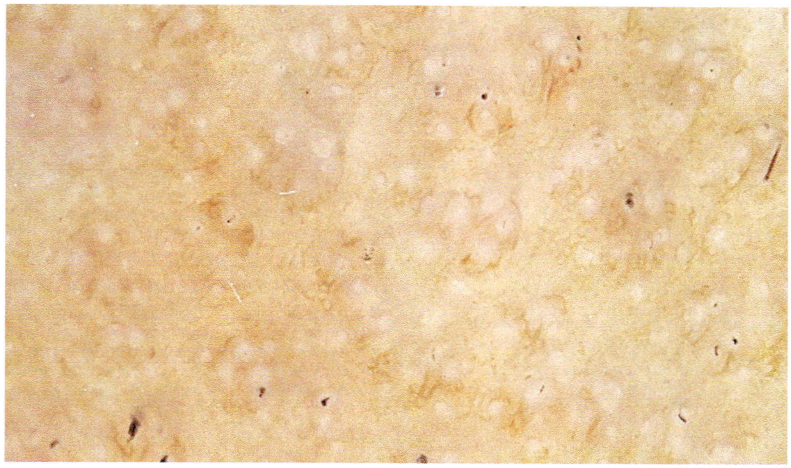

Fig. 4: Yellow dots in alopecia areata characteristically are regularly distributed. Their arrangements are also typical, in groups of two or three that reflects the number of hair shafts per follicular units.

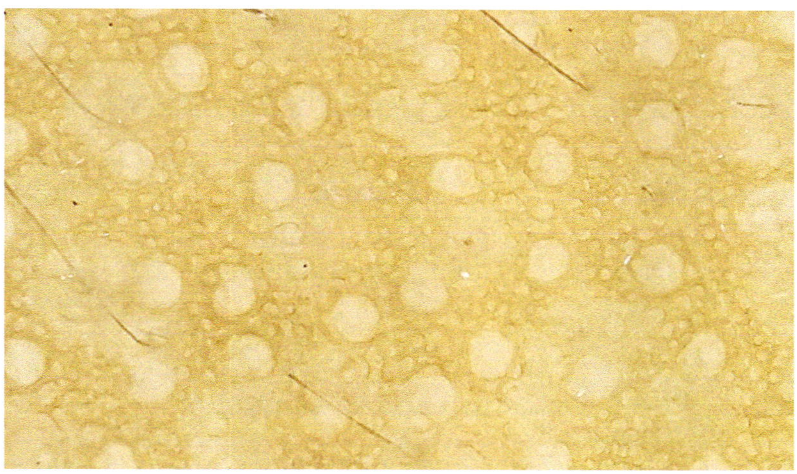

Fig. 5: Most of the yellow dots may have double margin.

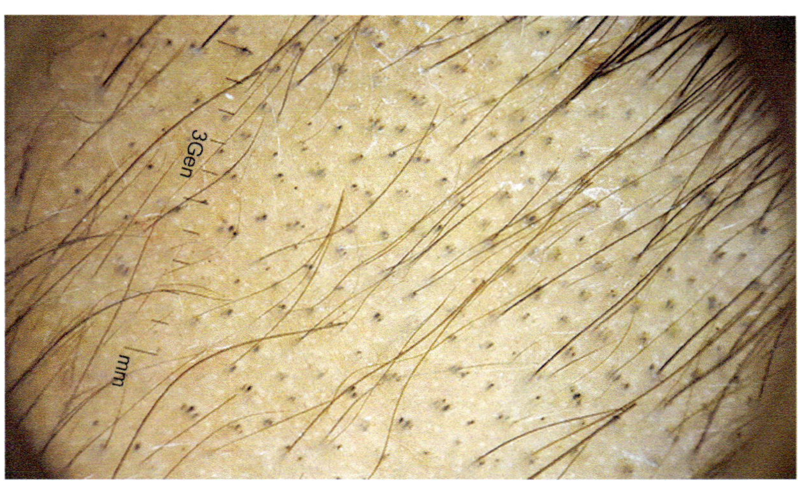

Fig. 6: The field is full of black dots which may be seen in alopecia areata and trichotillomania. In alopecia areata, the black dots are broken at the same level above the skin surface, whereas broken hair has a different length in case of trichotillomania.

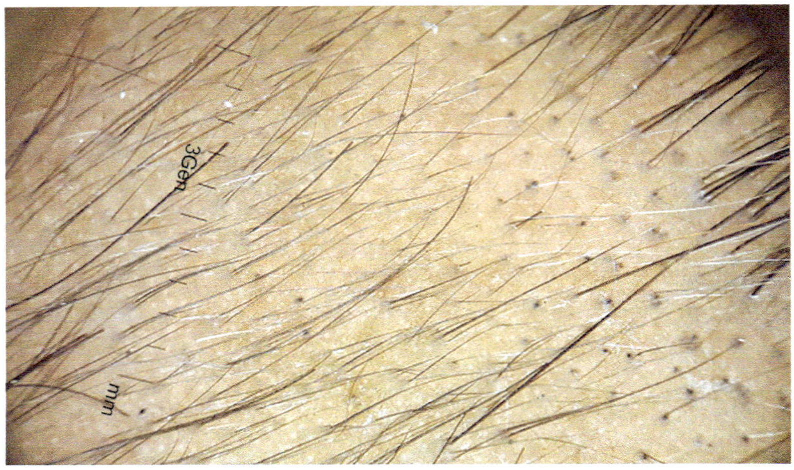

Fig. 7: Numerous vellus hairs seen in this field is indicative of remission phase of alopecia areata.

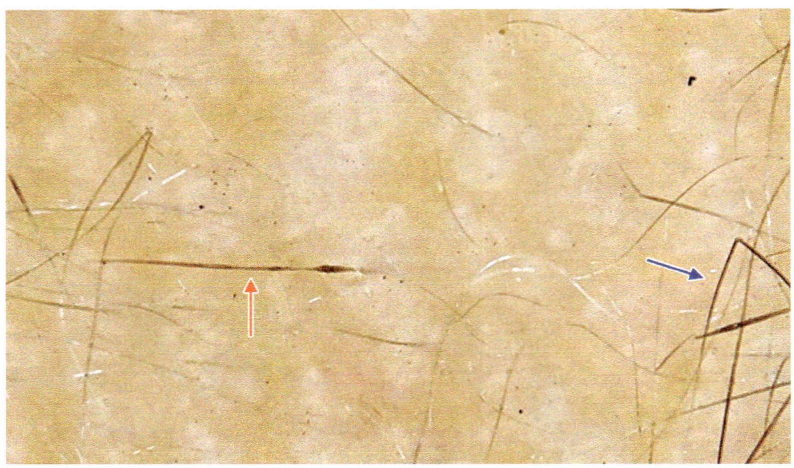

Fig. 8: *Monilethrix-like hairs* (red arrow). Formation of Pohl–Pinkus constrictions at repeated intervals during the course of alopecia areata result in the formation of monilethrix-like hairs. It indicates a variable activity of the disease in its course. It should be differentiated from monilethrix hairs. In monilethrix hairs, the nodes and internodes are at regular intervals whereas they are irregular in monilethrix-like hairs.
Note: *Zigzag hairs* in alopecia areata (blue arrow). They are commonly seen in recently occurred alopecia areata. Hair bends at different sites of the hair shaft, sometimes at the site of trichorrhexis nodosa or there may not be any true hair shaft abnormality.

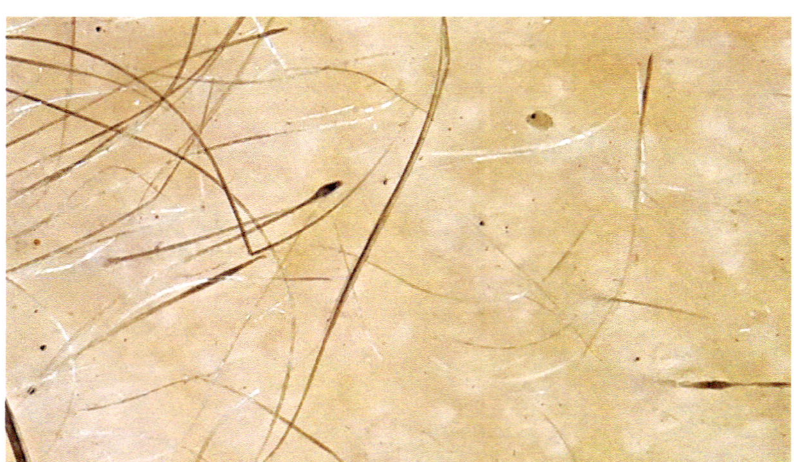

Fig. 9: Another case of monilethrix-like hairs in alopecia areata, visible at the lower extreme right.

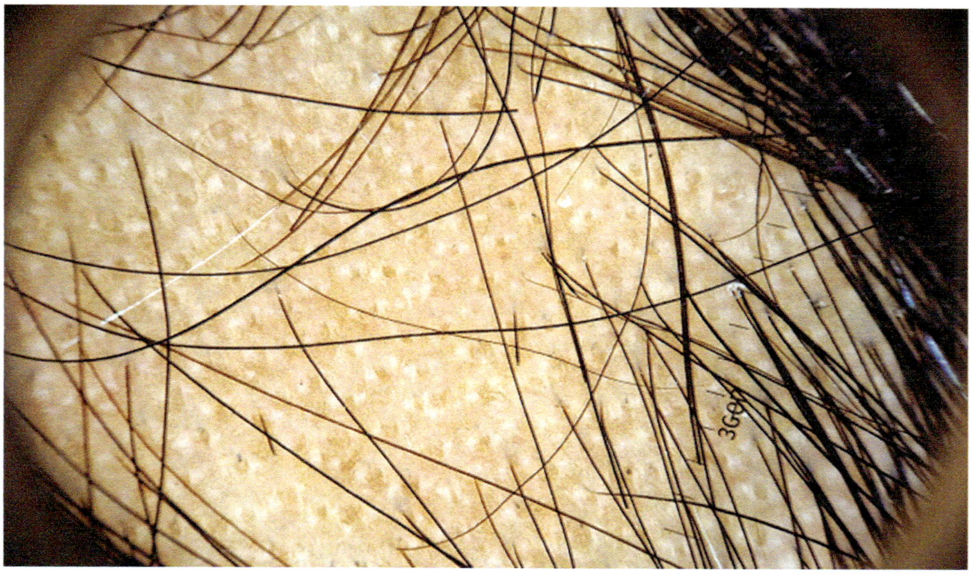

Fig. 10: This trichoscopic field has numerous yellow dots, marker of active alopecia areata. A characteristic feature in alopecia areata is there in regular distribution.

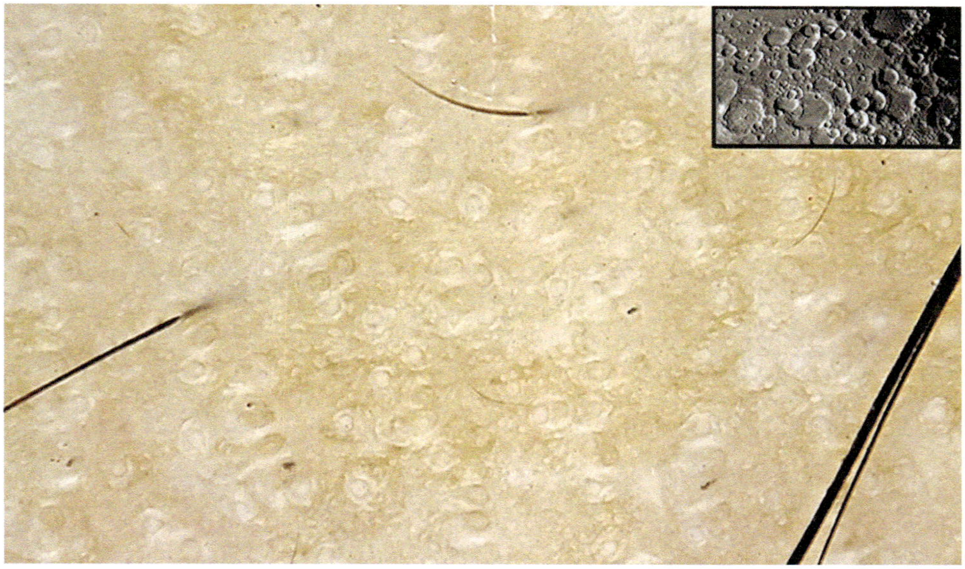

Fig. 11: The field is studded with yellow dots which form a special pattern termed "craters of the moon" appearance. This sign indicates severe alopecia areata. It serves as a poor prognostic marker. Inset showing moon craters.

REFERENCES

1. Mane M, Nath AK, Thappa DM. Utility of dermoscopy in alopecia areata. Indian J Dermatol. 2011;56:407-11.
2. Inui S, Nakajima T, Nakagawa K, et al. Clinical significance of dermoscopy in alopecia areata: Analysis of 300 cases. Int J Dermatol. 2008;47:688-93.
3. Malakar SS, Mehta PR, Malakar SS. Craters of the moon. A marker for disease severity in alopecia areata? Indian J Paediatr Dermatol. 2017;18:314-6.
4. Torres F, Tosti A. Trichoscopy: An update. G Ital Dermatol Venereol. 2014;149:83-91.
5. Inui S, Itami S. Emergence of trichoscopic yellow dots by topical corticosteroid in alopecia areata mimicking frontal fibrosing alopecia: case report. J Dermatol. 2012;39(1):39-41.

TRICHOTILLOMANIA

INTRODUCTION

The closest trichological mimic to alopecia areata is trichotillomania (TTM). As a result of this repetitive pulling action, the most frequent trichoscopic feature in TTM is broken hairs of varying lengths.[1,2] "Mace sign" is the newest trichoscopic sign described in TTM which differentiates it from alopecia areata. Due to the constant pulling action, the distal end of the hair shaft becomes rough and bulbous in texture resembling a mace. The entire shaft length in mace hair is hyperpigmented, and the distal end is rough in texture in comparison to the distal end of exclamation mark hair which is smooth in texture and hyperpigmented with its proximal end being hypopigmented.[3]

KEY TRICHOSCOPIC FEATURES

- Black dots
- Coiled hair
- Question mark hair
- Flame hair
- "MACE hair"
- Tulip hair
- i hair
- Block hair
- V sign
- Trichoptilosis.

DISCUSSION

Tulip hair is a short hair with the distal end being shaped like a tulip flower, which is attributed to the diagonal fracture to the hair shaft. When two hairs belonging to the same follicular unit break at the same level, it resembles the letter "V" and is the V sign. This V sign may be seen after regrowth of shaven hair where it will be present in all regrowing hair, whereas in TTM, the hair surrounding the "V" sign will be normal in length. Due to the destruction of the hair shaft as a result of constant manipulation, the hair residues that remain behind are called hair powder.[4,5] Of recent interest is the "burnt matchstick sign" described in TTM, wherein due to constant pulling action, the proximal end becomes dark and bulbous resembling a burnt match stick. The other trichoscopic features evident in TTM are black dots, coiled hair, or question mark hair which is a partially coiled hair, short hair with split ends (trichoptilosis) **(Figs. 12 to 20)**.

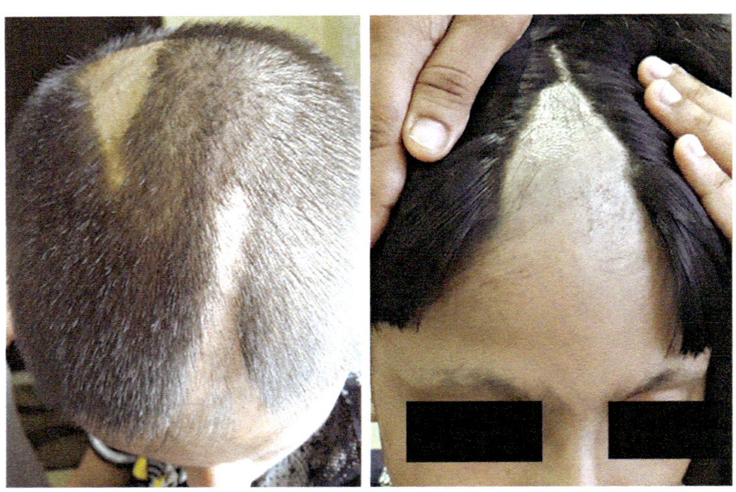

Fig. 12: Trichotillomania results from habitual, repetitive removal of own hair. The condition most commonly affects children between the ages of 9 years and 13 years. Patients present with patches of hairless areas or hairs with irregular length. The females are mostly affected.

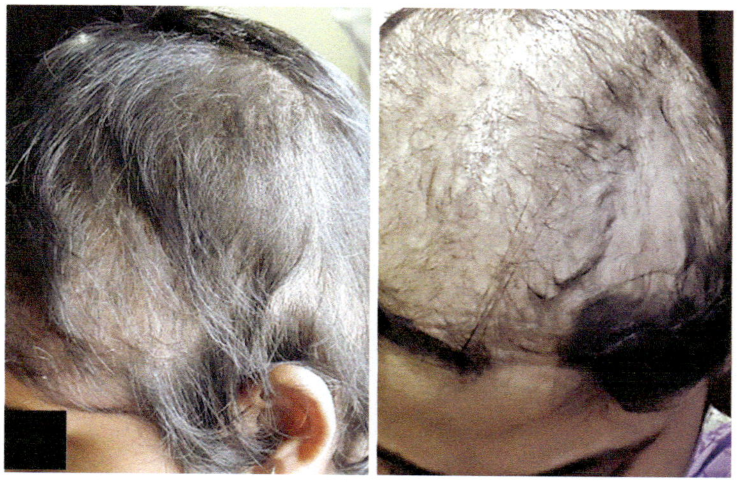

Fig. 13: Clinically trichotillomania (TTM) is characterized by irregular hair length and patchy decreased hair density. In the patient on the left hand side, the right side of scalp is affected because she is a right-handed child.
Friar Tuck sign: The sign refers to the Christian practice of shaving the mid-scalp hair and leaving peripheral circles of hair unshed. The clinical image on the right side shows Friar Tuck sign in a 14-year-old female patient with TTM.

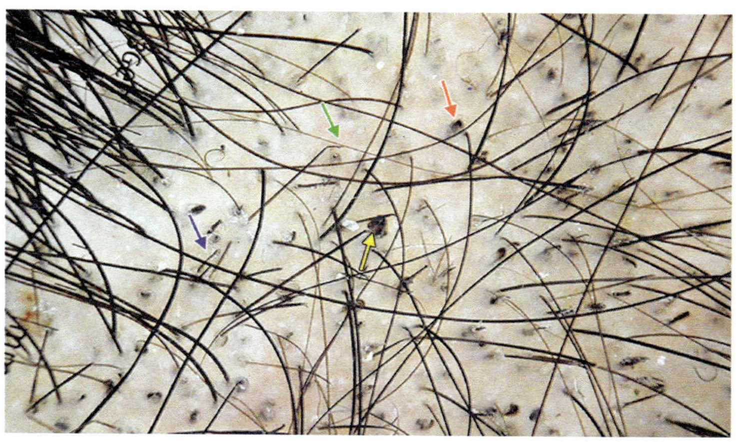

Fig. 14: Trichoscopically, a typical chaotic multicomponent pattern of trichotillomania. Flame hair (red arrow), coiled hair (yellow arrow), broken hairs (blue arrow), and question mark hair (green arrow) are seen.

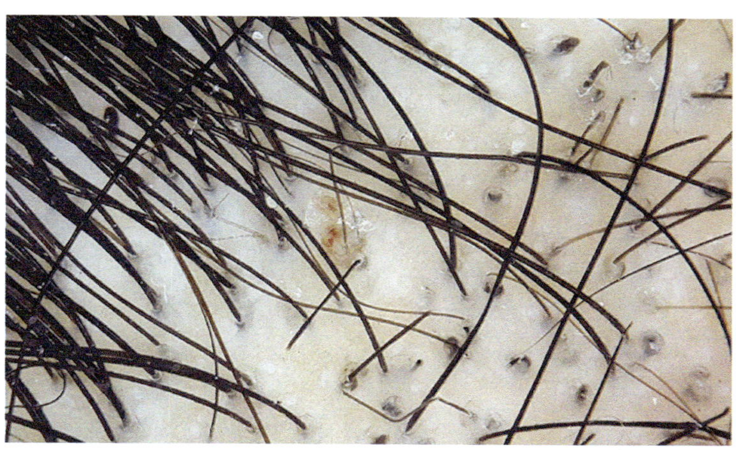

Fig. 15: This field shows multiple broken hairs, multiple flame hairs, and a bleeding area indicative of trauma by nail which is frequent in trichotillomania.

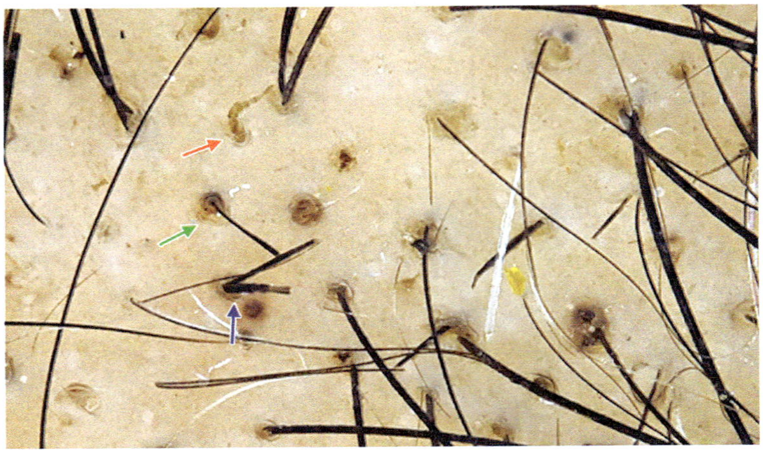

Fig. 16: The field shows flame hair (red arrow), mace hair (green arrow), and V hair (blue arrow). The additional features include black dots and yellow dots.

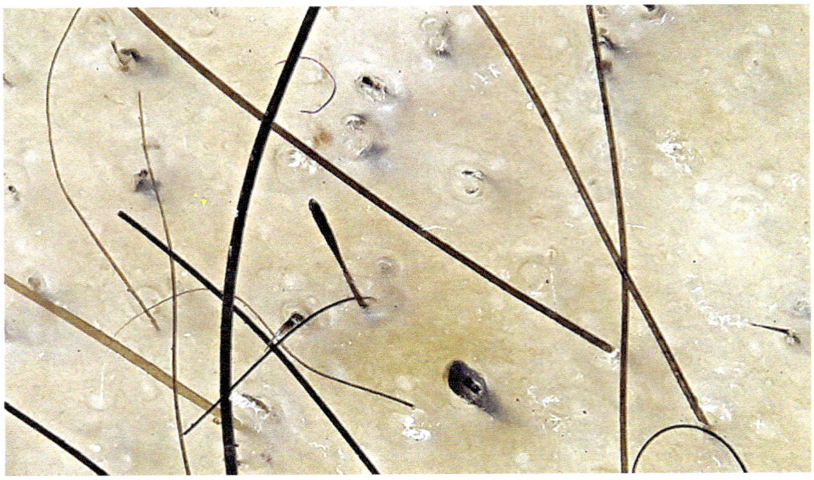

Fig. 17: Another case of trichotillomania showing "mace hair" and flame hair.

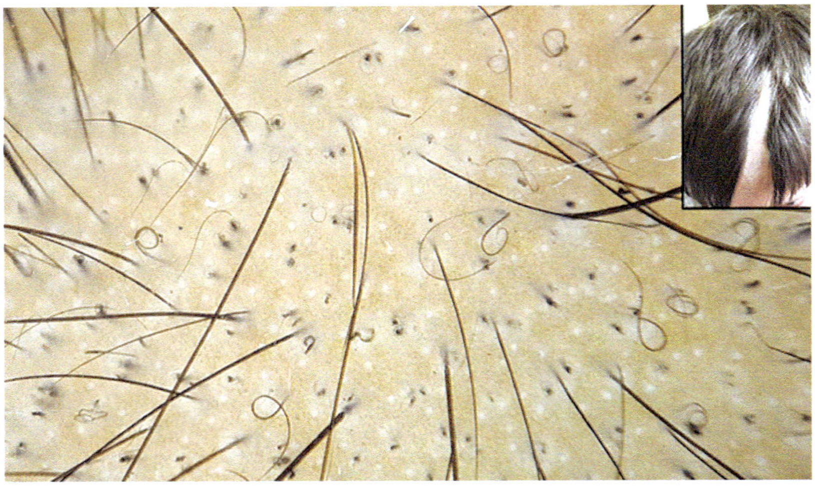

Fig. 18: This field full of flame hairs, black dots, and broken hair. In this figure, there are some pig tail hairs. They are nonspecific and shows coiling at its upper end like on pigtail.

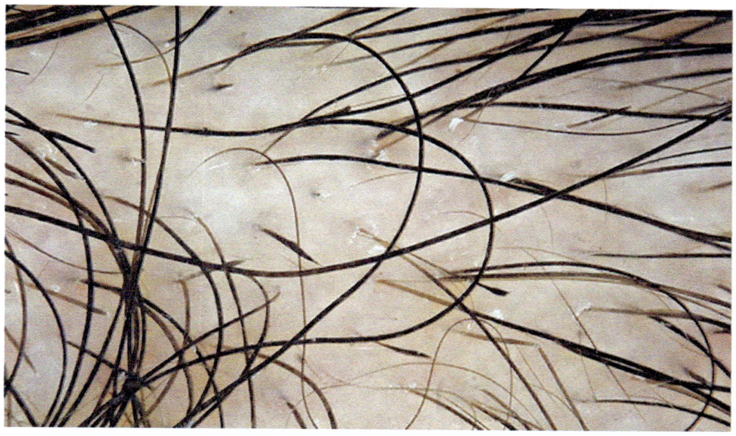

Fig. 19: Tulip hair resulting from an oblique fracture of the distal end of the hair shaft. It is a nonspecific feature seen in alopecia areata, trichotillomania.

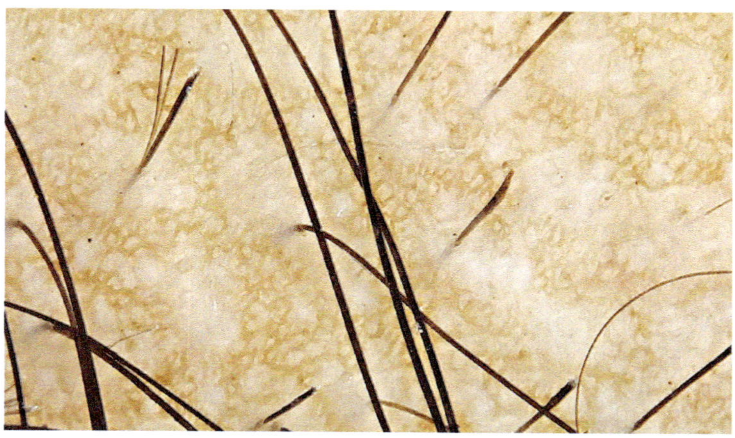

Fig. 20: "Mace hair" is characterized by the following: the distal end of the hair shaft becomes rough and bulbous, the entire shaft length in mace hair is hyperpigmented, and the distal end is rough in texture. In comparison, the distal end of exclamation mark hair is smooth in texture and hyperpigmented and its proximal end is hypopigmented.

REFERENCES

1. Sah DE, Koo J, Price VH. Trichotillomania. Dermatol Ther. 2008; 21:13-21.
2. Hautmann G, Hercogova J, Lotti T. Trichotillomania. J Am Acad Dermatol. 2002;46:807-21.
3. Malakar S, Mukherjee SS. 'Mace sign' - A definitive sign of trichotillomania? IDOJ. 2017;8:1-2.
4. Rudnicka L, Olszewska M, Rakowska A, et al. Trichoscopy update 2011. J Dermatol Case Rep. 2011;5:82-8.
5. Malakar S, Mukherjee SS. Burnt matchstick sign - A new trichoscopic finding in trichotillomania. Int J Trichology. 2017;9:44-6.

CONGENITAL TRIANGULAR ALOPECIA

INTRODUCTION

Congenital triangular alopecia (CTA) is a nonscarring, nonprogressive alopecia, which presents with a localized (triangular/oval/lanceolate) patch of hair loss mostly in the frontotemporal region. It may present at birth, in childhood, or rarely in adulthood. As it presents with a localized patch of hair loss, CTA can be clinically confused with other localized alopecias such as alopecia areata, trichotillomania especially in children. In such cases, trichoscopy is a helpful investigation to rule out mimics and obtain a diagnosis by exclusion.[1-3]

Histopathology shows miniaturized telogen hairs in the dermis along with the presence of normal number of hair follicles in the alopecic patch. However, scarring or perifollicular inflammation is absent.

KEY TRICHOSCOPIC FEATURES

- Short vellus hair with varying hair length diversity
- Intact follicular openings
- Carpet of vellus hair generally surrounded by terminal hair
- Absence of other features classical to localized alopecias.

KEY NOTES

Sometimes CTA may be confused with alopecia areata, androgenetic alopecia, tinea capitis, aplasia cutis congenita, etc. All of them have specific trichoscopic features and very easy to differentiate by trichoscopy **(Figs. 21 to 25)**.[4]

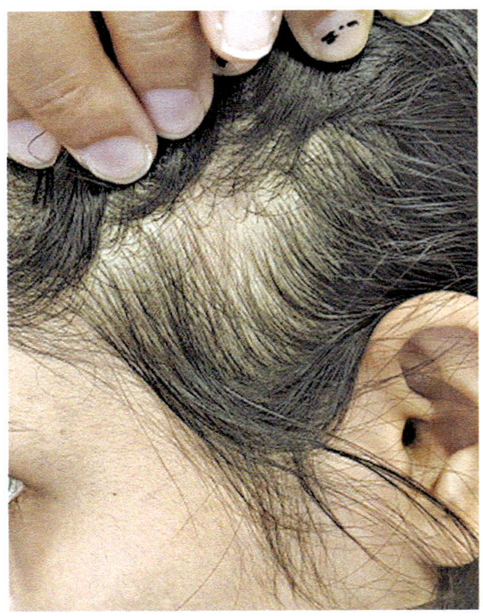

Fig. 21: A 10-year-old girl presenting with patchy alopecia (of unknown onset). Clinically, the possibilities of alopecia areata or trichotillomania come to mind.

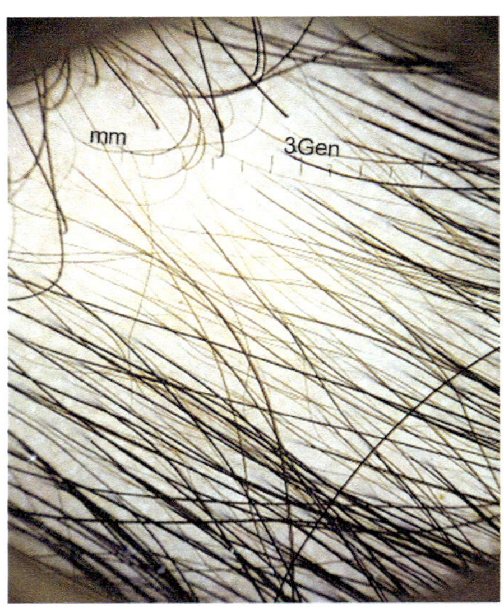

Fig. 22: Trichoscopy of the previous case shows vellus hair along with hair length diversity. Varying hair length diversity is classical of trichotillomania as well; however, broken hair is an important criterion for diagnosis of trichotillomania and is absent in this case.

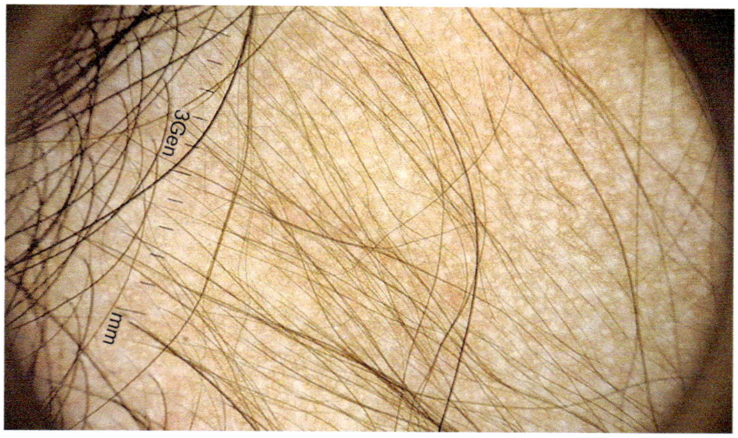

Fig. 23: Trichoscopy of another case of congenital triangular alopecia. A carpet of short vellus hair surrounded by terminal hair in this trichoscopic field is seen indicating toward a diagnosis of congenital triangular alopecia. The hair is of varying length but there is absence of broken hair (ruling out trichotillomania). Vellus hair in a clustered manner is a feature of alopecia areata too; however, the absence of yellow dots, tapering hair, black dots, and presence of intact ostia rules out alopecia areata.

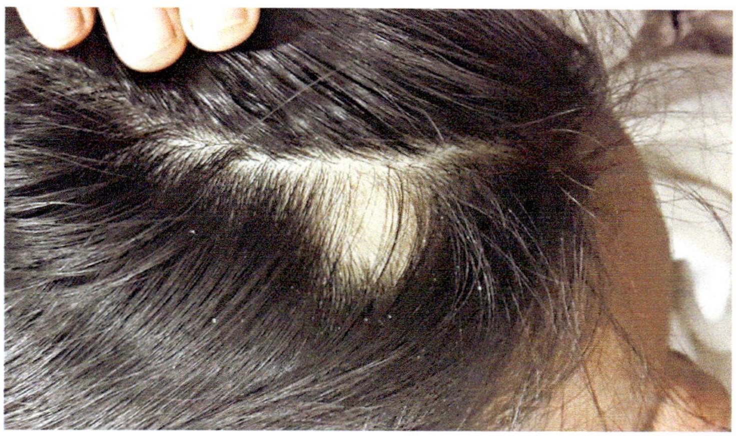

Fig. 24: Another case of patchy hair loss in an adolescent girl present since childhood, nonprogressive in nature and nonresponsive to treatment.

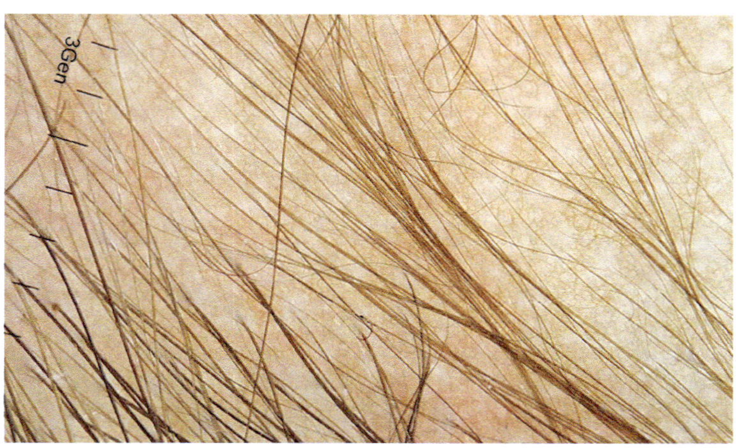

Fig. 25: Trichoscopy of the previous case demonstrates a carpet of vellus hair with a tuft of terminal hair and intact hair follicles. No evidence of empty follicles, yellow dots, black dots, or tapering hair ruling out alopecia areata. In these cases, a diagnosis of congenital triangular alopecia can be made by exclusion.

REFERENCES

1. Karadag Köse O, Güleç AT. Temporal triangular alopecia: significance of trichoscopy in differential diagnosis. J Eur Acad Dermatol Venereol. 2014;29(8):1621-5.
2. Shim WH, Jwa SW, Song M, et al. Dermoscopic approach to a small round to oval hairless patch on the scalp. Ann Dermatol. 2014;26:214-20.
3. Yin Li VC, Yesudian PD. Congenital triangular alopecia. Int J Trichol. 2015;7:48-53.
4. Mukherjee SS, Malakar S. Paediatric hair disorders. In: Malakar S, Chandrashekhar BS, Mukherjee S, Mehta P, Pradhan P (Eds). Trichoscopy - A Text and Atlas. Jaypee Brothers Medical Publishers; 2017. pp. 311-21.

TELOGEN EFFLUVIUM

INTRODUCTION

Telogen effluvium may be seen in the pediatric age group after prolonged febrile illness or as a result of nutritional deficiencies. Trichoscopy in telogen effluvium is of limited value as it fails to show key trichoscopic features.[1]

KEY TRICHOSCOPIC FEATURES

- Diagnosis of exclusion
- Short regrowing hairs
- Empty follicles.

DISCUSSION

Trichoscopically, it is mainly by diagnosis of exclusion **(Fig. 26)**.

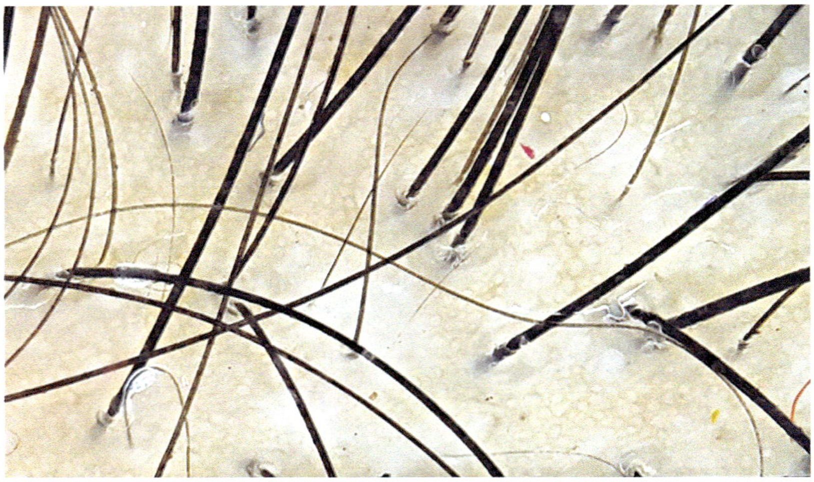

Fig. 26: Short regrowing hair is upright, uniformly pigmented and has a shaft tapering distally to end as a pointed tip.

REFERENCE

1. Telogen effluvium. In: Rakowska A, Olszewska M, Rudnicka L (Eds). Atlas of Trichoscopy. London: Springer; 2012. p. 238.

ANAGEN EFFLUVIUM

INTRODUCTION

Anagen effluvium is seen in the pediatric age group following chemotherapy.

KEY TRICHOSCOPIC FEATURES

- Black dots
- Yellow dots
- Tapering hair
- Pohl–Pinkus constriction
- Circle hair (author's observation)
- Tulipoid hairs (tulip hair-like structure) (author's observation)
- Peripilar sign (author's observation).

DISCUSSION

Tulipoid hair needs to be differentiated from tulip hair.

The proximal part of tulip hair is light colored, and the distal part is a dark tip due to oblique fracture of the hair shaft.

On the other hand, tulipoid hair is normal in color and thickness in its proximal portion, beyond which there is an acute constriction, and the shaft progressively narrows ultimately to end as a dark tip. The constriction of the tulipoid hair in anagen effluvium corresponds to induction of chemotherapy due to which the distal most part of the hair falls off resulting in a tulip-like tip. The proximal portion of the tulipoid hair signifies cessation of chemotherapy and resumption of follicular activity resulting in normal thickness of the shaft.[1]

Peripilar sign is brownish discoloration around the hair follicle and is attributed to perifollicular inflammation **(Figs. 27 and 28)**. It has been postulated that perifollicular inflammation in anagen effluvium is due to the effect of ultraviolet rays, chemical exposure, melanocytes, etc.[2]

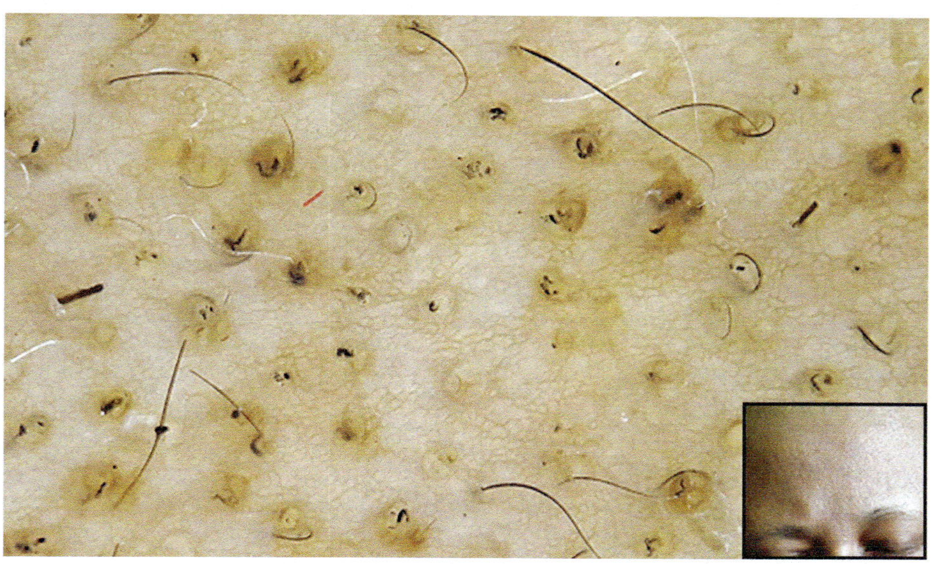

Fig. 27: The field shows black dots, yellow dots, and short regrowing hairs. Inset showing 16-year-old kid with chemotherapy-induced alopecia.

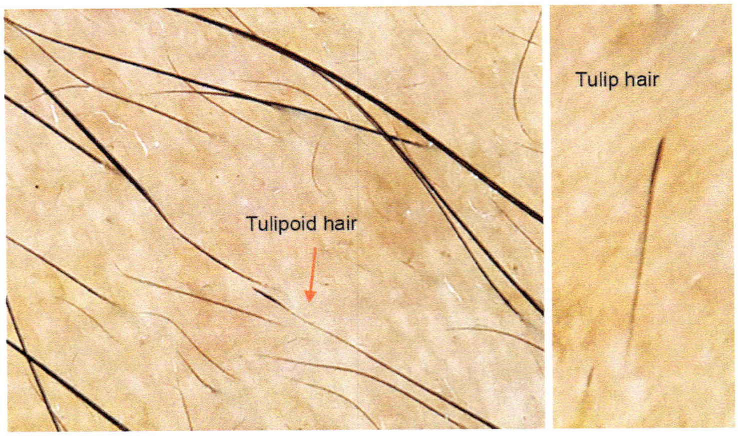

Fig. 28: The constriction of the tulipoid hair in anagen effluvium corresponds to induction of chemotherapy due to which the distal most part of the hair falls off resulting in a tulip-like tip. The proximal portion of the tulipoid hair signifies cessation of chemotherapy and resumption of follicular activity resulting in normal thickness of the shaft.

REFERENCES

1. Malakar S, Chowdhary B. Anagen effluvium. In: Malakar S, Chandrashekhar BS, Mukherjee S, Mehta P, Pradhan P (Eds). Trichoscopy: A Text and Atlas. New Delhi: Jaypee Brothers Medical Publishers; 2017. pp. 196-7.
2. Malakar S, Mehta P, Malakar S. Trichoscopy in anagen effluvium: Extensive peripilar sign. Our Dermatol Online. 2017;8:1-2.

CHAPTER 18

Scarring Alopecias

Subrata Malakar, Purva Mehta, Surit Malakar

LICHEN PLANOPILARIS

INTRODUCTION

Lichen planopilaris (LPP) is uncommon in children. However, if it occurs in children, it is important to establish the differential diagnosis with keratosis follicularis spinulosa decalvans (KFSD).

KEY TRICHOSCOPIC FEATURES

- Perifollicular scaling
- Peripilar casts
- Tufting of two to three hairs
- Perifollicular blue-gray dots in a target pattern
- Milky red areas
- Fibrotic white patches
- Absence of follicular openings
- Absence of vellus hair.

DISCUSSION

Milky red areas signify fibrosis of recent onset; whereas, fibrotic white dots are merging to form white patches that indicate inactive late stage LPP.[1] Frontal fibrosing alopecia lies within the spectrum of LPP but is not seen in children **(Figs. 1 to 4)**.[2,3]

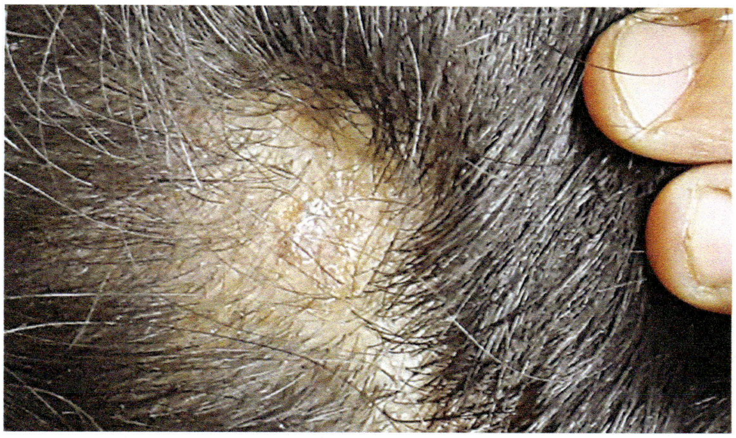

Fig. 1: Early lichen planopilaris showing mild scaling in the midpart. Itching may be constant.

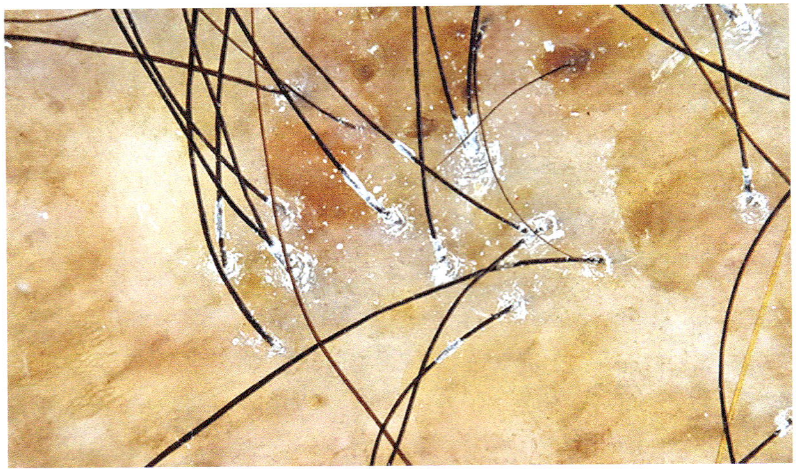

Fig. 2: *Perifollicular collar scaling*, which is a hallmark of lichen planopilaris. The scales migrate along the hair shaft and form a tubular structure that covers the proximal portion of hair shaft.

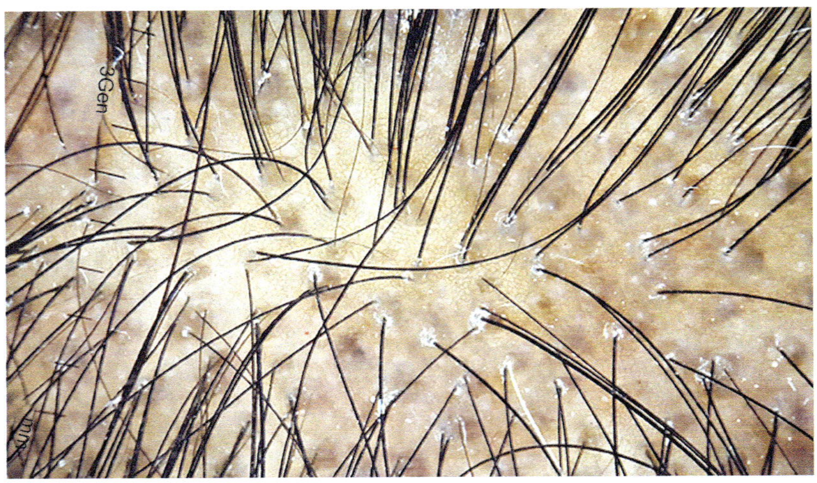

Fig. 3: Perifollicular blue-gray dots (targeted blue-gray dots) can be seen in entire field along with perifollicular scaling.

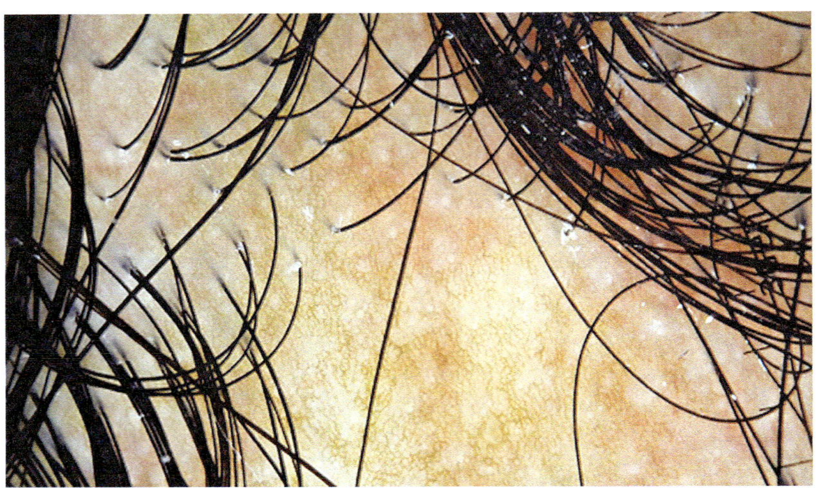

Fig. 4: Milky red area which corresponds to early fibrosis that lacks follicular openings.

KEYNOTE

If LPP occurs in children, it should be differentiated with KFSD. Though both have similar findings in trichoscopy, KFSD exhibits follicular pustules.

REFERENCES

1. Tosti A. Primary scarring alopecias. In: Tosti A (Ed). Dermoscopy of the Hair and Nails, 2nd edition. Boca Raton: Springer; 2016. pp. 50-1.
2. Heliana Freitas de Oliveira Góes, Maria Fernanda Reis Gavazzoni Dias, Simone de Abreu Neves Salles, et al. Lichen planopilaris developed during childhood. An Bras Dermatol. 2017;92(4):543-5.
3. Lencastre A, Tosti A. Role of trichoscopy in children's scalp and hair disorders. Pediatr Dermatol. 2013;30:674-82.

FOLLICULITIS DECALVANS

INTRODUCTION

Folliculitis decalvans (FD) is an inflammatory scalp disorder with recurrent follicular pustules finally leading to scarring alopecia.

Folliculitis decalvans is a neutrophilic cicatricial alopecia, which mainly affects vertex and occipital area of the scalp. The hallmark of FD is the presence of multiple hairs emerging from one single dilated follicular opening. These follicular tufts usually consist of 5–20 hairs. The disease has two phases. In active phase, recurrent follicular pustules, erythema, erosions, hemorrhagic crusts develop, eventually leading to small cicatricial patches. With disease progression, these small patches coalesce to form large areas of cicatricial alopecias.

KEY TRICHOSCOPIC FEATURES

- Tufting of six or more hair originating from a single follicle
- Starburst hyperplasia pattern **(Fig. 5)**.

DISCUSSION

These hair tufts are surrounded by yellow scales with collar formation and epidermal hyperplasia in the perifollicular region seen as a star burst pattern. Other trichoscopic features include yellowish follicular pustules, loop, and coiled vessels.[1]

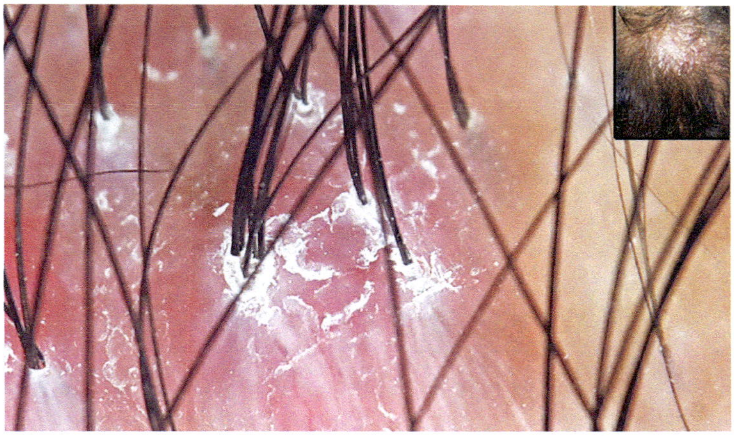

Fig. 5: Starburst hyperplasia surrounds a tuft containing six hairs. Note perifollicular hyperkeratosis and scaling. This corroborates with the combination of epidermal hyperplasia and hyperkeratosis with the underlying pan-dermal fibrosis in histopathology.

REFERENCE

1. Rakowska A, Stefanato C, Czuwara J, et al. Folliculitis decalvans. In: Rudnica L, Olszewska M, Rakowsa A (Eds). Atlas of Trichoscopy. London: Springer; 2012. pp. 319-20.

DISSECTING CELLULITIS

INTRODUCTION

Dissecting cellulitis (DC) is characterized clinically by the formation of pustules, nodules, abscesses, and sinuses that ultimately evolve into scarring alopecia. The disease usually starts at the vertex or occipital area.

In active phase of DC, a nonscarring alopecia develops over the nodules. Cervical **(Fig. 6)** or occipital lymphadenopathy may be present. The advanced stage of the disease is characterized by scarring alopecia.

Early DC presents as suppurative nodules and patchy hair loss thus mimicking nonscarring alopecia, and hence, trichoscopy is imperative to diagnose and monitor the disease.

KEY TRICHOSCOPIC FEATURES

- Keratotic follicular plugs
- Black dots
- Yellow dots
- Scalp erythema
- Broken hair **(Fig. 7)**.

DISCUSSION

As the disease progresses, yellow structureless areas are seen on trichoscopy and finally white areas signifying end-stage fibrosis **(Fig. 8)**.[1,2]

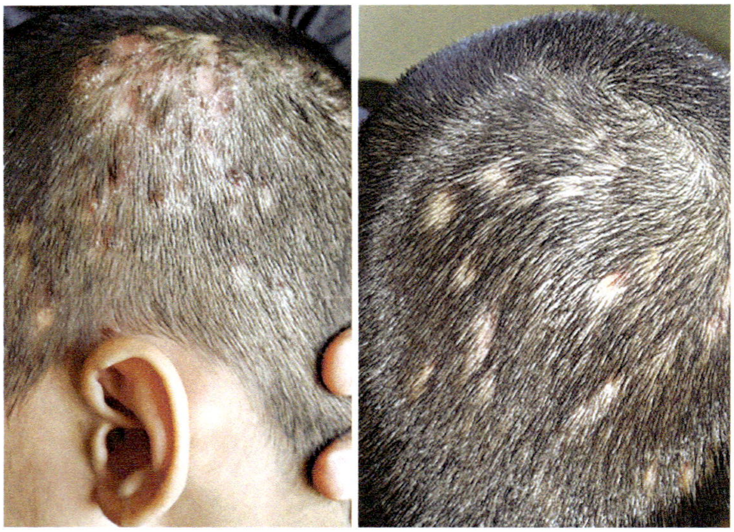

Fig. 6: The disease is very active in the occipital area. Note the prominent lymph nodes at the retroauricular area. Whereas in the vertex, the disease became silent.

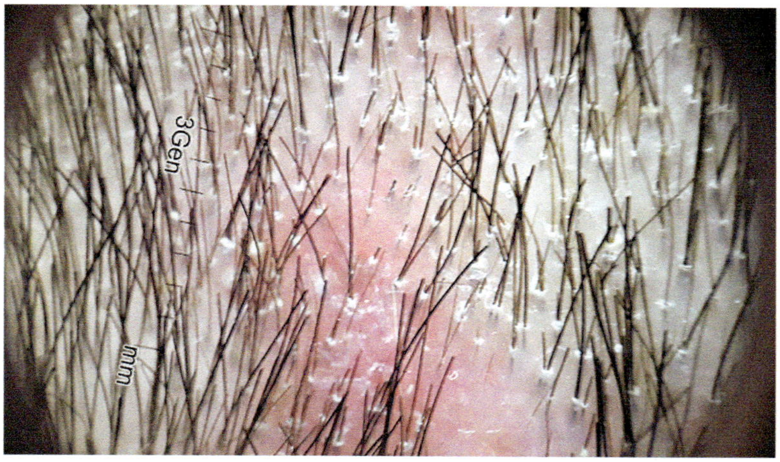

Fig. 7: The field shows plenty of broken hairs, follicular plugging. Note the scalp erythema.

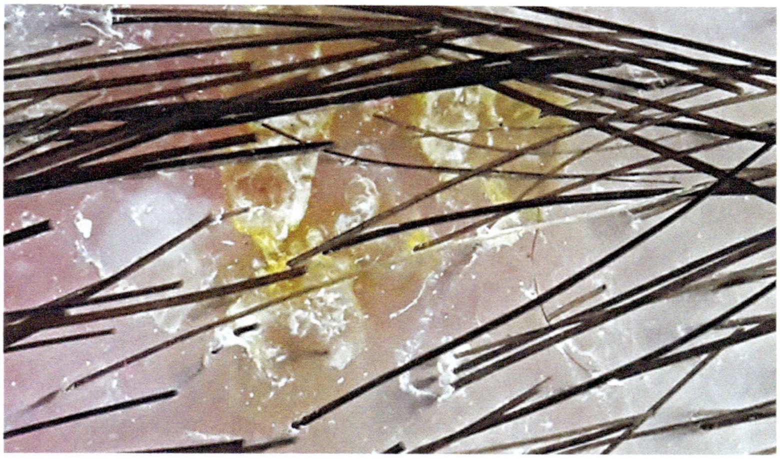

Fig. 8: Whitish area denoting fibrosis showing the end-stage of the disease. Note yellow scales full of pus.

REFERENCES

1. Tosti A. Primary scarring alopecias. In: Tosti A (Ed). Dermoscopy of the Hair and Nails, 2nd edition. Boca Raton: Springer; 2016. p. 46.
2. Rudnicka L. Dissecting cellulitis. In: Rudnicka L, Rakowska A, Olszewska M, Czuwara (Eds). Atlas of Trichoscopy. Springer; 2016. pp. 335-7.

CHAPTER 19

Hair Shaft Disorders Associated with Hair Fragility

Liane Zwetzich, Antonella Tosti

MONILETHRIX

Introduction

Monilethrix is a hair shaft disorder characterized by short, brittle hair and alopecia due to hair breakage. It is of autosomal dominant inheritance but the severity of the disease often varies between members of the same family. The genes most commonly involved are keratin genes *KRT81*, *KRT83*, or *KRT86* in the hair cortex. The hair is normal at birth but within months the child develops papules, alopecia, and shortening of the hair. The alopecia is more severe on scalp regions that are more exposed to friction such as the occipital and temporal area. The patient can also develop asymptomatic, keratotic papules on the scalp along with breakage of hair as well as itchy hyperkeratotic papules on the neck, shoulders, arms, and thighs with progressive alopecia. Monilethrix is not limited to scalp hair but can affect the eye brows, eye lashes, and axilla **(Fig. 1)**.

Key Trichoscopic Feature

"Regularly beaded ribbon" appearance of the shaft.

Discussion

The word "Monilethrix" comes from the Latin word for necklace (monile) and its characteristic feature is the beaded "necklace" appearance of individual strands of hair. This can be appreciated with dermatoscopy. The hair shaft reveals

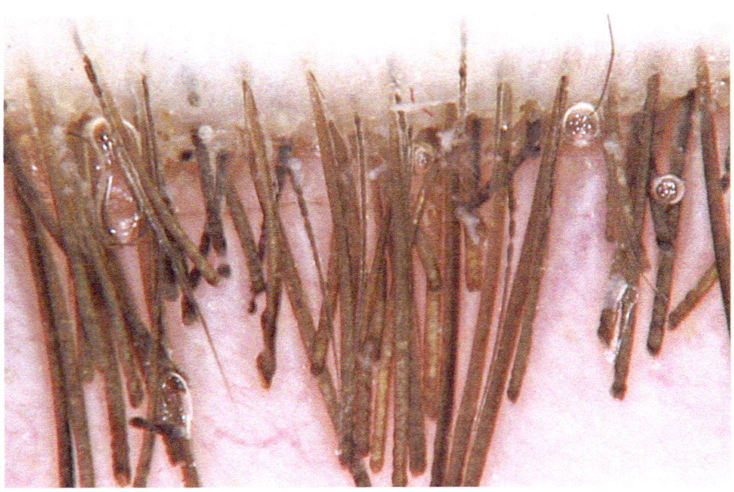

Fig. 1: Monilethrix—eyelashes.

uniform constrictions separated by elliptical nodes of normal thickness at regular intervals giving it a "regularly beaded ribbon" appearance **(Fig. 2)**. The beaded hair has a tendency to break in the internodes where the medulla is absent, so the hair shaft may seem to bend in different directions, which is described as the "regularly bended ribbon sign". Hair with normal morphology can be seen intermixed within these beaded hair.

Since the extent of monilethrix can vary enormously from few hair shaft abnormalities to numerous broken hairs including vellus hair, dermatoscopy is a great tool to quickly assess the extent of involvement of the disorder in the patient as well as their family members **(Figs. 3 and 4)**. It also allows distinguishing monilethrix from pseudomonilethrix seen in alopecia areata **(Fig. 5)**.

TRICHORRHEXIS INVAGINATA (NETHERTON SYNDROME)

In trichorrhexis invaginata, also known as "bamboo hair", the hair shaft invaginates on itself at several points along the shaft demonstrating a "ball and socket" like morphology.

Trichorrhexis invaginata occurs in Netherton syndrome, which is a rare autosomal recessive disease caused by a mutation in the serine protease inhibitor of *SPINK5* gene that may play an important role in inflammation of epithelial and lymphoid tissues. The syndrome presents as a triad of ichthyosis, atopy, and trichorrhexis invaginata. Hair abnormalities such as pili torti, trichorrhexis nodosa, and helical curls can occasionally be seen but are not specific for this disorder.

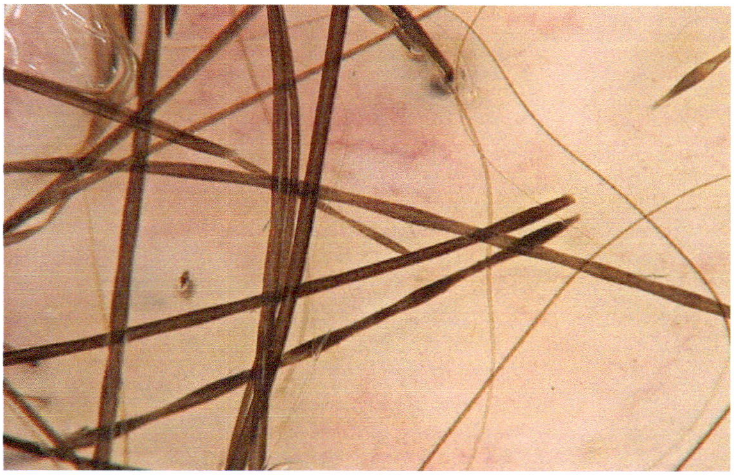

Fig. 2: Monilethrix—"regularly beaded ribbon" on dermatoscopy.

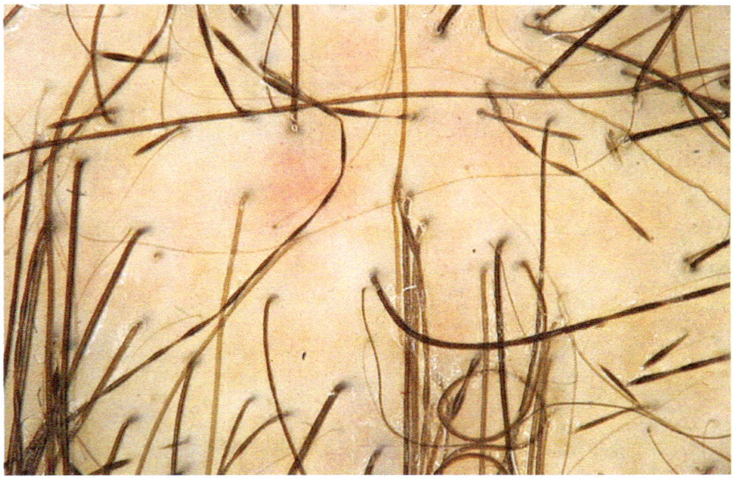

Fig. 3: Monilethrix.

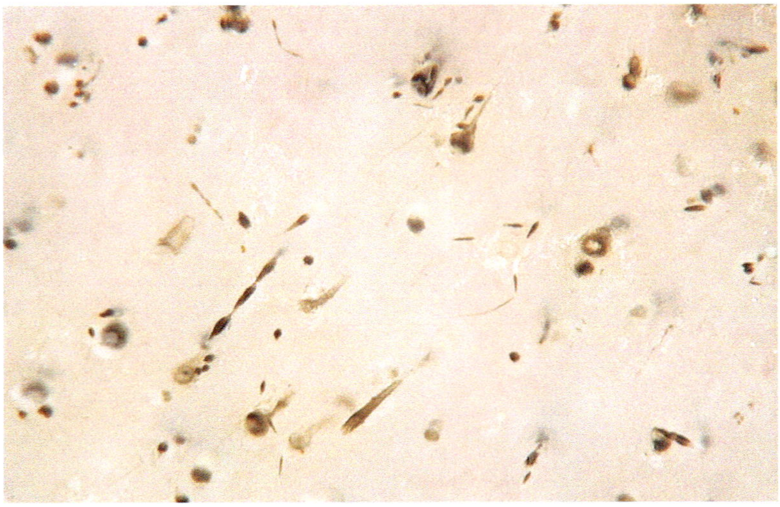

Fig. 4: Monilethrix—severe case.

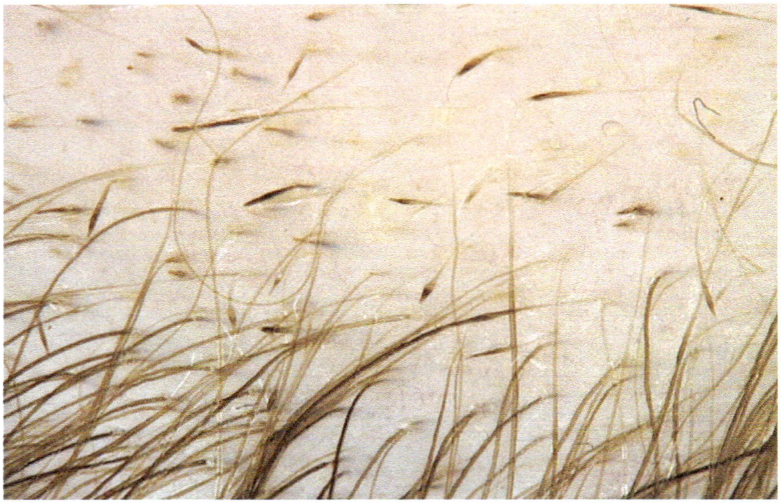

Fig. 5: Pseudomonilethrix in alopecia areata.

Trichorrhexis invaginata manifests as short, dry, spiky and brittle hair on the scalp and eye brows. On dermoscopy, the hair shaft shows multiple nodular swellings along the shaft at irregular intervals. On higher magnification, you can see an intussusception of the distal portion into the proximal portion of the hair shaft resembling the "ball and socket" appearance. Breakage along the ball and socket intussusception results in the formation of broken shafts with a "ball-shaped "- end (matchstick hairs) and with a ragged cupped end (golf tee hairs) **(Fig. 6)**.

The lateral eyebrows are a good location to detect the abnormal hairs because of their higher hair density compared to scalp hair. Eyelashes may also show trichoscopy features and can be used.

In some patients, the alopecia on the scalp may improve with age and appear normal; however, eyelashes and eyebrows usually show stable trichoscopy features without recovery.

TRICHORRHEXIS NODOSA

Trichorrhexis nodosa presents as fracture of the hair at nodes with characteristic splaying **(Fig. 7)**. It is the most common defect of the hair shaft.

Trichorrhexis nodosa may be inherited or acquired. In the inherited form, it is seen in multisymptom syndromes such as Kabuki syndrome and Menkes disease. In children below 6 months, trichorrhexis nodosa is associated with underlying metabolic disorder, hypothyroidism, and ectodermal dysplasia, which should get immediate investigation. The hair shaft

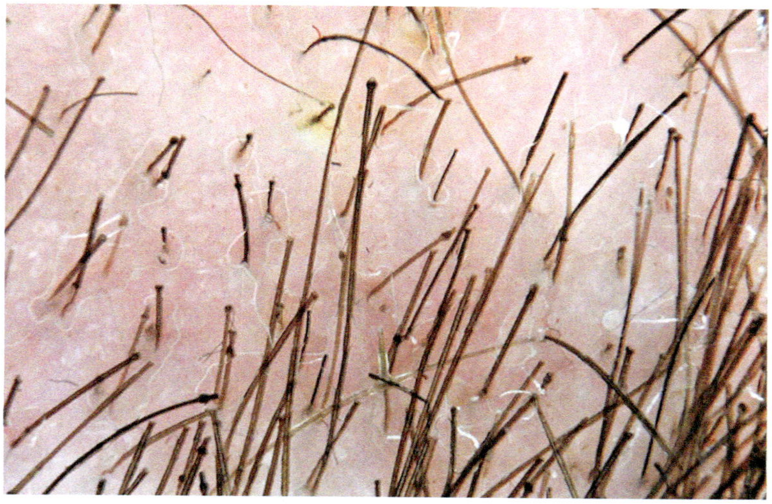

Fig. 6: Netherton—matchstick hair and golf tee hair.

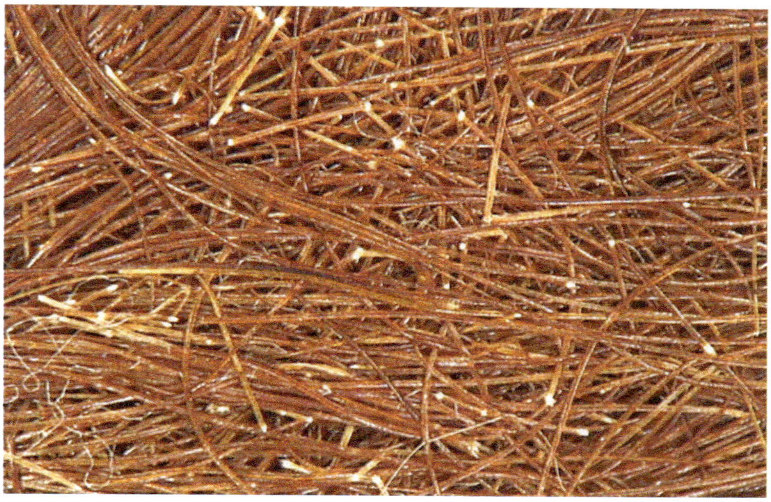

Fig. 7: Trichorrhexis nodosa.

fragility can also be acquired and induced by external factors such as heat from blow drying, chemicals for hair styling as well as scratching from conditions like scalp dysesthesia.

Clinically, the patient with trichorrhexis nodosa has short, sparse hair that has a tendency to break at different lengths. Dermoscopy can show different images depending on the magnification. At low magnification, nodular thickness may be seen along the hair shaft due to loss of cuticle and cortical fibers. The hair may appear to bend on sharp angles with rounded edges, which presents the hair breaking on the site of the nodule. This causes a slightly thickened hair shaft end.

At higher magnification, you can appreciate small numerous fibers, resembling two brooms or brushes pushed together. On the site of the breakage, brush-like ends with small fibers at the distal end of the hair shaft can be seen **(Fig. 8)**.

TRICHOTHIODYSTROPHY

Trichothiodystrophy is an autosomal recessive disorder that presents as short brittle hair with low sulfur content. This unique characteristic is given the disorder its Greek name, which is derived from—tricho, thio, dys, and trophe meaning hair, sulfur, faulty, and nourishment, respectively.

Clinical symptoms of trichothiodystrophy vary widely in phenotype and severity. While some patients only have isolated brittle hair defect, others can have multiple neuroectodermal symptoms which include ichthyosis, impaired intelligence, decreased fertility, and short stature. Patients can also present with photosensitivity which is believed to be due to mutations in the transcription factor IIH (TFIIH) and consequent defective DNA repair.

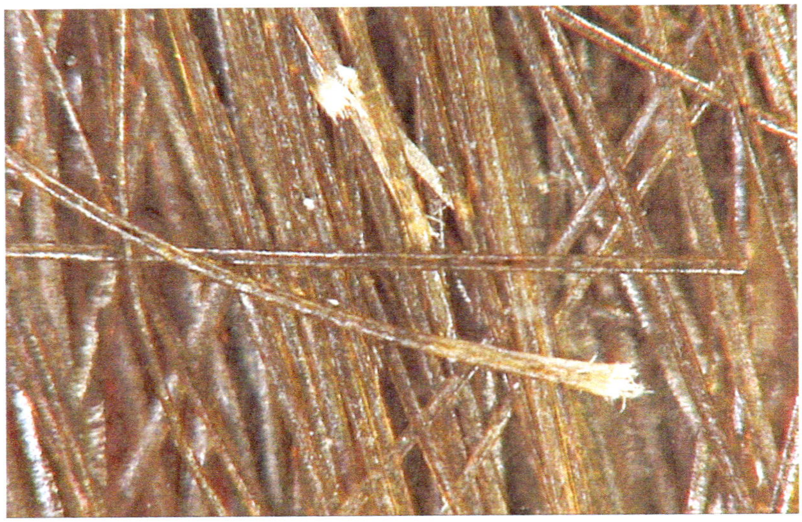

Fig. 8: Trichorrhexis nodosa—brush-like ends.

The hallmark of the disease however is the brittle hair; clinically, the scalp hair, eyebrows, and eyelashes are fragile, sparse, thin, and of variable lengths. In addition, hair loss can be observed with periodic cyclicity or during infections.

On light microscopy and dermoscopy, the hair shaft has an irregular, undulating contour and transverse fractures called trichoschisis. Pili torti are commonly observed. Final diagnosis requires polarized light microscopy that shows alternating light and dark bands along the hair shaft. This is called the "tiger-tail" pattern and is the characteristic phenomena of the disorder. A new technique, called *polarized transilluminating dermoscopy*, has recently been proposed for the diagnosis of trichothiodystrophy. The technique is performed either using two dermatoscopes and a light source or one dermatoscope and a mirror. In this way, the hair shaft is "transilluminated" by the polarized light, allowing the visualization of the typical "tiger-tail" pattern. Dermoscopy is also useful to select the hairs with a nonhomogeneous structure resembling "grains of sand" that should be examined on the microscope. Amino acid analysis confirms diagnosis.

PILI TORTI

Pili torti are irregularly twisted hair. It is a rare hair fragility disorder that presents as short, lustless, brittle, and sparse hair involving scalp and the eyebrows.

A few pili torti can be observed in a normal scalp but others can be associated with various conditions that are inherited of acquired. Pili torti often occurs in patients with cicatricial alopecia, particularly lichen planopilaris and frontal fibrosing alopecia. The abnormality is caused by destruction of the inner root sheaths but the genetic background is not known and may be multifactorial. Acquired forms may result from oral retinoid treatment, repetitive trauma, and conditions such as anorexia nervosa.

Congenital conditions associated with pili torti include Menkes syndrome, ectodermal dysplasias, and Björnstad and Crandall syndrome, where sensory neural deafness is also a feature. Clinically, the hair is brittle and dry and usually breaks before it grows long. There is hypopigmentation of the hair and children with congenital pili torti often have light blonde or light brown dull hair that grows poorly.

Under dermoscopy, you can see a flattening of the hair shaft at irregular intervals with a twist at an angle of 180° along the axis **(Fig. 9)**. Only part of the hair length is affected, while other parts appear normal.

PILI ANNULATI

This is an autosomal dominant disorder characterized by alternating light and dark bands of the hair shaft, giving the hair a shiny and speckled appearance **(Fig. 10)**.

Pili annulati is generally classified as a hair shaft disorders without fragility but there are reports of breakage and weathering in some cases of pili annulati.

Trichoscopy shows alternating light and dark bands along a hair shaft **(Fig. 11)**. A variable amount of hairs may be affected. The light bands correspond to air cavities within the shaft.

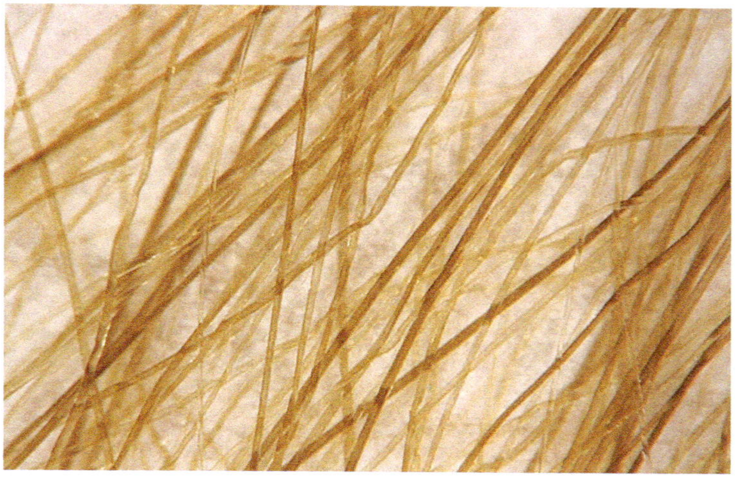

Fig. 9: Pili torti.

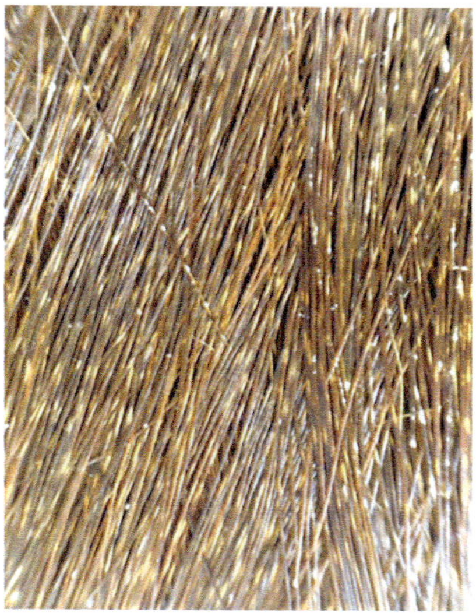

Fig. 10: Pili annulati.

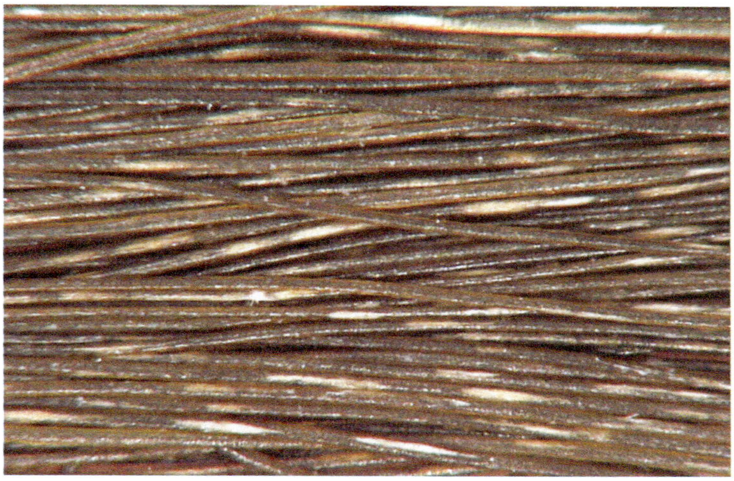

Fig. 11: Pili annuli—high magnification.

LOOSE ANAGEN HAIR SYNDROME

Loose anagen syndrome is a nonscarring hair loss disorder that manifests with increased hair shedding due to poorly anchored anagen hairs.

The condition can be sporadic or of autosomal dominant inheritance with variable expressivity and incomplete penetrance. It is believed to result from defects in keratinization of the inner root sheath. Instead of normal anagen follicles that have dense and well-oriented cells of the inner root sheath, the hair in loose anagen syndrome shows dysmorphic changes and intercellular edema in the hair shaft which causes poor anchoring of the hairs.

It can present in children of various ethnicity and hair type but is often found in blonde, female children between 2 years and 6 years of age. Due to short hair preference, boys are often undiagnosed.

Cutaneous examination shows thin and sparse hair over the scalp that is easily removed during everyday activities or hair pulling. Diagnosis requires a trichogram showing more than 70% of anagen roots devoid of sheats. The dermatoscope can be used to look for loose anagen roots, which shows ruffling of the cuticle and a deformed pigmented anagen bulb **(Fig. 12)**. Scalp trichoscopy shows rectangular black granular structures, solitary yellow dots, and major predominance of follicular units with single hairs **(Fig. 13)**.

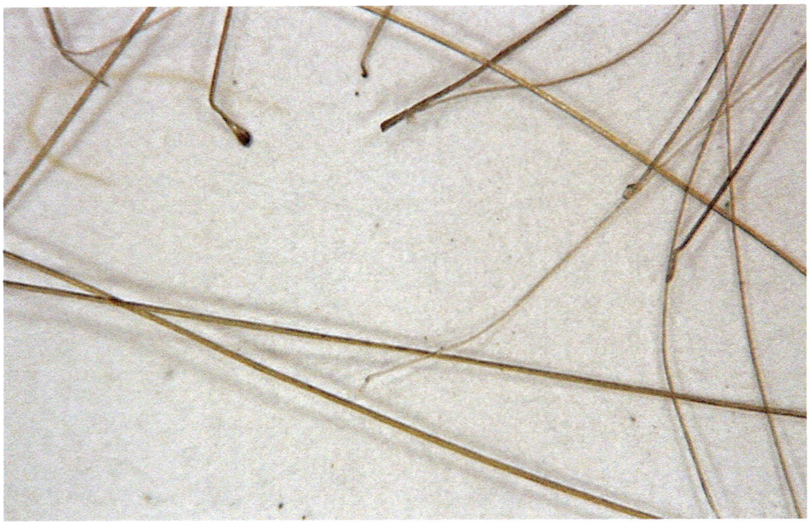

Fig. 12: Loose anagen—roots.

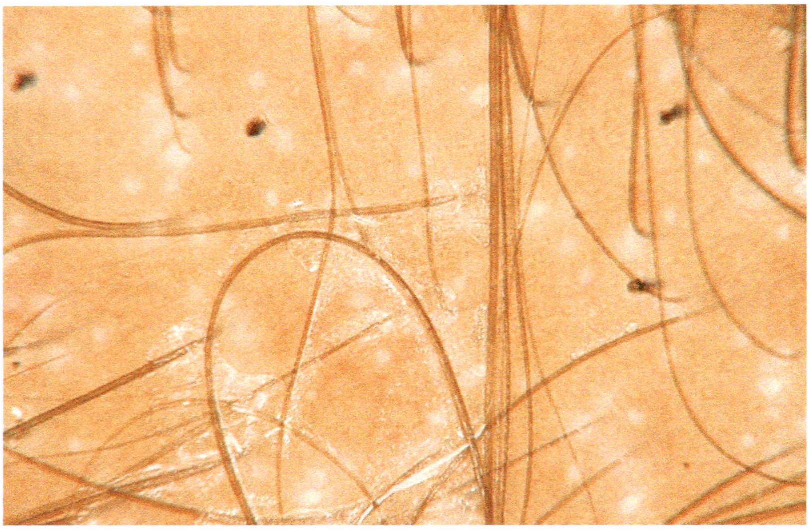

Fig. 13: Loose anagen—rectangular structures.

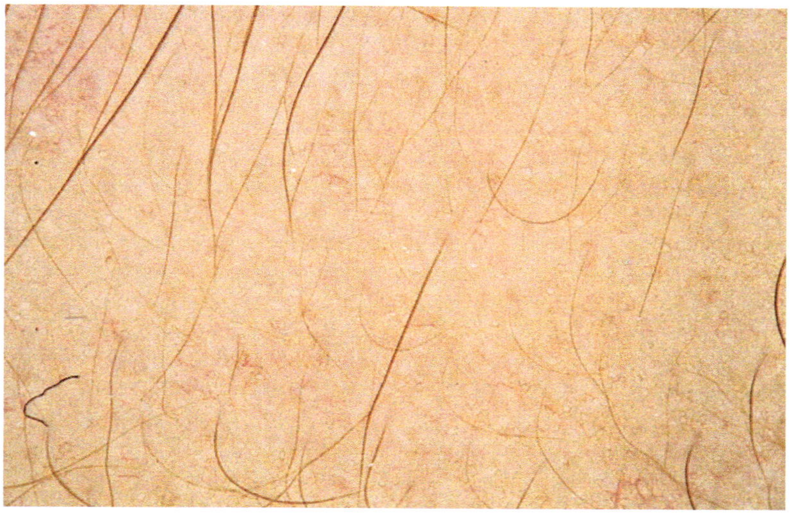

Fig. 14: Congenital triangular alopecia.

SHORT ANAGEN HAIR SYNDROME

In short anagen syndrome, children present with short, thin hair due to decreased period of the anagen phase in the hair cycle.

While the normal duration of scalp hair anagen phase is 2–6 years, in patients with short anagen syndrome, it is only 4–13 months. The anagen to telogen ratio of the hair is significantly reduced with only 20% of hairs in anagen phase compared to 90% in normal hair. This increase in telogen hair causes an abnormally short scalp hair. The growth and development of the child is otherwise normal.

Clinically, the hair is short and sparse, fine in texture, and has overall normal or reduced density. The hair does not grow and is only couple centimeters long at its maximum length.

The hair pull test is characteristic for short telogen hairs with pointed tips. On dermoscope, the short hair shaft shows normal anatomy and tapered tip showing that it was not cut.

CONGENITAL TRIANGULAR ALOPECIA

This condition is not rare and usually diagnosed in childhood. Patient complains of a triangular or oval patch of alopecia, most commonly involving the temporal region. The patch may show evident vellus hair and remains stable in time. The condition may be bilateral. The dermoscopic feature of triangular alopecia is the presence of vellus hairs. This has been described as a carpet of vellus hairs. This is highly suggestive for diagnosis and can avoid unnecessary biopsies **(Fig. 14)**.

APLASIA CUTIS CONGENITA

Aplasia cutis congenita is characterized by the absence of a skin fragment at birth. The defect can be limited to the skin or involve the skull. Most lesions occur on the scalp vertex laterally to the midline and appear as a patch of scarring alopecia. Trichoscopy shows radially arranged hair bulbs visible through the translucent atrophic epidermis, described as starburst hair follicles pattern.

SUGGESTED READING

1. Bartels NG, Blume-Peytavi U. Hair loss in children. In: Blume-Peytavi U, Tosti A, Whiting D, Trueb R (Eds). Hair Growth and Disorders. Leipzig, Germany: Springer; 2008. pp. 277-8.
2. Burk C, Hu S, Lee C, et al. Netherton syndrome and trichorrhexis invaginata: a novel diagnostic approach. Pediatr Dermatol. 2008;25(2):287-8
3. Cantatore-Francis JL, Orlow SJ. Practical guidelines for evaluation of loose anagen hair syndrome. Arch Dermatol. 2009;145:1123.
4. Cruz RD, Horev L, Green J, et al. A novel monilethrix mutation in coil 2A of KRT86 causing autosomal dominant monilethrix with incomplete penetrance. Br J Dermatol. 2012;166(Suppl 2):20.

5. Ferrando J, Mir-Bonafé JM, Cepeda-Valdés R, et al. Further insights in trichothiodystrophy: a clinical, microscopic, and ultrastructural study of 20 cases and literature review. Int J Trichology. 2012;4:158.
6. Hashimoto S, Egly JM. Trichothiodystrophy view from the molecular basis of DNA repair/transcription factor TFIIH. Hum Mol Genet. 2009;18:R224.
7. Hays SB, Camisa C. Acquired pili torti in two patients treated with synthetic retinoids. Cutis. 1985;35:466.
8. Herskovitz I, de Sousa IC, Simon J, et al. Short anagen hair syndrome. Int J Trichol. 2013;5(1):45-6.
9. Humphrey SR, Hu X, Adamson K, et al. A practical approach to the evaluation and treatment of an infant with aplasia cutis congenita. J Perinatol. 2018;38:110.
10. Lencastre A, Tosti A. Role of trichoscopy in children's scalp and hair disorders. Pediatr Dermatol. 2013;30(6):674-82.
11. Liu CI, Hsu CH. Rapid diagnosis of monilethrix using dermoscopy. Br J Dermatol. 2008;159(3):741-3.
12. Lurie R, Danziger Y, Kaplan Y, et al. Acquired pili torti: a structural hair shaft defect in anorexia nervosa. Cutis. 1996;57:151.
13. Meltem Akkurt Z, Tuncel T, Ayhan E, et al. Rapid and easy diagnosis of Netherton syndrome with dermoscopy. J Cutan Med Surg. 2014;18:280.
14. Nam CH, Park M, Choi MS, et al. Pili annulati with multiple fragile hairs. Ann Dermatol. 2017;29:254.
15. Netherton EW. A unique case of trichorrhexis nodosa; bamboo hairs. AMA Arch Derm. 1958;78:483.
16. Price VH. Treatment of hair loss. N Engl J Med. 1999;341:964.
17. Rakowska A, Maj M, Zadurska M, et al. Trichoscopy of focal alopecia in children—new trichoscopic findings: hair bulbs arranged radially along hair-bearing margins in aplasia. Skin Appendage Disord. 2016;2(1-2):1-6.
18. Rakowska A, Slowinska M, Czuwara J, et al. Dermoscopy as a tool for rapid diagnosis of monilethrix. J Drugs Dermatol. 2007;6(2):222-4.
19. Rakowska A, Slowinska M, Kowalska-Oledzka E, et al. Trichoscopy in genetic hair shaft abnormalities. J Dermatol Case Rep. 2008;2(2):14-20.
20. Robinson GC, Johnston MM. Pili torti and sensory neural hearing loss. J Pediatr. 1967;70:621.
21. Selvaag E. Pili torti and sensorineural hearing loss. A follow-up of Bjørnstad's original patients and a review of the literature. Eur J Dermatol. 2000;10:91.
22. Silengo MC, Davi GF, Bianco R, et al. Distinctive hair changes (pili torti) in Rapp-Hodgkin ectodermal dysplasia syndrome. Clin Genet. 1982;21:297.
23. Sun JD, Linden KG. Netherton syndrome: a case report and review of the literature. Int J Dermatol. 2006;45:693.
24. Tosti A, Whiting D, Iorizzo M, et al. The role of scalp dermoscopy in the diagnosis of alopecia areata incognita. J Am Acad Dermatol. 2008;59(1):64-7.
25. Van Steensel M, Vreeburg M, Urbina MT, et al. Novel KRT83 and KRT86 mutations associated with monilethrix. Exp Dermatol. 2015;24:222.
26. Verzì AE, Lacarrubba F, Micali G. Starburst hair follicles: a dermoscopic clue for aplasia cutis congenita. J Am Acad Dermatol. 2016;75(4):e141-2.
27. Yang YW, Yarbrough K, Mitkov M, et al. Polarized transilluminating dermoscopy: bedside trichoscopic diagnosis of trichothiodystrophy. Pediatr Dermatol. 2018;35:147.
28. Yin NC, Tosti A. A systematic approach to Afro-textured hair disorders: dermatoscopy and when to biopsy. Dermatol Clin. 2014;32:145.
29. Zitelli JA. Pseudomonilethrix: an artifact. Arch Dermatol. 1986;122:688-90.

CHAPTER 20

Dermoscopy of Chemotherapy Alopecia in Pediatric Age Group

Gabriella Fabbrocini, Maria Carmela Annunziata, Mariateresa Cantelli

INTRODUCTION

Chemotherapy-induced alopecia (CIA) is a frequent complication in patients with cancer, with an incidence of 65%.[1] Although the majority of CIA is reversible, the hair loss has a strong negative impact on body image and self-esteem. CIA has been studied in adult patients, but little is known about pediatric CIA.[2] In the majority of the pediatric patients, the scalp alopecia after treatment is a transient alopecia. When the hair regrew after chemotherapy was terminated, most patients experienced changes in the density, color, and texture of their hair. The reasons for such phenotypic changes are unknown.

Although the majority of CIA is reversible, pediatric case of permanent alopecia are reported.[3]

Transient alopecia generally occurs after 3–4 weeks after the first dose of chemotherapy and hair regrowth will be complete after 1–3 months from the end of the therapy.[3]

Permanent CIA is defined as absent or incomplete hair regrowth at 6 months postchemotherapy.[2]

In pediatric patient, as well as in the adult one, it is important to better identify chemotherapy alopecia's features by dermoscopy. There are no studies in literature about dermoscopic features in pediatric CIA **(Figs. 1 to 3)**.

KEY TRICHOSCOPIC FEATURES

Case 1: **Figures 4 and 5**

Case 2: **Figures 6 and 7**

Permanent CIA usually occurs after high-dose chemotherapy and subsequent hematopoietic stem cell transplantation (HSCT). Hematopoietic malignancies, which are common malignancies in children, are the main indication for HSCT.[3] Although permanent CIA is not uncommon among pediatric patients, its prevalence and features are not well-studied. To date, only two studies on permanent CIA in pediatric patients has been reported.[1-4]

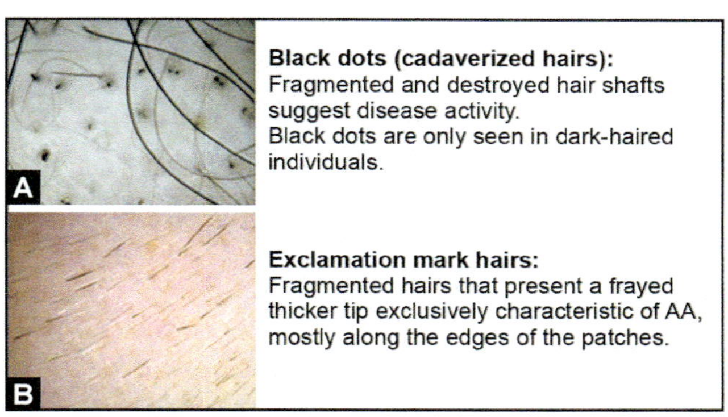

Figs. 1A and B: (A) *Black dots (cadaverized hairs)*: Fragmented and destroyed hair shafts suggest disease activity; (B) *Exclamation mark hairs*: Fractured hairs that present a frayed thicker tip exclusively characteristic of alopecia areata, mostly along the edges of the patches.

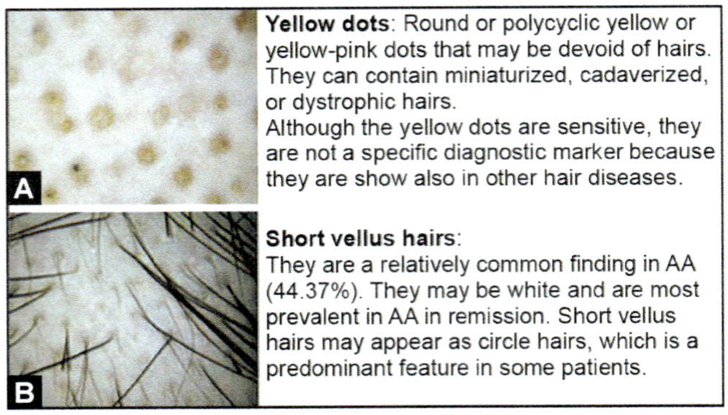

Figs. 2A and B: (A) *Yellow dots*: Round or polycyclic yellow or yellow-pink dots that may be devoid of hairs. They can contain miniaturized, cadaverized, or dystrophic hairs. Although the yellow dots are sensitive, they are not a specific diagnostic marker because they are shown also in other hair diseases; (B) *Short vellus hairs*: They are a relatively common finding in alopecia areata (AA) (44.37%). They may be white and are most prevalent in AA in remission. Short vellus hairs may appear as circle hairs, which is a predominant feature in some patients.

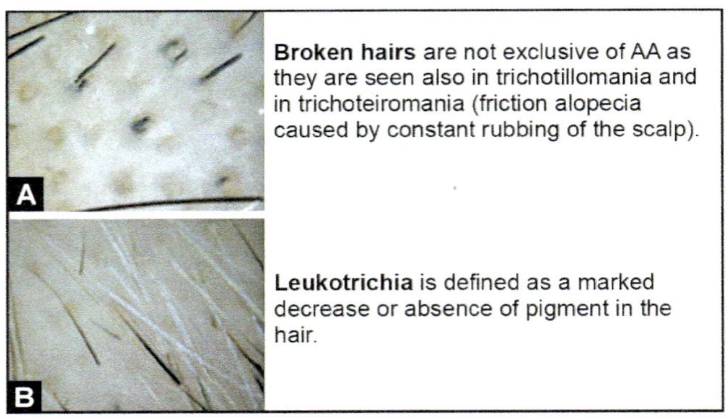

Figs. 3A and B: (A) *Broken hairs*: These are not exclusive of alopecia areata as they are seen also in trichotillomania and in trichoteiromania (friction alopecia caused by constant rubbing of the scalp); (B) *Leukotrichia*: It is defined as a marked decrease or absence of pigment in the hair.

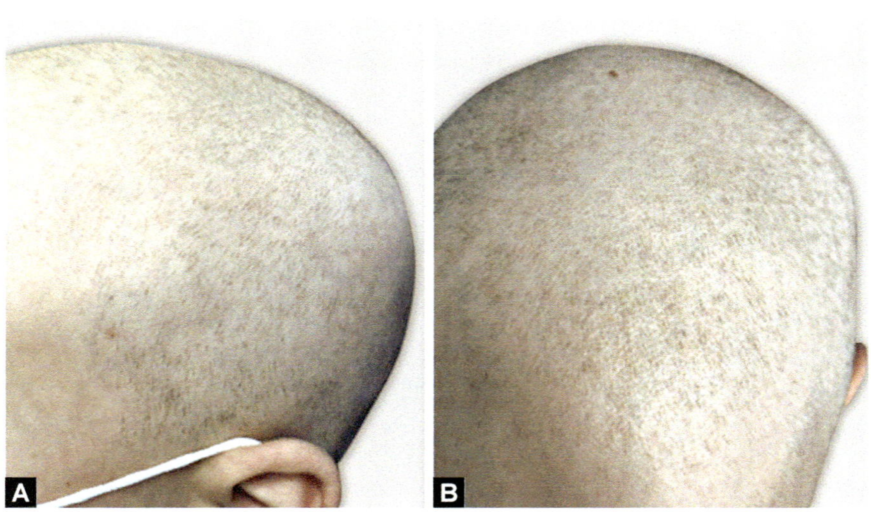

Figs. 4A and B: Male, 11-year-old, affected by leukemia in treatment with methotrexate, cyclophosphamide, and cytarabine. Presence of diffuse scalp alopecia since 1 month.
Courtesy: Department of Pediatric Hematology and Oncology; Santobono-Pausilipon Children's Hospital, Naples, Italy.

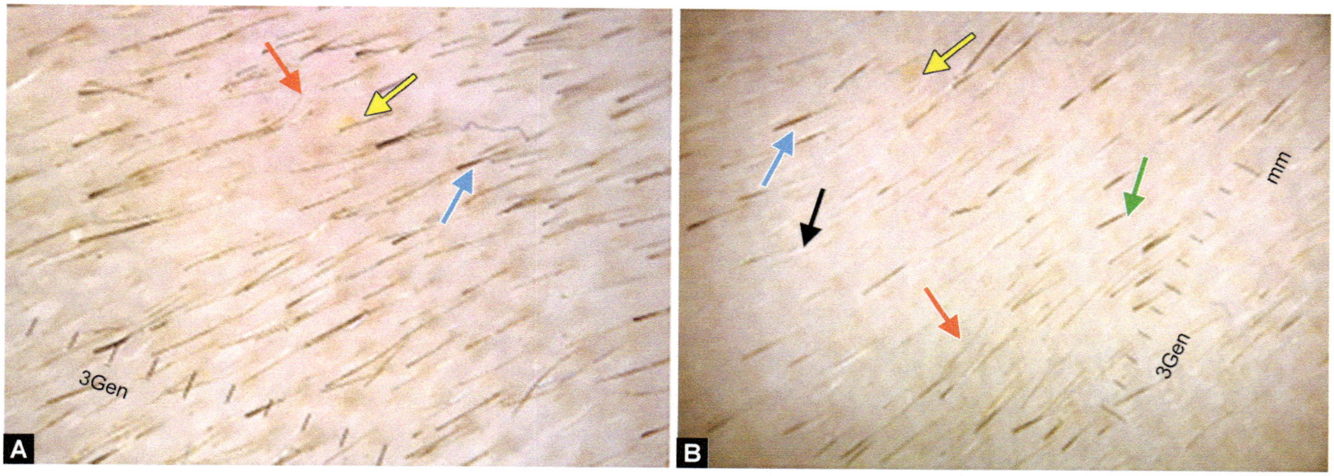

Figs. 5A and B: The dermoscopy pattern is characterized by: broken hair (green arrow), vellus hair (red arrow), yellow dots (yellow arrow), exclamation marks (blue arrow), and leukotrichia (black arrow).

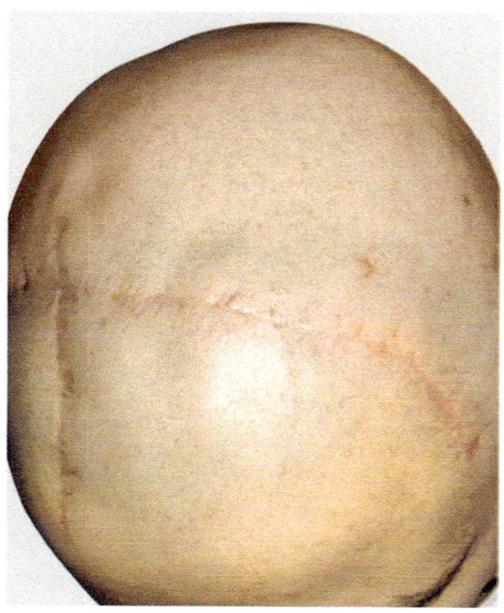

Fig. 6: Male, 15-year-old, affected medulloblastoma treated by surgical excision and treatment with etoposide, ifosfamide, and platinum derivatives. Presence of diffuse scalp alopecia since 2 months.
Courtesy: Department of Pediatric Hematology and Oncology; Santobono-Pausilipon Children's Hospital, Naples, Italy.

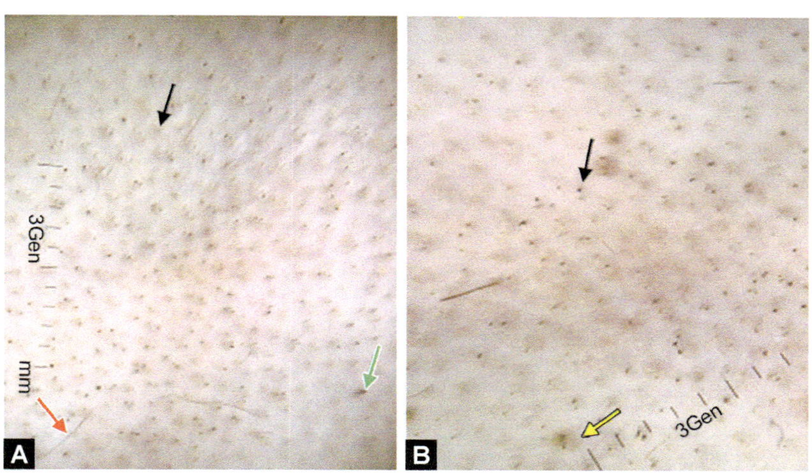

Figs. 7A and B: The dermoscopy pattern is characterized by: broken hair (green arrow), vellus hair (red arrow), yellow dots (yellow arrow), and numerous black dots (black arrows).

THE OLSEN CIA SCALE

The Olsen CIA scale was used to evaluate the CIA severity in oncological patients.

Briefly, this uses a five-grade scale:[5]

- Minimal = Grade 1 (1–24% loss, compared with the pretreatment state)
- Moderate = Grade 2 (25–49% loss), or grade 3 (50–74% loss)
- Extensive = Grade 4 (75–99% loss)
- Complete = Grade 5 (100% loss).

Permanent CIA is common after high-dose conditioning chemotherapy for bone marrow transplantation.[6]

Case 3: **Figures 8 and 9**

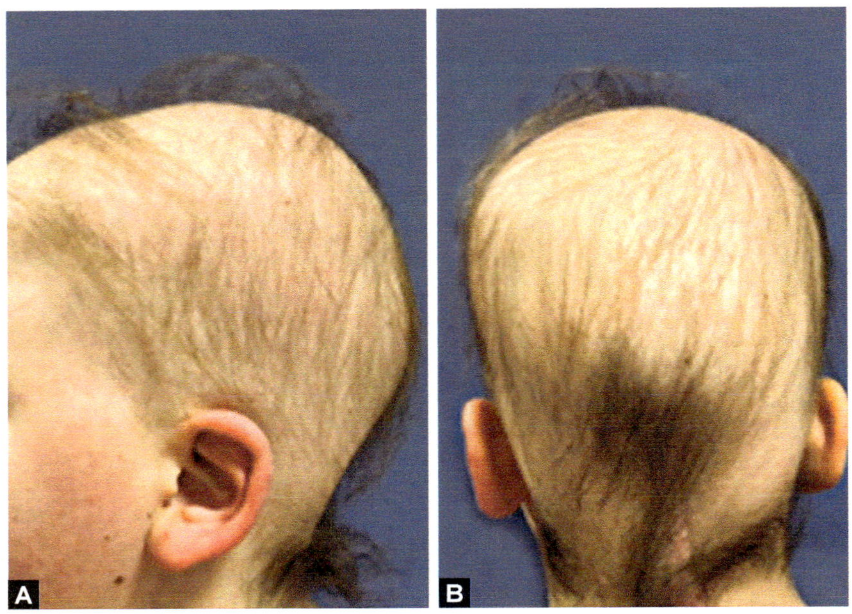

Figs. 8A and B: Female, 10-year-old, affected by medulloblastoma and treated by surgery, etoposide, platinum derivatives, and radiotherapy. *Courtesy*: Department of Pediatric Hematology and Oncology; Santobono-Pausilipon Children's Hospital, Naples, Italy.

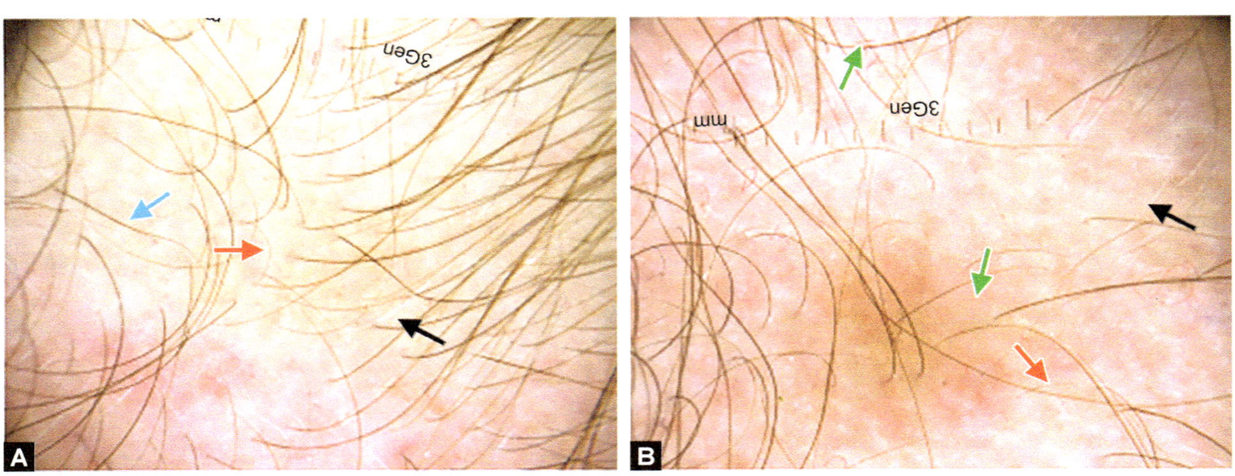

Figs. 9A and B: The dermoscopy pattern is characterized by: broken hair (green arrows), vellus hair (red arrow), exclamation marks (blue arrow), and leukotrichia (black arrows).

REFERENCES

1. Cash TF. The psychology of hair loss and its implications for patient care. Clin Dermatol. 2001;19:161-6.
2. Choi M, Kim MS, Park SY, et al. Clinical characteristics of chemotherapy induced alopecia in childhood (Mira Choi). 2014;70(3): 499-505.
3. Gratwohl A, Baldomero H, Aljurf M, et al. Hematopoietic stem cell transplantation: a global perspective. JAMA. 2010;303:1617-24.
4. Vowels M. Factors affecting hair regrowth after bone marrow transplantation. 1993;12(4):347-50.
5. Olsen EA. Chemotherapy-induced alopecia: overview and methodology for characterizing hair changes and regrowth. In: Oliver IN, Multinational Association of Supportive Care in Cancer (Eds). The MASCC Textbook of Cancer Supportive Care and Survivorship. New York: Springer; 2011. pp. 381-8.
6. Baker BW, Wilson CL, Davis AL, et al. Busulphan/cyclophosphamide conditioning for bone marrow transplantation may lead to failure of hair regrowth. Bone Marrow Transplant. 1991;7:43-7.

SECTION 4

Onychoscopy

CHAPTER

- Dermoscopy of Pediatric Nail Diseases: Pediatric Onychoscopy

CHAPTER 21

Dermoscopy of Pediatric Nail Diseases: Pediatric Onychoscopy

Chander Grover, Deepak Jakhar

INTRODUCTION

Nail disorders presenting in pediatric age group can be challenging to diagnose. This is largely because of the small size of children's nail. An altered appearance of nails in children may have a profound psychosocial impact due to ridicule from the peer group. Additionally, the use of standard diagnostic techniques like nail clipping or nail biopsy may not be acceptable to the patient or even the parents. Hence, dermoscopy of nail (onychoscopy) assumes an important role in aiding nail diagnoses in the pediatric age group. This chapter describes and demonstrates the dermoscopic features of various physiological and pathological conditions affecting nails in children.

A number of afflictions of the pediatric nail are known. Many of these are benign, physiological alterations, which nevertheless arouse anxiety in parents. Knowledge of onychoscopic features can thus help the dermatologist allay their anxiety and reassure them without resorting to any more invasive modalities.

At the same time, there are some pathological nail changes which tend to present and behave differently as compared to adults. A knowledge and familiarity with the onychoscopic features for these is thus a helpful skill for the dermatologist dealing with them. Salient pediatric nail afflictions according to the age groups in which they present are discussed below.

PEDIATRIC LONGITUDINAL MELANONYCHIA

Introduction

Longitudinal melanonychia refers to the presence of a pigmented longitudinal streak along the nail plate. It results from an increased melanin production and deposition within the nail plate. The prevalence is much higher in children with pigmented skin.

Longitudinal pigmented bands can be a cause for concern in the pediatric age group. A thick brown-black pigmented band arising from proximal and extending to the distal nail plate may be seen uncommonly, but causes deep parental anxiety. It is commonly the result of a benign melanocyte hyperplasia (nevus or lentigo in three-fourth cases) or benign melanocyte activation (one-fourth cases). Nail melanoma is extremely rare in this age group; nevertheless, it needs to be assessed reliably to offer sound advice.

It is popular perception that a nail matrix biopsy should be avoided as far as possible, so as to prevent permanent nail dystrophy. Unless specifically indicated, like in cases with increasing width, progressive darkening, pigment variegation, periungual pigmentation or nail plate changes, a histopathologic examination is generally avoided. Even though risk for melanoma is low in pediatric age group, lesions should be closely monitored for these changes. A prolonged follow-up, even up to adulthood may be required, as melanoma of the nail apparatus in adults with a history of longitudinal melanonychia beginning in childhood has been reported.

Key Dermoscopic Features

Melanonychia has been extensively studied by onychoscopy. The International Study Group on Melanonychia published evidence-based guidelines (2013) on its use in detection and management of nail pigmentation. The group suggested the use of the same dermoscopy instrument during follow-up of the patients. The best immersion fluid suggested was ultrasound gel.

The suggested step-wise algorithm first involves distinguishing the nature of the pigment, whether it is blood or melanin. Subungual hemorrhage is suggested by the presence of globules, with or without distal streaks. There could be a range of colors varying from red to brown to black.

If the pigment appears to be melanin, then the cause could be either *melanocyte activation or melanocyte proliferation.* Both can be discerned to a large extent on onychoscopy.

- *Benign melanonychia* due to melanocyte activation (ethnic or drug-induced) appears as homogeneous gray bands with thin, longitudinal gray lines. The color can however vary depending on the pigment location and nail plate thickness.
- *Benign melanocyte proliferation* is suggested by a brown background, associated with regular parallel lines of identical color, spacing, and width. The underlying cause in such a case is usually a nevus or a lentigo. However, this regularity may be disrupted in children. For example, it is possible to see converging dark bands in children, which are otherwise benign in origin. Hence, this simple flowchart may not be applicable to pediatric nails.
- *Malignant melanoma* is suggested by a brown background with irregular lines; the irregularity being in terms of color, width, spacing, or parallelism. Individual lines tend to show irregular color or width along their length. A dark background with different hues of pigmentation is suggestive of a melanoma even in the absence of irregular lines.

Onychoscopic examination of the nail plate is not enough. For a holistic evaluation, an examination of the *distal edge* should always be done as it suggests the possible locus of origin in the matrix. If the band is located more dorsally, it probably originates from proximal nail matrix, whereas a ventrally placed band originates from distal matrix. However, this may not be a reliable marker in very thin nail plates or with very dark or very light pigment bands.

Onychoscopy should also focus on the *proximal nail fold and hyponychium* to assess for any spread of pigment (Hutchinson's or micro-Hutchinson's sign). *Hutchinson's sign* refers to an extension of brown-black pigment onto the cuticle or the nail folds, suggesting a subungual melanoma. If such a spread is not visible to naked eye but picked up only on magnification, it is called *micro-Hutchinson sign*. On the other hand, *pseudo-Hutchinson sign* refers to a homogeneous linear pigmentation visible through the translucent cuticle and proximal nail fold. This is common in children due to the thin nail folds and should be carefully distinguished to avoid unnecessary apprehension.

Case Details

Case 1: A 12-year-old male child presented with discoloration and darkening of the right index nail of recent onset. Melanonychia involved the proximal nail bed as well as the proximal nail fold as visible to naked eye. Onychoscopy showed a proximal blackish discoloration with variegation of color suggestive of a subungual hematoma. Magnified examination showed the presence of globular structures and streaks suggestive of blood, confirming the diagnosis of a subungual hematoma **(Figs. 1A to C)**.

Case 2: A 5-year-old male child presented with noticeable darkening of little fingernail noticed since 4–5 months. The parents were very apprehensive about the thick bands. Onychoscopy showed a black band with slight lightening at the edges. No distinct lines were identified, and there was no distortion of regularity. Examination of proximal nail fold showed that the pigment was visible through the cuticle only *(pseudo-Hutchinson sign)*, with no involvement of skin **(Figs. 2A and B)**.

Case 3: Another 5-year-old child presented with recent onset, black band for a few months. Onychoscopy showed a variegated coloration, with slight irregularity. The examination of distal edge showed the band to be darker on the ventral aspect of the nail plate. This suggested that the origin could be in more distal matrix. Examination of proximal nail fold showed that the pigment was visible through the cuticle as well as through skin. This is possible in young children at times, due to a very thin skin. However, a nail matrix biopsy was done for confirmation, and it revealed a benign nail matrix nevus **(Figs. 3A to C)**.

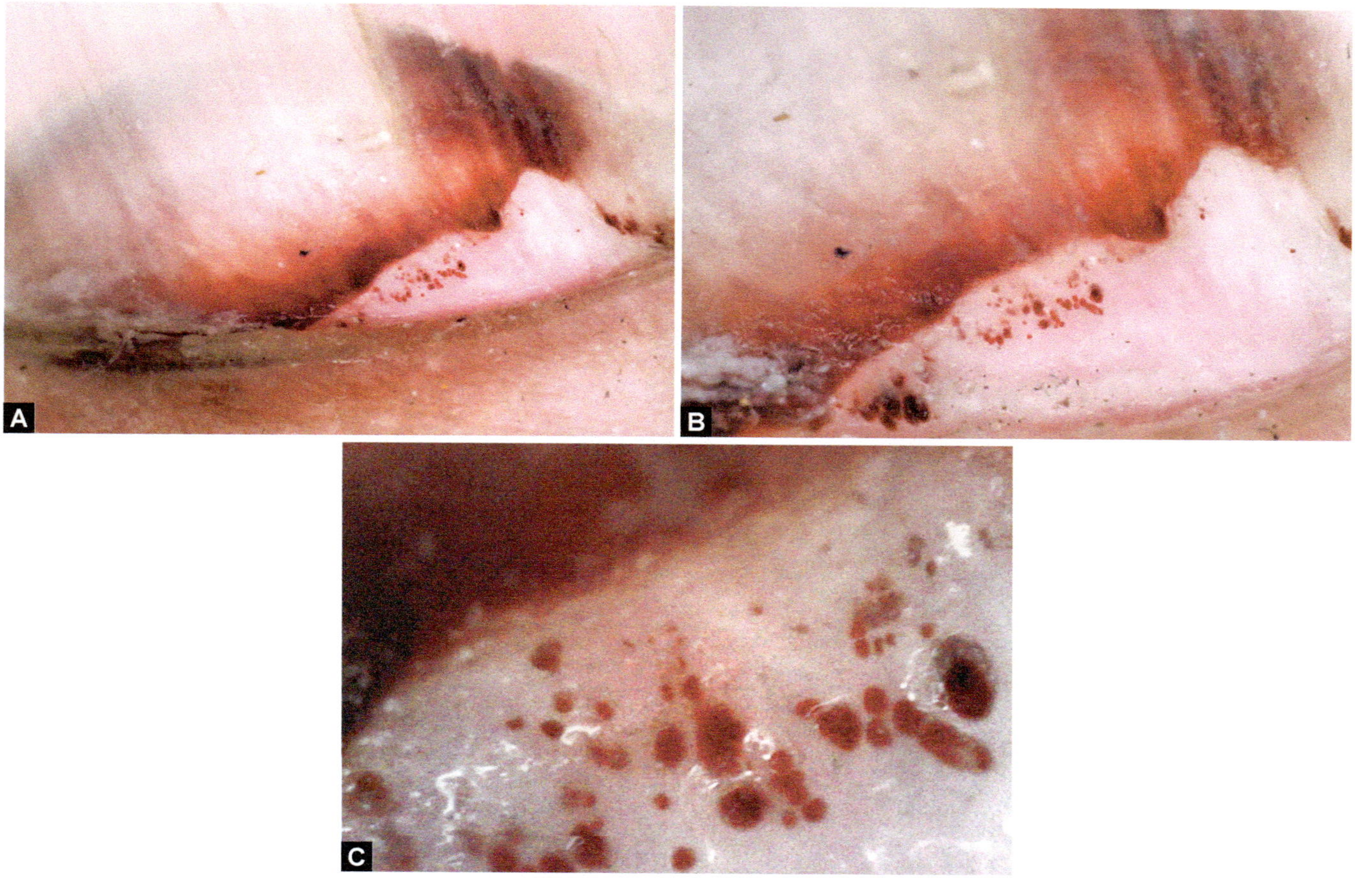

Figs. 1A to C: (A) Onychoscopic examination of the proximal nail plate of a suspicious discoloration in a young child. Note the variegation of color and globule like pigment (Dinolite AM7115MZT polarized view with linkage fluid, 20×); (B) On higher magnification, there are smaller globules recognized at the proximal end (Dinolite AM7115MZT polarized view with linkage fluid, 50×); (C) Still higher magnification shows this discoloration to be organized as globules and streaks suggestive of subungual hematoma. (Dinolite AM7115MZT polarized view with linkage fluid, 100×).

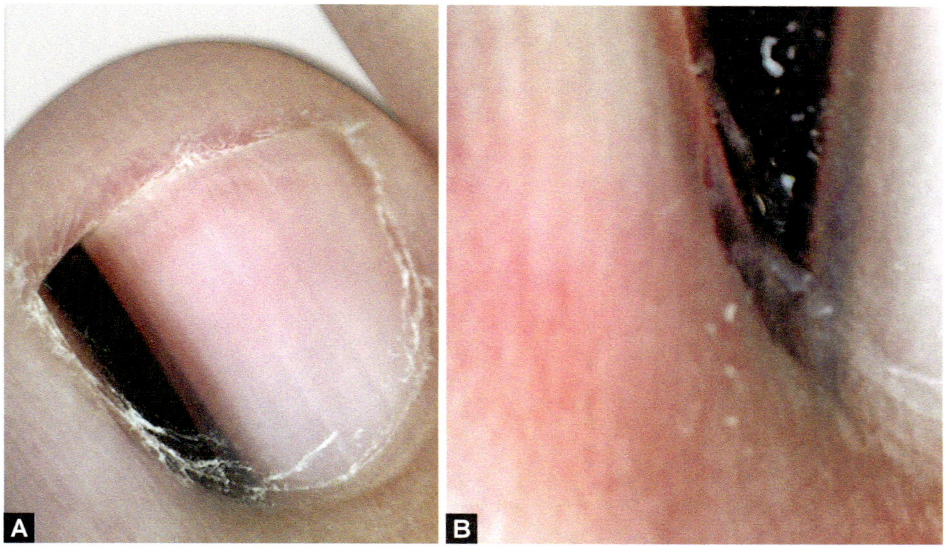

Figs. 2A and B: (A) Uniform, thick dark band, place laterally, fading medially (Dinolite AM7115MZT polarized view with linkage fluid, 10×); (B) Pseudo-Hutchinson sign (Dinolite AM7115MZT polarized view with linkage fluid, 50×).

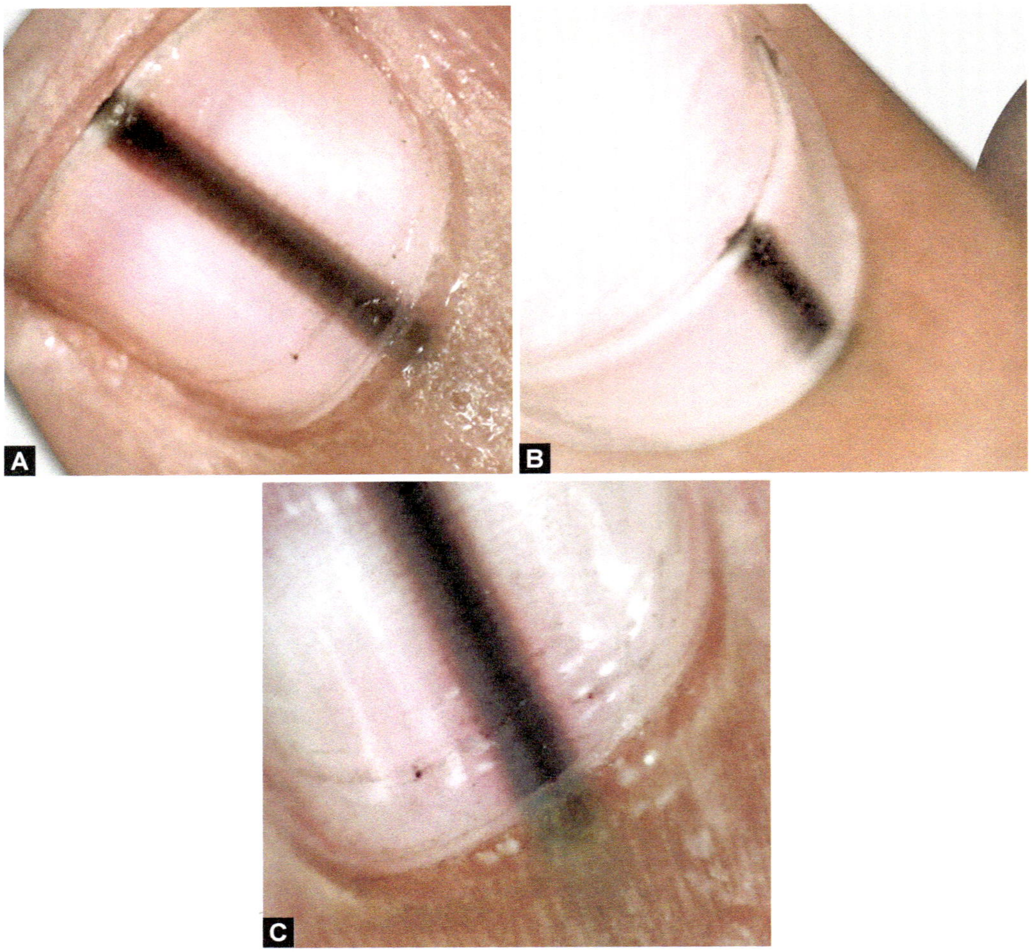

Figs. 3A to C: (A) Dark band with peripheral fading and mild tapering toward the center. (Dinolite AM7115MZT polarized view with linkage fluid, 20×); (B) Distal edge shows the pigmentation to be predominant in the ventral part of the nail plate. (Dinolite AM7115MZT polarized view with linkage fluid, 20×); (C) The band is visible through the cuticle as well as the thin skin of the child. But there is no lateral spread of pigment (Dinolite AM7115MZT polarized view with linkage fluid, 50×).

Suggested Reading

1. Burleigh A, Lam JM. Pediatric longitudinal melanonychia. CMAJ. 2017;189(34):E1093.
2. Goettmann-Bonvallot S, André J, Belaich S. Longitudinal melanonychia in children: a clinical and histopathologic study of 40 cases. J Am Acad Dermatol. 1999;41(1):17-22.

LEUKONYCHIA

Introduction

It is a commonly seen physiological alteration, which could present in various patterns including punctate or transverse leukonychia. It is common in toddlers as they frequently play using their hands, causing microtrauma to the matrix. This can affect both fingernails and toenails.

Key Dermoscopic Features

Leukonychia appears as white cloud-like structures. Onychoscopy can be especially useful in differentiating true leukonychia from apparent leukonychia. *True leukonychia* has well-defined borders, and arises within the nail plate structure due to defective keratinization. The borders are indistinct in *apparent leukonychia*, as it arises because of discoloration in nail bed. Additionally, pressure can induced blanching in apparent leukonychia, making it further indistinct, whereas true leukonychia persists as it is. *Pseudoleukonychia* has an external origin; hence, the changes will be seen "on" the surface of the nail plate.

Case Details

A 4-year-old child brought with white spots in nails. The mother was very worried regarding possible nutritional deficiencies. Onychoscopic examination was done and multiple punctate, well-defined spots were identified in nails. The spots were serially arranged and had distinct margins. The mother was reassured that they will grow out serially and are a result of minor daily traumas **(Figs. 4A to C)**.

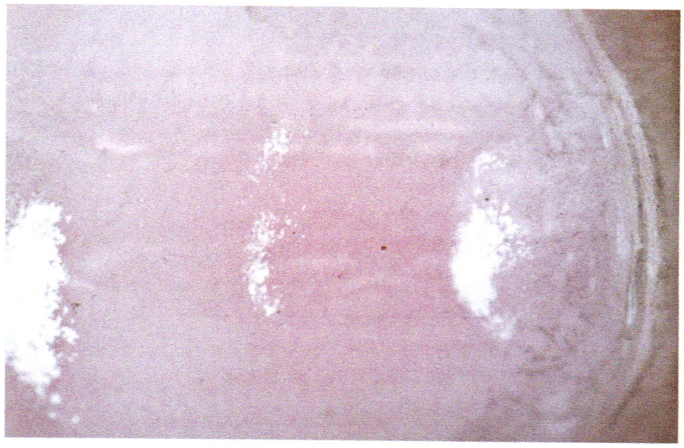

Fig. 4A: Well-defined spots of leukonychia, involving the nail plate in a young child. The spots are clearly present within the nail plate structure. The nail plate surface is smooth and shiny. (Dinolite AM7115MZT polarized view with linkage fluid, 50×).

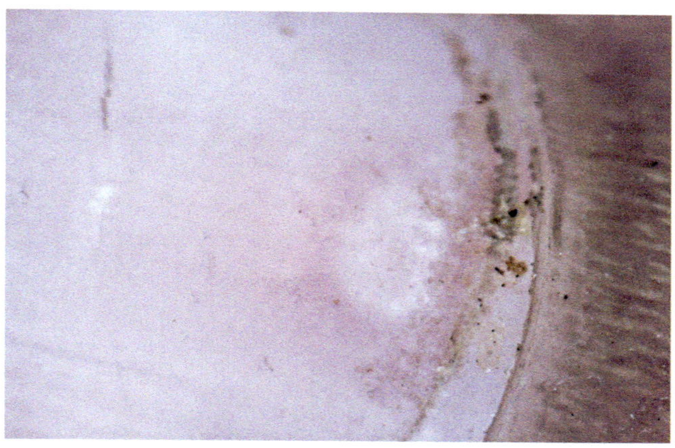

Fig. 4B: Leukonychia with more indistinct margins as seen in an older child. (Dinolite AM7115MZT polarized view with linkage fluid, 50×).

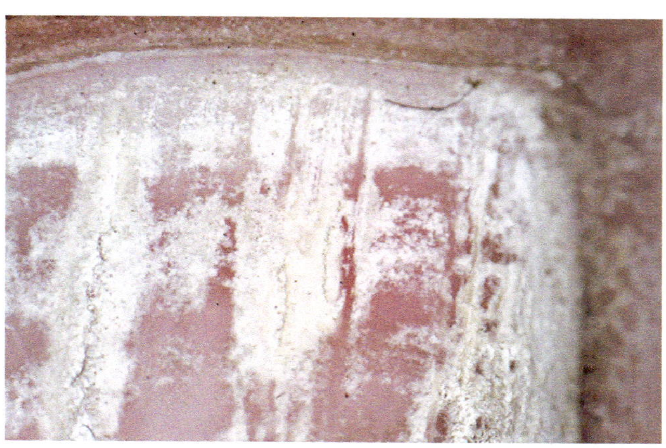

Fig. 4C: Pseudoleukonychia due to superficial white onychomycosis. It shows a rough nail plate surface. (Dinolite AM7115MZT polarized view with linkage fluid, 100×).

Suggested Reading

1. Alessandrini A, Starace M, Piraccini BM. Dermoscopy in the evaluation of nail disorders. Skin Appendage Disord. 2017;3(2):70-82.
2. Bel B, Jeudy G, Vabres P. Dermoscopy of longitudinal leukonychia in Hailey-Hailey disease. Arch Dermatol. 2010;146(10):1204.

CHEVRON (HERRINGBONE NAILS)

Introduction

It is a physiological alteration, commonly presenting at 5–7 years of age. The nail plate may show oblique, longitudinal ridges converging distally and medially to form a "V" shape. The etiopathogenesis is undetermined and the condition tends to resolve in early adulthood. Superficial longitudinal ridges in *herringbone pattern* may persist in infancy and normalize gradually. It reflects as a gradual change in the maturation of the matrix.

Key Dermoscopic Features

Chevron nail is better appreciated on nonpolarizing onychoscopy. It appears as oblique, longitudinal ridges converging at the distal end of nail plate. Superficial longitudinal ridges in *herringbone pattern* may persist in infancy and normalize gradually.

Case Details

The parents of a 3-year-old child brought in their child for "rough" nail plate surface. Onychoscopy revealed longitudinal ridges converging toward the distal end **(Fig. 5)**.

Suggested Reading

1. Starace M, Alessandrini A, Piraccini BM. Nail disorders in children. Skin Appendage Disord. 2018;4:217-29.

PACHYONYCHIA CONGENITA

Introduction

It is a genodermatosis presenting with a distal prominent thickening of nails and hypercurvature (due to prominent nail bed hyperkeratosis). Other clinical features include painful palmoplantar blisters, cysts, follicular hyperkeratosis, and oral leukokeratosis. It is an autosomal dominant condition with variable penetrance and expressivity. The nails are generally normal at birth, but within a few weeks, the classical changes begin to develop in the form of smooth but hard nail plate with massive subungual hyperkeratosis.

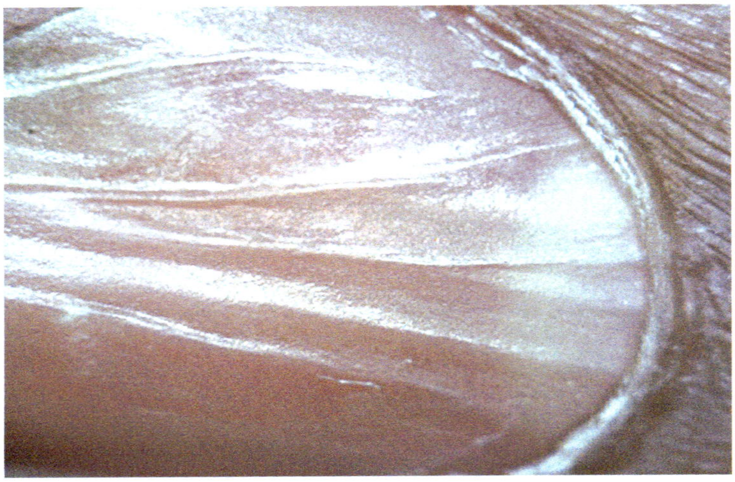

Fig. 5: Herringbone pattern appearing as oblique, longitudinal ridges converging at the distal end of nail plate. (Dinolite AM7115MZT nonpolarized view with linkage fluid, 20×).

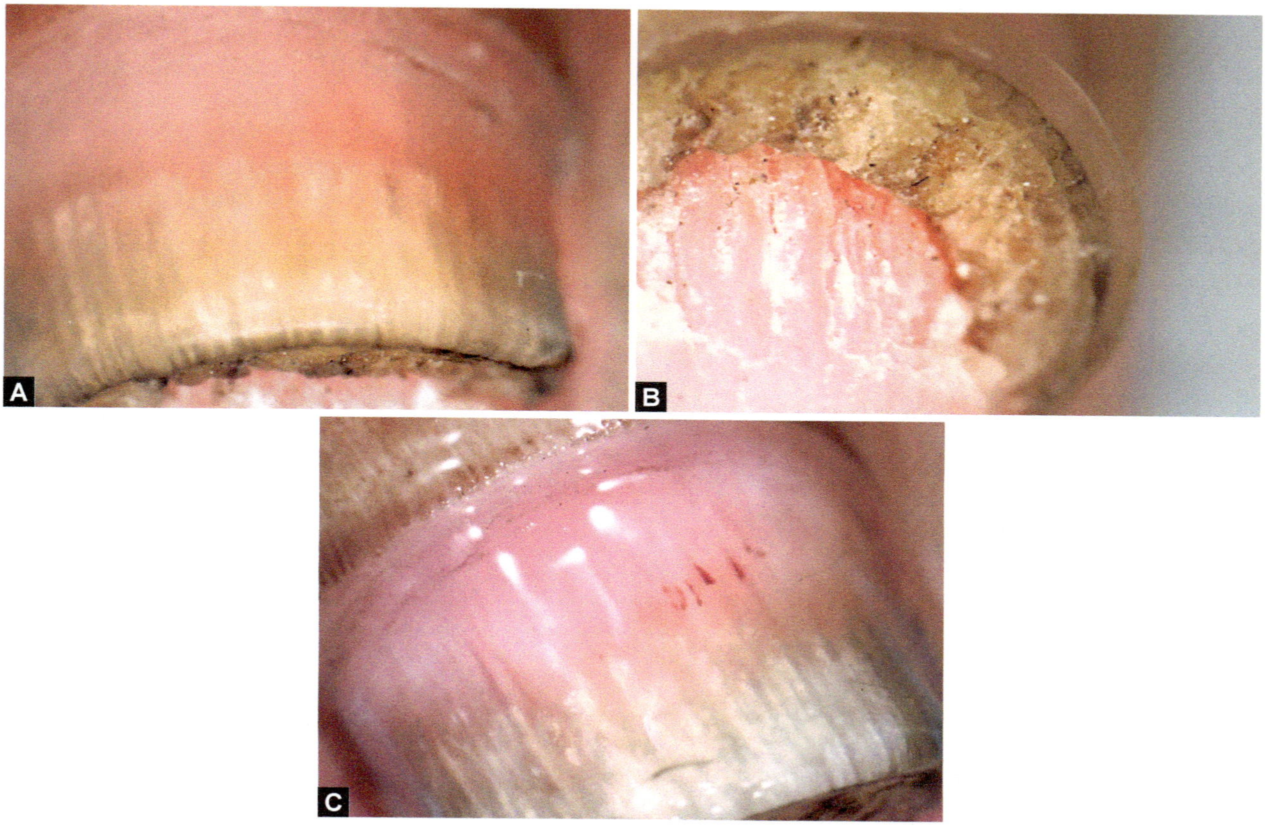

Figs. 6A to C: (A) Thickening and yellowish discoloration of the distal nail plate structure. (Dinolite AM7115MZT polarized view with linkage fluid, 20×); (B) Distal view shows thick subungual hyperkeratosis which is very compact. (Dinolite AM7115MZT polarized view with linkage fluid, 20×); (C) Dorsal view of another nail in the same patient shows splinter hemorrhages. (Dinolite AM7115MZT polarized view with linkage fluid, 20×).

Key Dermoscopic Features

It is characterized by massively thickened nails, which may or may not be discolored. In addition there is substantial subungual hyperkeratosis, which is quite compact as compared to the "ruin appearance" seen in onychomycosis. Also, there may be occasional presence of splinter hemorrhages or hematomas, primarily because of the functional disability such patients face.

Case Details

A 13-year-old girl presented with progressive thickening and lifting up of the distal nail plates. She was conscious of her discolored nails as well as complained of difficulty in writing as well as cutting her own nails. The changes had been slowly progressing for the past many years. The child had received oral antifungal therapy for the previous 2 years; however, there had been no improvement **(Figs. 6A to C)**.

Suggested Reading

1. Alessandrini A, Starace M, Piraccini BM. Dermoscopy in the evaluation of nail disorders. Skin Appendage Disord. 2017;3(2):70-82.

ANONYCHIA

Introduction

Anonychia can be a partial or complete loss of the nail plate. It can present as an isolated abnormality or maybe associated with complex syndromes like epidermal dysplasia, nail patella syndrome, etc.

Key Dermoscopic Features

Clinical distinction between partial or complete anonychia is sometimes difficult. Onychoscopy can be a useful tool to differentiate between partial or complete anonychia. A partial anonychia will show a dull refractile nail plate remnant. At times, the pseudohyperkeratotic nail plate remnant may be clinically mistaken for a crumbling nail plate. Polarizing onychoscopic examination with linkage fluid can differentiate a pseudohyperkeratotic nail bed from nail plate. Dermoscopy can be thus be used as a tool to prognosticate the parents regarding the future possibilities of nail plate formation.

Case Details (Figs. 7A to C)

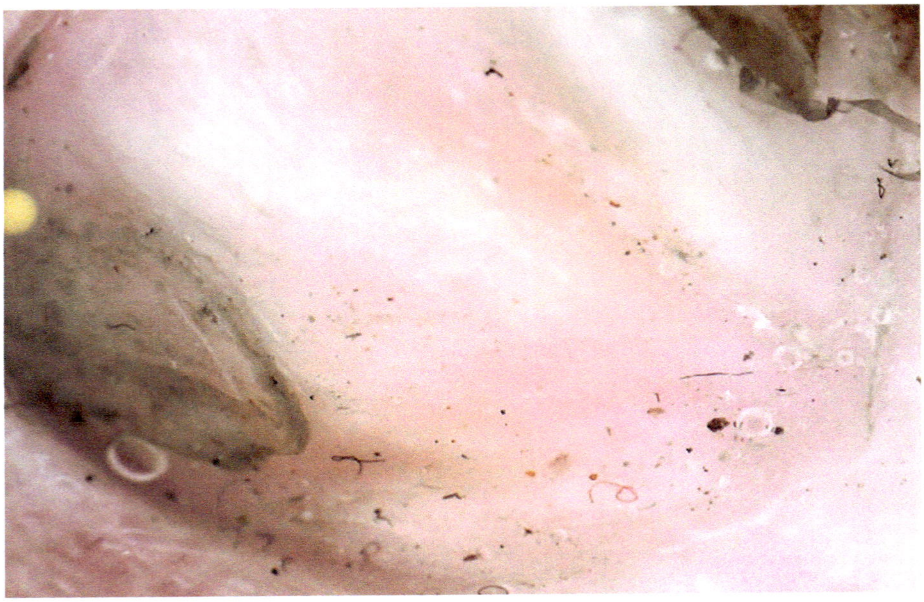

Fig. 7A: A patient with loss of nails (anonychia) post severe drug reaction (toxic epidermal necrolysis). The onychoscopic examination shows small remnants of nail plate in the lateral sulci. (Dinolite AM7115MZT polarized view with linkage fluid, 20×).

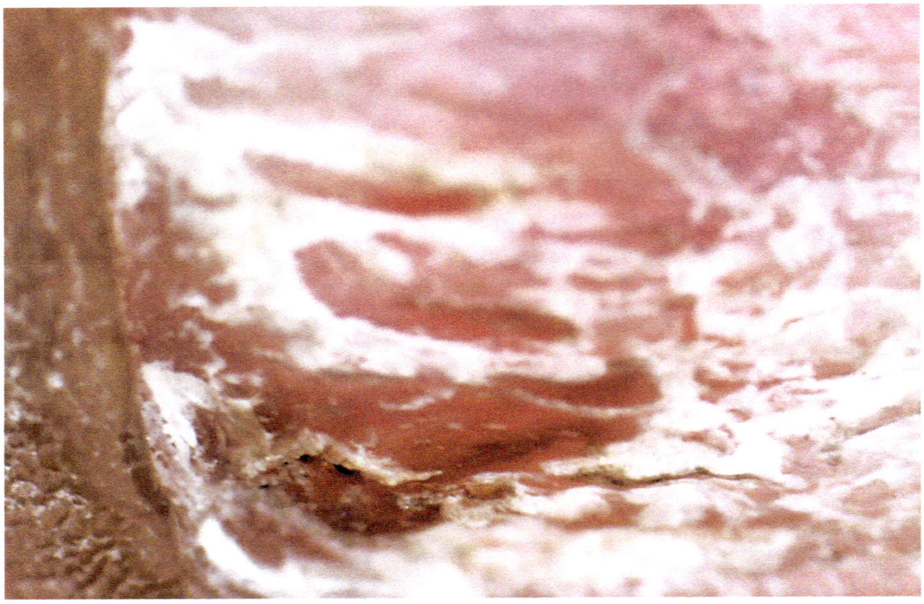

Fig. 7B: Thickening and hyperkeratosis of the nail plate with a crumbled appearance in a 14-year-old male with psoriatic erythroderma. (Dinolite AM7115MZT polarized view without linkage fluid, 20×).

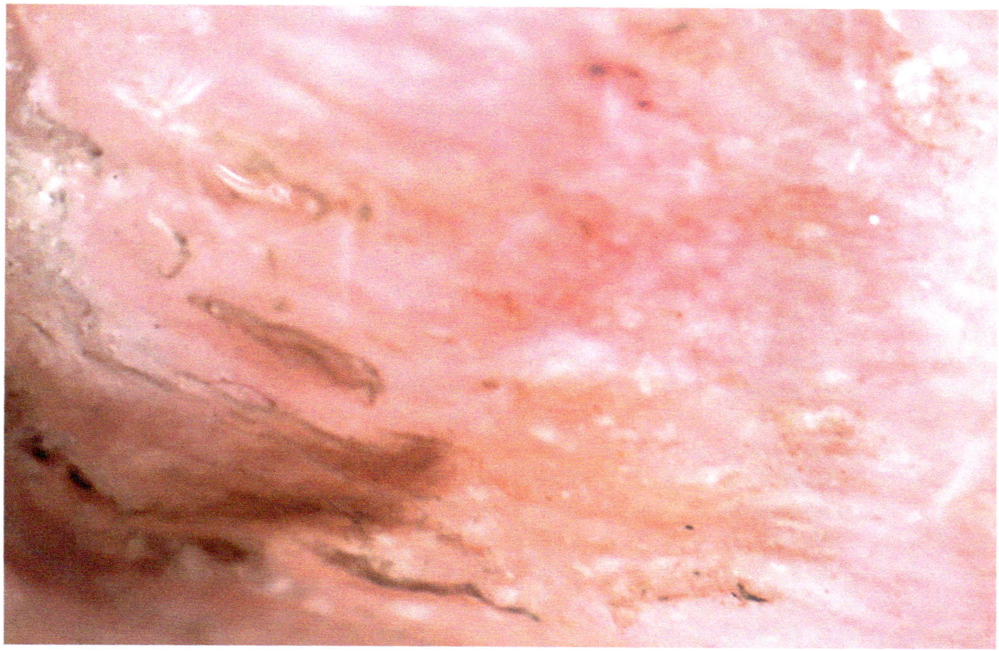

Fig. 7C: The same view, taken again after using linkage fluid, shows a total absence of nail plate structure (anonychia). An exposed nail bed undergoes squamous epidermalization to produce a pseudohyperkeratosis or pseudo-nail plate. (Dinolite AM7115MZT polarized view with linkage fluid, 20×).

Suggested Reading

1. Starace M, Alessandrini A, Piraccini BM. Nail disorders in children. Skin Appendage Disord. 2018;4:217-29.

INFECTIONS

Infections affecting the nail unit are mostly associated with a habit of finger sucking or nail biting, both of which are common in children. Commonly seen infections include bacterial, viral, or fungal infections. These include *blistering distal dactylitis* (localized infection of the volar fat-pad of distal phalanx, caused by hemolytic *Streptococcus or Staphylococcus aureus); Acute paronychia or chronic paronychia* (often a result of finger sucking or chronic manipulation); and herpetic *whitlow* (herpes virus infection), etc. Nail biting also increases the susceptibility to develop ungual warts, which start as small firm, keratotic, papules on nail fold progressing to involve more areas.

ONYCHOMYCOSIS

Introduction

It is rare before 6 years of age, though candidal infection can rarely present as onychomycosis in premature or immunodeficient children. In children, a possibility of chronic mucocutaneous candidiasis should be ruled out. Dermoscopic features of onychomycosis are similar to those seen in adults.

Key Dermoscopic Features

Onychoscopy shows onycholysis with jagged edges, spikes within the onycholytic area, longitudinal striations, and aurora borealis pattern (longitudinal striations of varying colors). The subungual hyperkeratosis and "ruin pattern" (distal to proximal longitudinal spikes in subungual keratosis) are the other features seen. Fungal melanonychia is characterized by brown to black longitudinal or transverse bands with pigmented globules or clumps. Dermatophytoma appears as round, yellow to orange color patches within the nail plate, connected to the distal nail plate by narrow channels. Onychoscopic features of onychomycosis are typical. These help differentiate onychomycosis from common differentials like psoriasis and traumatic onycholysis.

Case Details

A 7-year-old child presented with thickened and dystrophied nail plate of finger and toe nails since 6 months. There was history of multiple courses of oral and topical antifungal medications in the past. The child was a known case of nephrotic syndrome **(Figs. 8A to F)**.

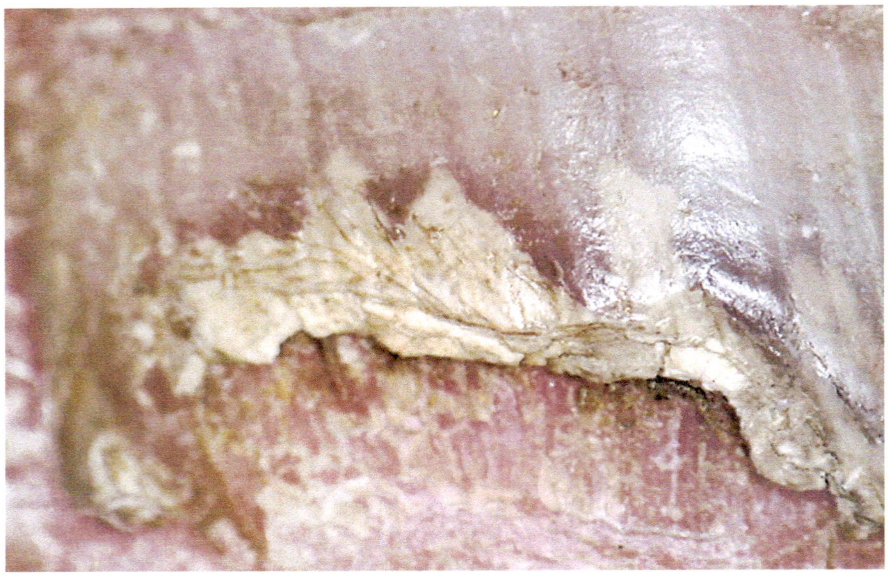

Fig. 8A: The proximal border of onycholysis in this young child was seen to be jagged with multiple spikes. (Dinolite AM7115MZT nonpolarized view without linkage fluid, 20×).

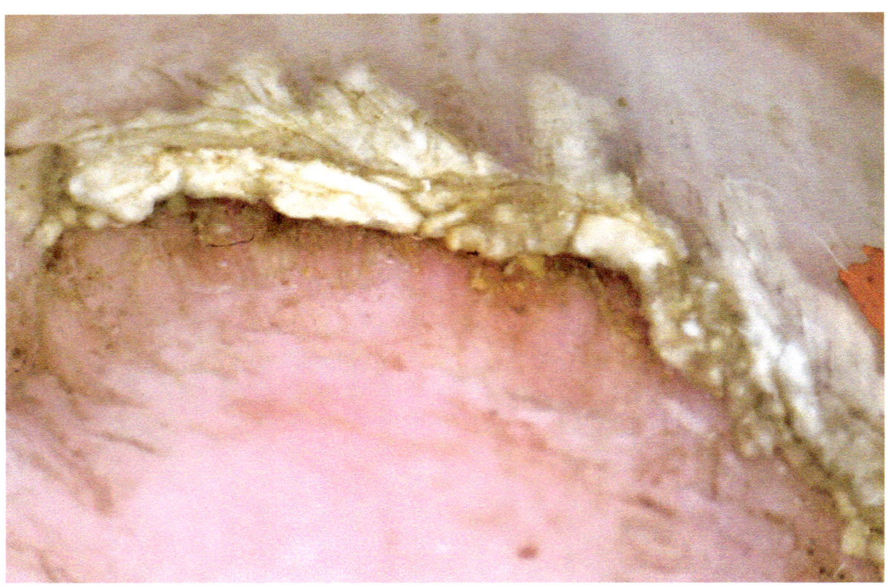

Fig. 8B: The same nail when examined distally showed a "loose" subungual hyperkeratosis with sparse debris. This is known as a subungual "ruin" appearance. (Dinolite AM7115MZT nonpolarized view without linkage fluid, 20×).

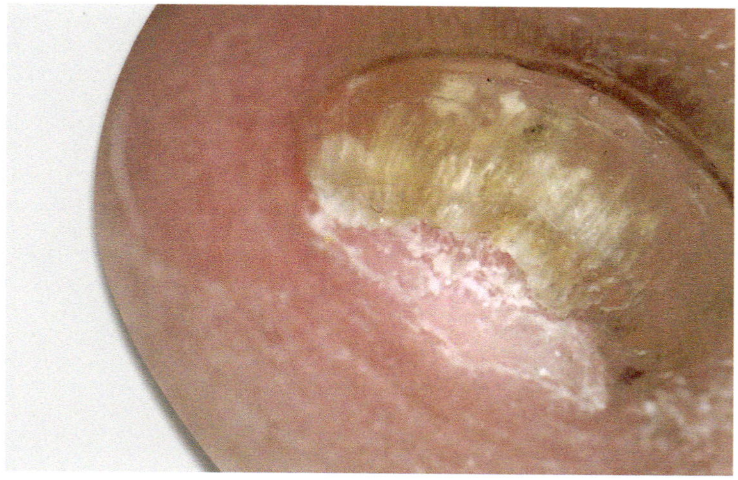

Fig. 8C: Another child with a similar distal lateral subungual onychomycosis, with involvement of almost the total nail. (Dinolite AM7115MZT polarized view without linkage fluid, 20×).

Fig. 8D: Color changes seen in cases with onychomycosis, varying from green, yellow to brown. This is known as "Aurora borealis" pattern. (Dinolite AM7115MZT polarized view with linkage fluid, 50×).

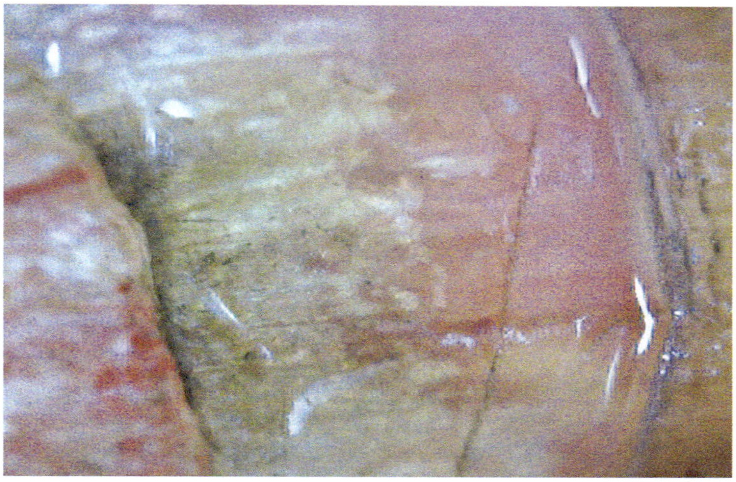

Fig. 8E: Striations seen within the area of onycholysis. It is a characteristic feature of onychomycosis. (Dinolite AM7115MZT polarized view with linkage fluid, 50×).

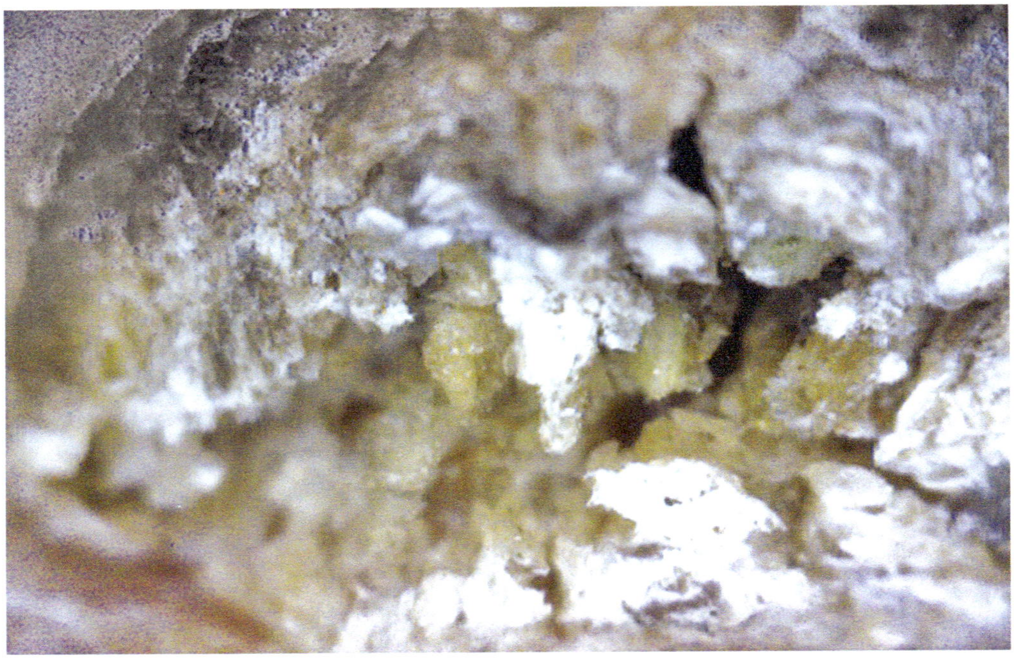

Fig. 8F: Another case with subungual debris. The "ruin pattern" is seen. (Dinolite AM7115MZT polarized view with linkage fluid, 50×).

Suggested Reading

1. Grover C, Jakhar D. Diagnostic utility of onychoscopy: Review of literature. Indian J Dermatopathol Diagn Dermatol. 2017;4:31-40.
2. Grover C, Jakhar D. Onychoscopy: A practical guide. Indian J Dermatol Venereol Leprol. 2017; 83:536-49.

PERIUNGUAL WARTS

Introduction

Periungual warts are facilitated by the common habit of nail biting in children. They are usually present on the nail folds and can sometimes become subungual causing onycholysis.

Key Dermoscopic Features

Onychoscopy of a wart shows a whitish homogeneous, hyperkeratotic mass with red dots, indicative of thrombosed blood vessels. As dermoscopic features of warts are quite distinctive, it facilitates an early recognition of suspicious small lesions in the subungual or periungual location. This is essential to halt the progression and spread of wart. The detection of subungual spread of wart is an added advantage of onychoscopy.

Case Details

A 5-year-old girl presented with an asymptomatic hyperkeratotic mass near the hyponychium. Similar lesions were also present in the mother's thumb nail **(Figs. 9A and B)**.

Suggested Reading

1. Grover C, Jakhar D. Diagnostic utility of onychoscopy: Review of literature. Indian J Dermatopathol Diagn Dermatol. 2017;4:31-40.
2. Grover C, Jakhar D. Onychoscopy: A practical guide. Indian J Dermatol Venereol Leprol. 2017; 83:536-49.

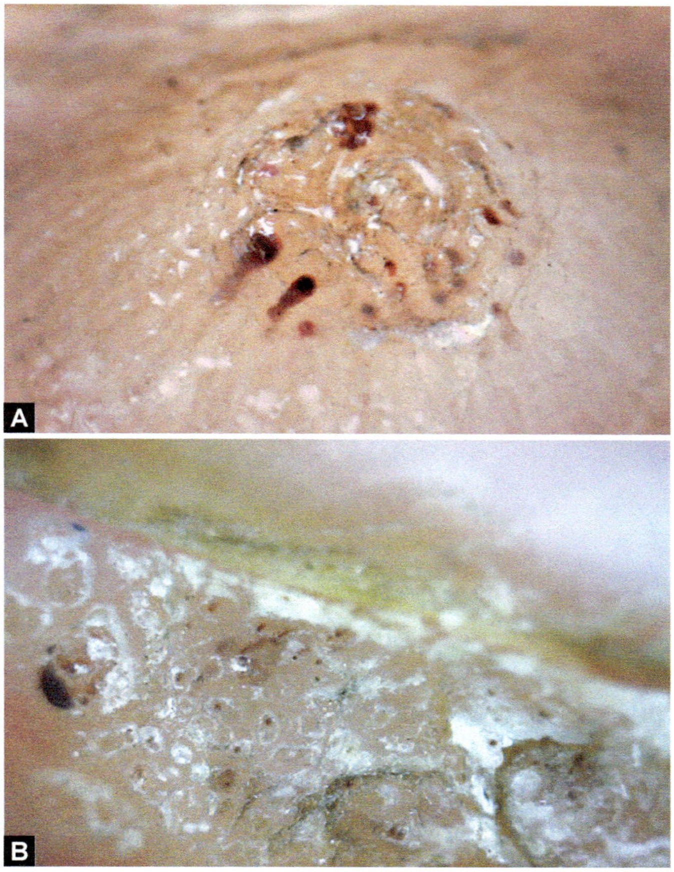

Figs. 9A and B: (A) Onychoscopy of the small mass from the distal aspect shows a periungual wart showing dark red-colored dots indicating hemorrhages in the stratum corneum. (Dinolite AM7115MZT polarized view without linkage fluid, 50×); (B) Another patient with a hyperkeratotic lesion along the lateral nail fold. Onychoscopy shows a whitish hyperkeratosis, studded with red-colored dots indicating hemorrhages. The picture is suggestive of a periungual wart. (Dinolite AM7115MZT polarized view without linkage fluid, 50×).

INFLAMMATORY NAIL DISORDERS

NAIL PSORIASIS

Introduction

Nail involvement in psoriasis is not very frequent; however, a minority of cases may present as isolated nail psoriasis only. Onychoscopy is useful in delineating the underlying cause especially in such cases, as onychoscopic features of nail psoriasis are fairly distinctive. Nail psoriasis can produce numerous nail alterations such as pitting, onycholysis, or subungual hyperkeratosis. At times, nail features may offer a valuable diagnostic clue toward cutaneous disease. Nail changes are evident in 10% cases of pediatric psoriasis.

Key Dermoscopic Features

Onychoscopic features of nail psoriasis depend on the part of nail unit involved. The salient features observed onychoscopically are summarized in **Table 1**. What one must remember is that the final diagnosis is mostly dependent on a combination of the features seen.

Case Details

A 12-year-old child presented with guttate psoriasis with involvement of scalp since 1 year. Nail examination revealed multiple coarse pits and salmon patches **(Figs. 10A to G)**.

Table 1: Salient onychoscopic features of nail psoriasis.

Part of nail unit affected by psoriasis	*Onychoscopic feature*	*Description*
Nail matrix	Pitting	• Depressions are irregular in size and shape; sometime surrounded by a whitish halo • Indentations over nail plate, irregular in size and shape • Large, deep, and irregular distributed cupuliform depressions
	Leukonychia	White irregular areas within the substance of nail plate
Nail bed	Salmon patch	• Red to orange patch, irregular in size and shape • Red brown-colored area • Yellowish-red discoloration appearing as irregular translucent area
	Splinter hemorrhages	• Longitudinal red, brown-to-black marks • Longitudinal purple-to-black streaks • Longitudinal fusiform streaks and serpentine hemorrhages
	Onycholysis	• Area either homogeneously white or having longitudinal striations, often surrounded by reddish-to-orange proximal border • Reddish orange to brown color band separating the area of onycholysis from the normal nail (this feature helps differentiate psoriatic onycholysis from traumatic onycholysis) • Erythematous border encircling white onycholytic area
	Nail bed vessels	Fusiform dilatation of vessels surrounded by prominent halo, as seen close to the onychodermal band
Proximal nail fold	Capillary density and architecture	• Reduced capillary density • Reduced capillary density, drop outs, coiled vessels
Hyponychium	Capillary architecture	• Dilated and irregularly distributed long and tortuous capillaries • Dilated, tortuous, and glomerulus-shaped capillaries • Correlates with severity of disease
Other findings	Pseudofiber sign	Red-black filamentous structures located along the cuticle or underneath the distal free edge of hyponychium

Source: Adapted from Grover C, Jakhar D. Diagnostic utility of onychoscopy: Review of literature. Indian J Dermatopathol Diagn Dermatol. 2017;4:31-40.

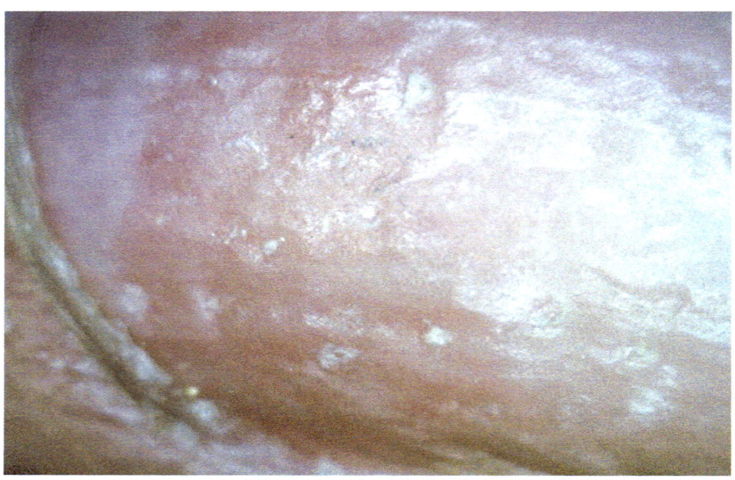

Fig. 10A: Nonpolarizing dermoscopy of the nail plate showing large, deep and irregular depressions. (Dinolite AM7115MZT nonpolarized view without linkage fluid, 20×).

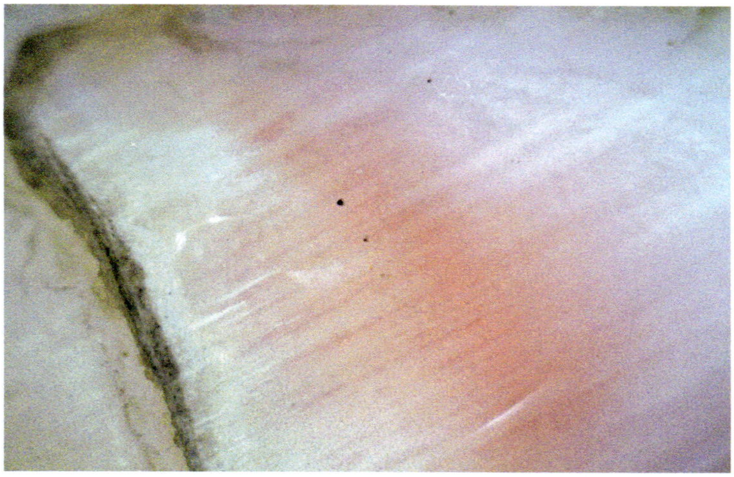

Fig. 10B: Onychoscopy showing distal onycholysis with a proximal erythematous band. (Dinolite AM7115MZT polarized view without linkage fluid, 50×).

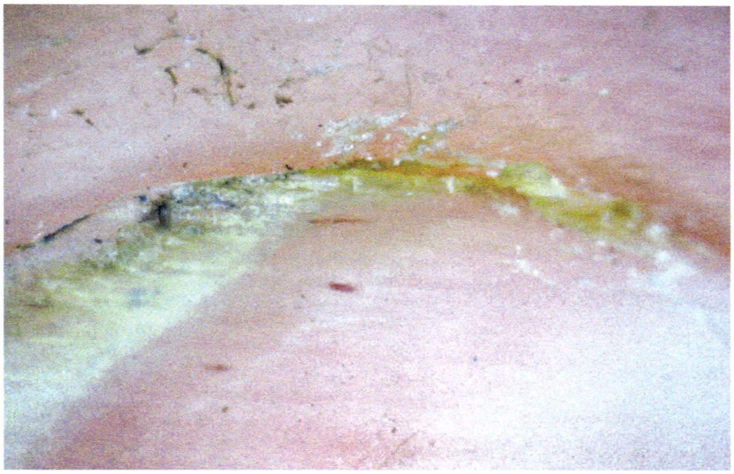

Fig. 10C: Onychoscopy showing multiple splinter hemorrhages near the area of distal onycholysis. (Dinolite AM7115MZT polarized view with linkage fluid, 50×).

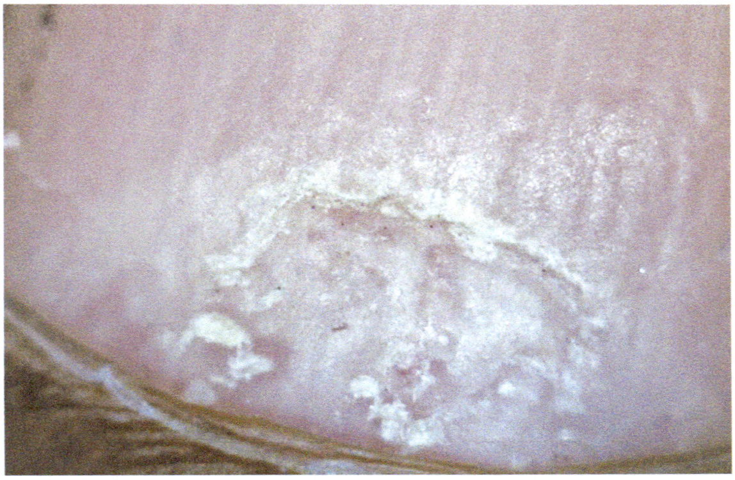

Fig. 10D: Onychoscopy showing multiple small, irregular pits, in the proximal part, overlying the lunula. The pits are all irregular in shape and size. They are surrounded by whitish keratotic rim, suggestive of a psoriatic scale. (Dinolite AM7115MZT nonpolarized view without linkage fluid, 50×).

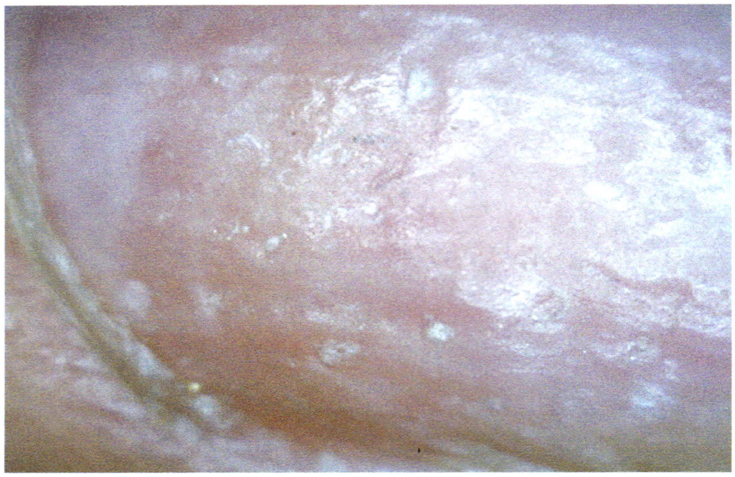

Fig. 10E: Another patient with multiple pits, irregular in distribution, over the nail plate. (Dinolite AM7115MZT nonpolarized view without linkage fluid, 50×).

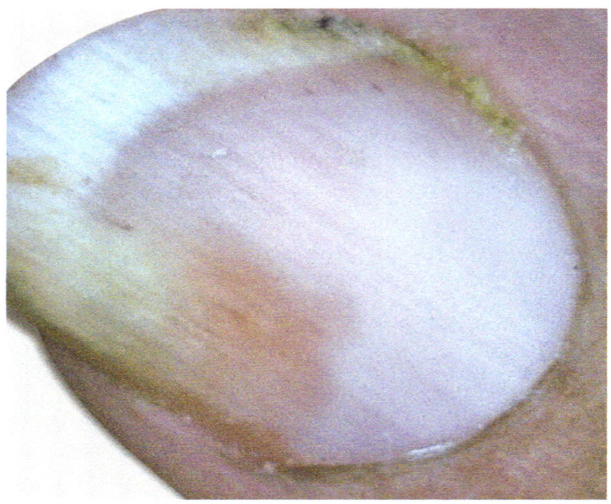

Fig. 10F: Onychoscopy showing a prominent salmon patch involving the nail bed. The characteristic psoriatic onycholysis can be seen. (Dinolite AM7115MZT polarized view with linkage fluid, 20×).

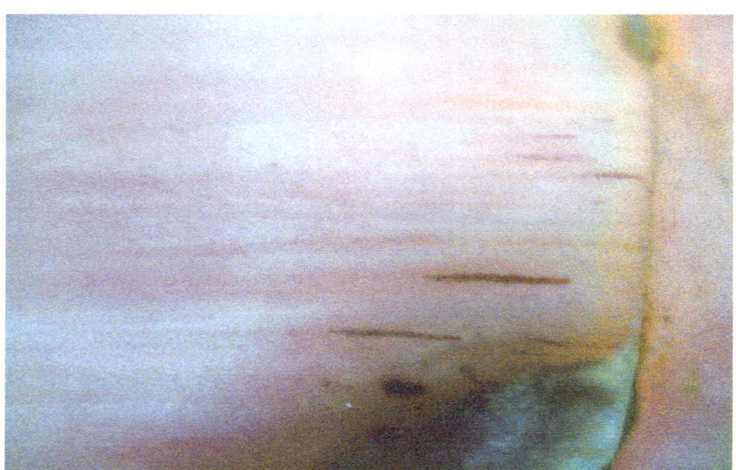

Fig. 10G: Another nail with multiple linearly arranged splinter hemorrhages near an area of onycholysis. (Dinolite AM7115MZT polarized view with linkage fluid, 50×).

Suggested Reading

1. Farias DC, Tosti A, Chiacchio ND, et al. Dermoscopy in nail psoriasis. An Bras Dermatol. 2010;85:101-3.
2. Grover C, Jakhar D. Diagnostic utility of onychoscopy: Review of literature. Indian J Dermatopathol Diagn Dermatol. 2017;4:31-40.
3. Yorulmaz A, Artuz F. A study of dermoscopic features of nail psoriasis. Postepy Dermatol Alergol. 2017;34:28-35.

NAIL LICHEN PLANUS

Introduction

Nail lichen planus is more prevalent in children as compared to cutaneous disease. The dreaded complication, pterygium, however develops rarely. It can also present as trachyonychia or permanent atrophy of nails. Early treatment is necessary in view of a high risk of progression to irreversible scarring.

Key Dermoscopic Features

Nail changes in lichen planus are described to be those of nail matrix origin, nail bed origin or those of the nail folds. Nail matrix changes included trachyonychia, pitting, pterygium, and red lunula; while nail bed changes included chromonychia, nail fragmentation, splinter hemorrhages, onycholysis, and subungual keratosis. Onychoscopy is a useful adjunct in diagnosis as it even helps detect early nail changes. It also helps in detecting nails at risk of imminent scarring, signified by converging longitudinal ridges. Linear dyschromias of the nail bed are commonly seen in nails which may even appear clinically uninvolved. Other features reported include paronychia, longitudinal streaks, and anonychia. Capillaroscopic changes are largely not observed, though proximal nail fold pigmentation can be prominent.

Onychoscopy in nail lichen planus is important to differentiate it from nail lichen striatus and other causes of trachonychia.

Case Details

An 11-year-old child was brought with recent onset thinning and roughening of multiple nails. He had no skin lesions, but a few violaceous plaques in the oral cavity. Changes were suggestive of nail lichen planus and a nail matrix biopsy confirmed the diagnosis **(Figs. 11A to F)**.

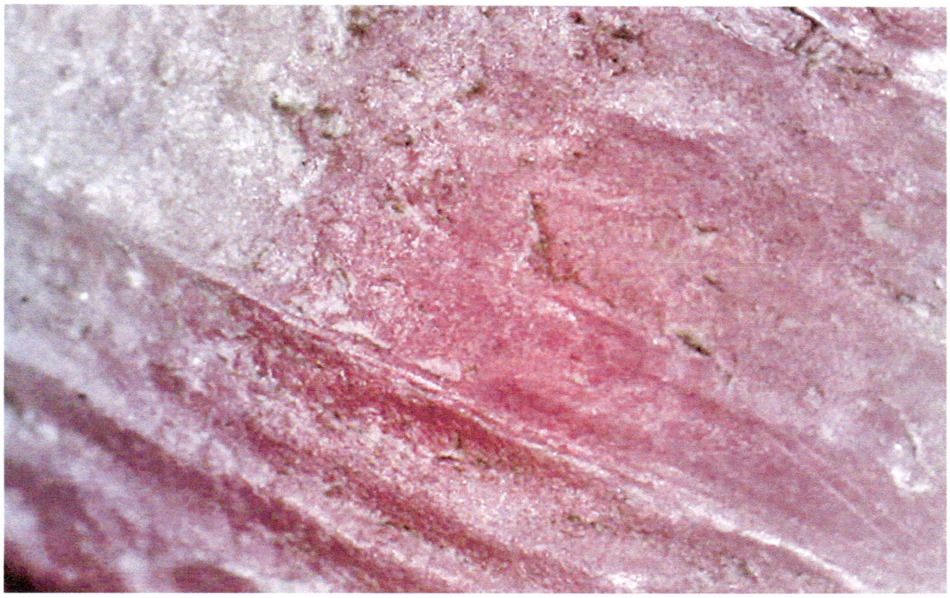

Fig. 11A: Onychoscopy showed multiple linear ridges over the nail plate surface (onychorrhexis). There were few minute pits also seen proximally. The nail plate overall was much thinned, as evidenced by the prominently visible lunula and nail bed. (Dinolite AM7115MZT nonpolarized view without linkage fluid, 50×).

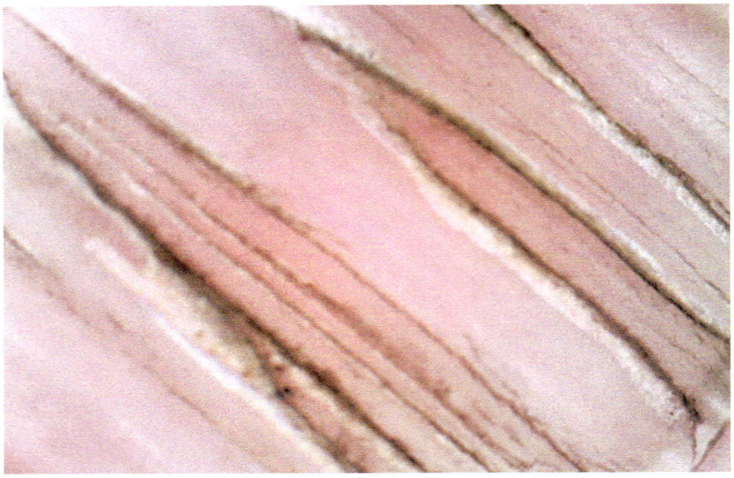

Fig. 11B: Another nail showed onychorrhexis, here in the form of linear splits. The splits were converging at places, which are considered to signify worse prognosis. (Dinolite AM7115MZT polarized view with linkage fluid, 50×).

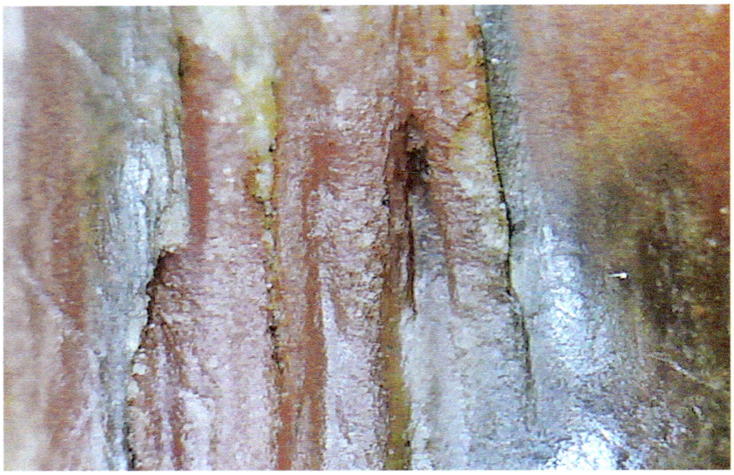

Fig. 11C: Chromonychia with prominent color changes involving the nail plate and bed. (Dinolite AM7115MZT nonpolarized view without linkage fluid, 50×).

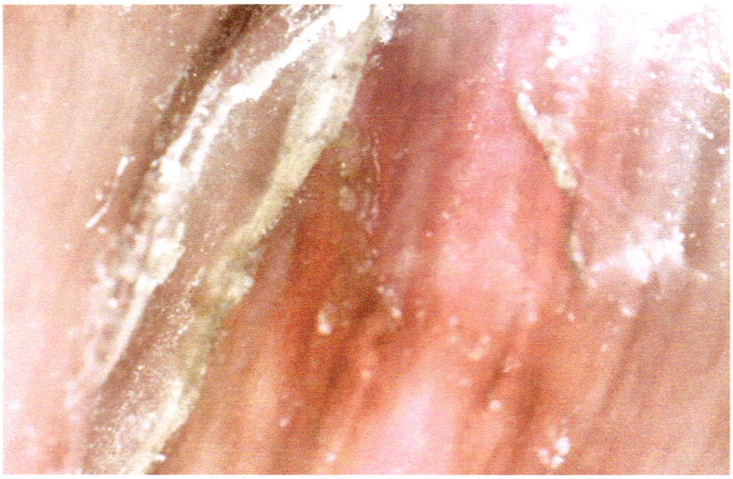

Fig. 11D: This picture with a polarized view shows the nail bed chromonychia through a thinned out nail plate. (Dinolite AM7115MZT polarized view with linkage fluid, 50×).

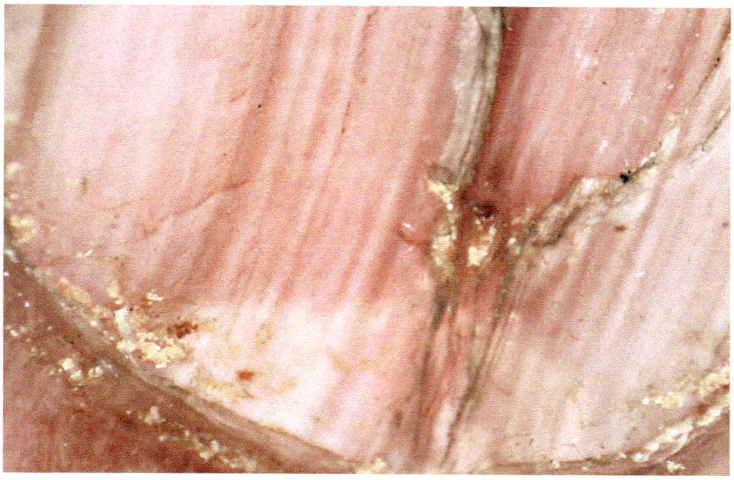

Fig. 11E: Prominent erythematous nail bed with linear dyschromic bands (linear nail bed dyschromia). Overlying nail plate also shows onychorrhexis with nail plate splitting. (Dinolite AM7115MZT polarized view with linkage fluid, 50×).

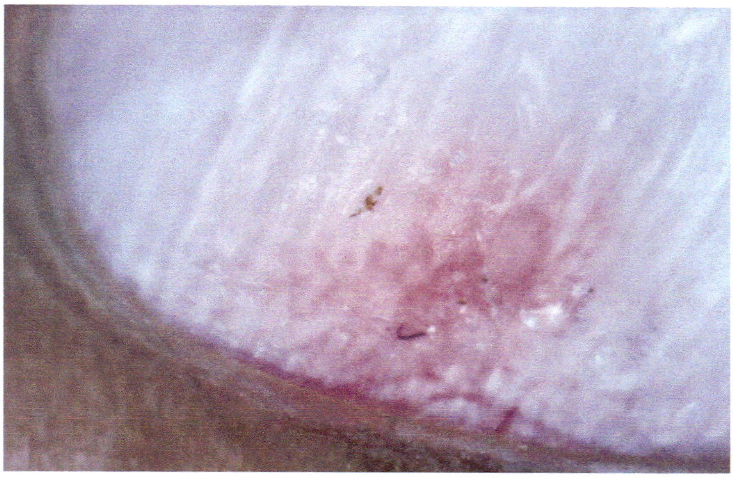

Fig. 11F: An apparently normal nail of the same patient, but onychoscopy showed an erythematous lunula indicating subclinical involvement. (Dinolite AM7115MZT polarized view with linkage fluid, 50×).

Suggested Reading

1. Grover C, Kharghoria G, Bhattacharya SN. Linear nail bed dyschromia: a distinctive dermoscopic feature of nail lichen planus. Clin Exp Dermatol. 2019;44(6):697-9.
2. Nakamura R, Broce AA, Palencia DP, et al. Dermatoscopy of nail lichen planus. Int J Dermatol. 2013;52:684-7.

NAIL LICHEN STRIATUS

Introduction

It is a condition almost exclusively seen in children, either in isolation or associated with cutaneous disease. Lichenoid changes involve a single digit or limb and regress spontaneously. Nail involvement may not be very common, but when present, is quite characteristic in the form of lateral involvement of the nail plate.

Key Dermoscopic Features

Onychoscopy reveals onychoschizia, longitudinal ridging, and distal nail splitting with nail bed erythema in the affected region. Nail lichen striatus may also show longitudinal erythematous bands disrupting the appearance of lunula and

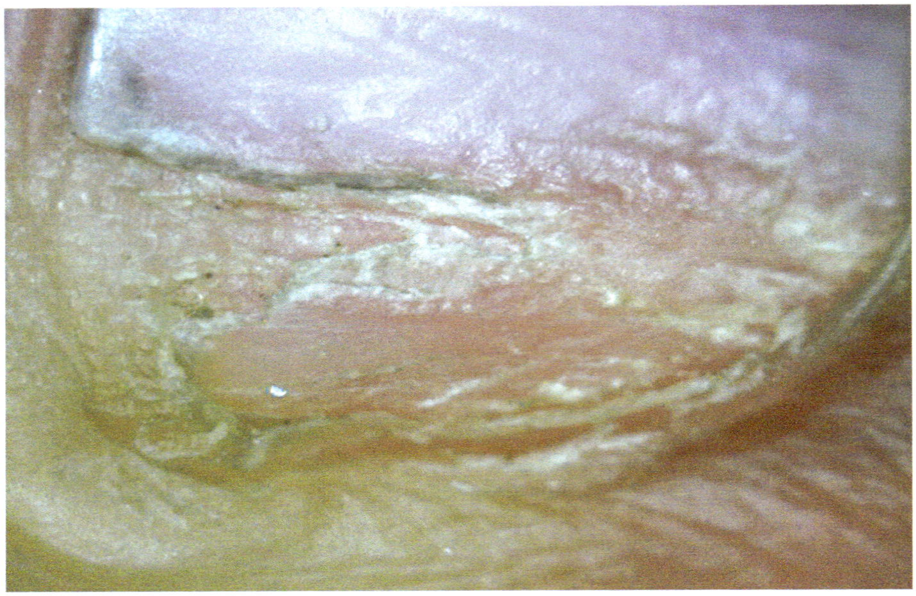

Fig. 12: Onychoscopy of the involved nail showing distal nail bed splitting, onychoschizia, and longitudinal splitting. (Dinolite AM7115MZT nonpolarized view without linkage fluid, 50×).

extending proximally beneath the proximal nail fold. Nail changes can occur before, simultaneously or after the appearance of cutaneous lesions in lichen striatus. Nail lichen striatus may be difficult to differentiate from nail lichen planus clinically. Characteristic onychoscopic features may aid in the diagnosis. Dermoscopy of cutaneous lesions of lichen striatus may be a useful aid which shows brownish to grayish granular pigmentation with dotted vessels and white scales.

Case Details

A 10-year-old child presented with erythematous to violaceous papules over the right hand in a linear distribution. On examination, the lesions were extending on the ring finger with involvement of the nail. Nail examination revealed longitudinal ridging, splitting, and nail plate thinning **(Fig. 12)**.

Suggested Reading

1. Jakhar D, Kaur I. Onychoscopy of nail involvement in lichen striatus. Indian Dermatol Online J. 2018;9:360-1.

TRACHYONYCHIA

Introduction

This condition is commonly seen in the pediatric age group. Trachyonychia presents as a rough, sand paper-like appearance of nail plate resulting from mild inflammation of the proximal nail matrix. It usually presents at 2–7 years of age, affecting single or all nails [twenty-nail dystrophy(TND)]. Idiopathic TND generally improves spontaneously while TND associated with skin diseases may have a longer course.

Twenty-nail dystrophy is a term popularized by Hazelrigg et al. in their initial report of children with acquired trachyonychia of all 20 nails. *Trachyonychia* or *sand-blasted nails* refers to nails with closely spaced longitudinal striations, onychorrhexis, onychoschizia, distal chipping and a dull, opalescent appearance giving them a rough appearance. This term describes a reaction pattern rather than a specific disease. The onset is insidious, either simultaneously in all nails or in individual nails, progressing gradually over many months. According to some reports, the appearance of the nail plate may vary from rough, lusterless, sand-papered appearance to a shiny appearance with numerous, small, superficial pits.

Most commonly, TND is seen as an isolated nail abnormality (spongiotic trachyonychia); however, many associations have been attributed including lichen planus, alopecia areata, eczematous changes, IgA deficiency, ichthyosis vulgaris, primary biliary cirrhosis, pemphigus, vitiligo, etc. Most of these cases resolve spontaneously over several years.

Key Dermoscopic Features

Trachyonychia presents as rough nails. It can either be idiopathic or caused by inflammatory disorders such as alopecia areata, lichen planus, or psoriasis. Onychoscopy shows multiple fine and superficial longitudinal fissures covered by thin scales in the nail plate. In the "shiny" variant, the nail shows superficial ridging and small geometrical pits. In cases secondary to inflammatory disorders, the characteristic changes of the underlying pathology may also be seen.

Case Details

A 7-year-old child was brought with progressive roughening of his finger and toe nails. On examination there was darkening and an opaque appearance of his nails **(Figs. 13A and B)**.

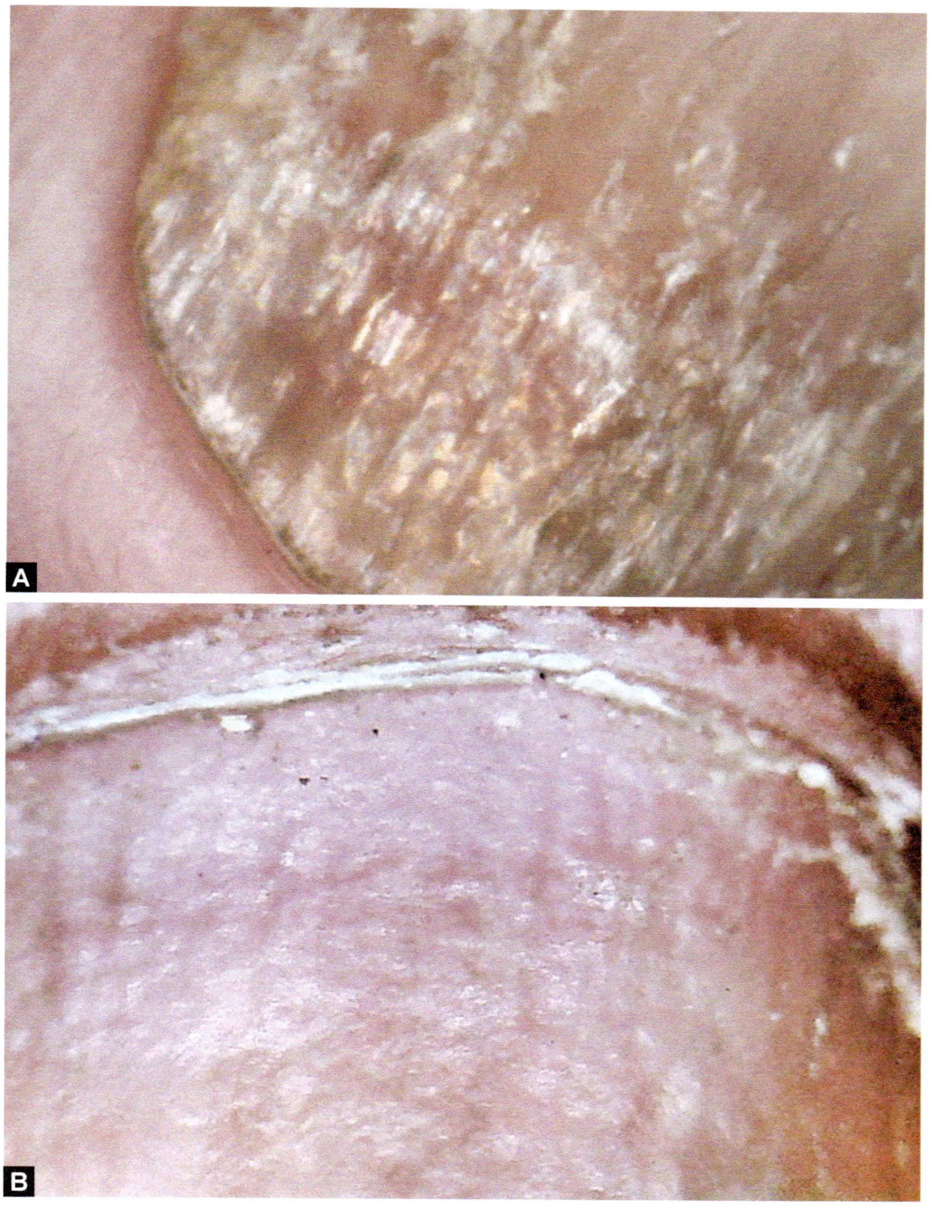

Figs. 13A and B: (A) "Opaque trachyonychia" with rough sand-paper appearance of fingernails. (Dinolite AM7115MZT nonpolarized view without linkage fluid, 50×); (B) "Shiny trachyonychia" in another child with rough appearance of fingernails. The nails are however not pigmented or opaque. The surface changes are seen to be a combination of fine pits and longitudinal ridges. (Dinolite AM7115MZT nonpolarized view without linkage fluid, 50×).

Suggested Reading

1. Alessandrini A, Starace M, Piraccini BM. Dermoscopy in the evaluation of nail disorders. Skin Appendage Disord. 2017;3(2):70-82.

ONYCHOPHAGIA

Introduction

It refers to chronic nail biting affecting about 30–50% children. Features seen include permanent shortening of nails, oral carriage of *Escherichia coli* (leading to tooth decay), and various infections such as ungual warts, herpetic whitlow, etc.

Key Dermoscopic Features

There is a decreased length of the nail with exposed distal nail bed to varying extent. Onychoscopy shows onychoschizia, pitting, splinter hemorrhages, Beau's lines, periungual erythema or hemorrhages, and hang nails. Onychoschizia is seen typically at the distal nail plate. Onychophagia leads to traumatic nail abnormalities, apart from increasing the spread of warts and infectious agents. Also long-term onychophagia can induce melanonychia.

Case Details

Parents of a 10-year-old child were concerned about his nail biting habit. On examination, the nails had dull nonrefractile irregular surface with hang-nails in the nail folds. The child had no other obsessive compulsive habit **(Figs. 14A to C)**.

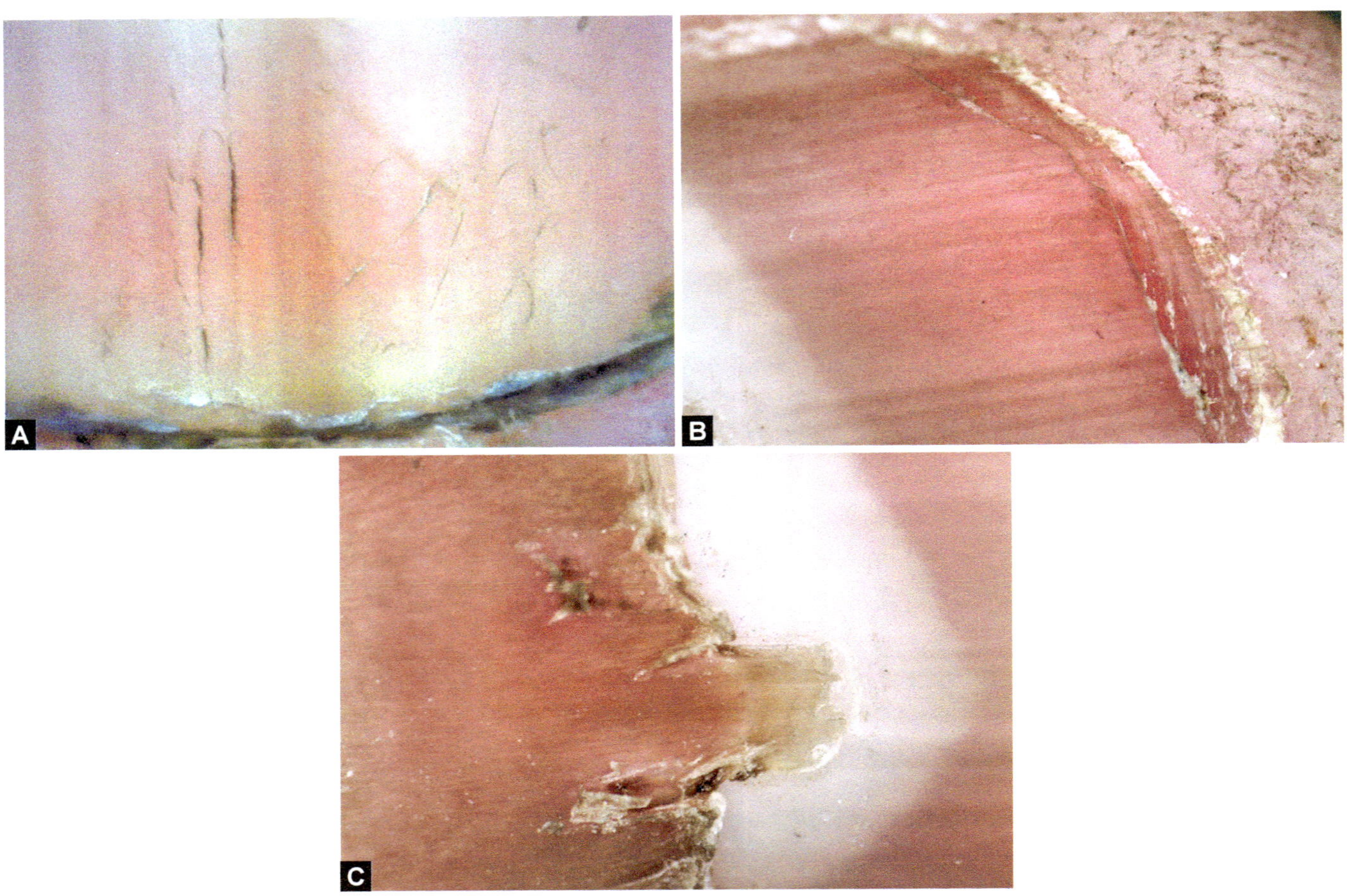

Figs. 14A to C: (A) Onychoscopy showing distal nail plate onychoschizia. (Dinolite AM7115MZT polarized view without linkage fluid, 50×); (B) Distinct shortening of the nail plate with distally visible nail fold. (Dinolite AM7115MZT polarized view with linkage fluid, 50×); (C) Onychoscopy showing distal nail plate onychoschizia. (Dinolite AM7115MZT polarized view without linkage fluid, 50×).

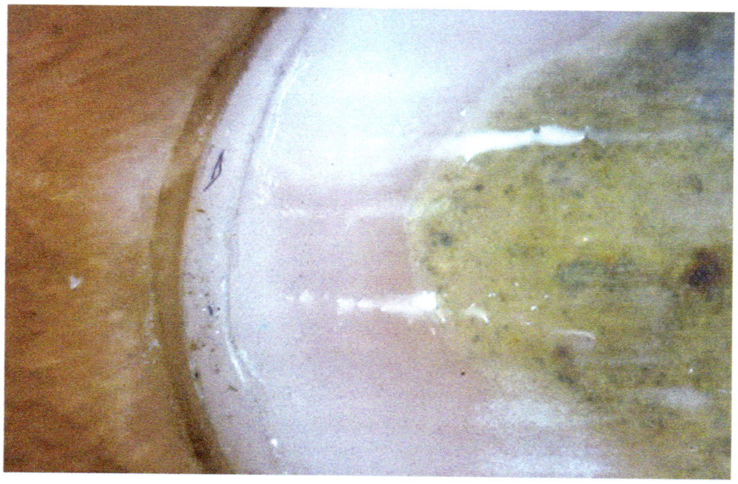

Fig. 15: Onychoscopy of traumatic onycholysis showing the onycholytic band without proximal erythematous band or striations.

Suggested Reading

1. Fıçıcıoğlu S, Korkmaz S. Onychophagia-induced melanonychia, splinter hemorrhages, leukonychia, and pterygium inversum unguis concurrently. Case Rep Dermatol Med. 2018;2018:3230582.

TRAUMATIC ONYCHOLYSIS

Introduction

Onycholysis (distal separation of the nail plate from the nail bed) can occur due to various causes. The most common cause is trauma, either acute or low-grade chronic trauma. Due to a high physical activity among the children, they are prone to develop trauma-induced onycholysis.

Key Dermoscopic Features

On onychoscopy, a smooth proximal border of onycholytic band without proximal erythema and jagged edges is highly suggestive of traumatic onycholysis. Splinter hemorrhages and/or subungual hematoma may be found in the vicinity of the onycholysis, indicating trauma. As highlighted above, onychoscopy is useful in differentiating onycholysis caused secondary to trauma, psoriasis, and onychomycosis.

Case Details

A young child presented with onycholysis of the finger nails. There was no other nail deformity. Rest of the mucocutaneous examination was noncontributory **(Fig. 15)**.

Suggested Reading

1. Grover C, Jakhar D. Diagnostic utility of onychoscopy: Review of literature. Indian J Dermatopathol Diagn Dermatol. 2017;4:31-40.

SECTION 5

Interesting Cases and Differentials

CHAPTER

- **Case Scenarios**

CHAPTER 22

Case Scenarios

Subrata Malakar, Harshal Ranglani, Surit Malakar

CASE 1

History: A 6-year-old boy presented with a unilateral patch over the left forehead above left eyebrow, blue-gray in color. Parents noticed it 5 months back. They have applied some ointments without any improvement.

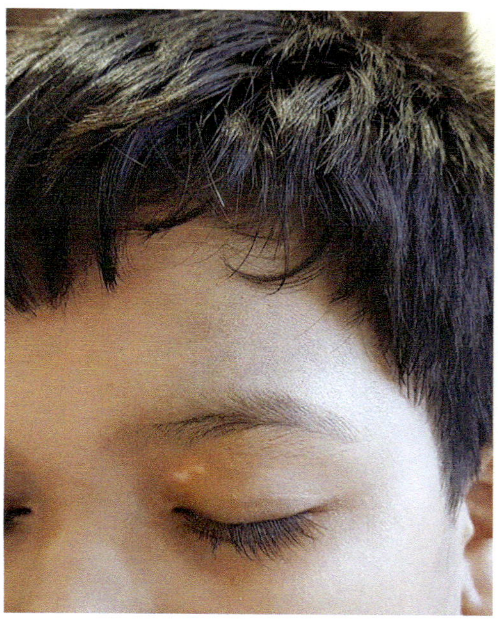

What are your differentials?

a. Nevus of Ota
b. Congenital melanocytic nevus
c. Frictional melanosis
d. None of the above

Answer:

d. None of the above

Dermoscopy shows *dirty dotted particles* acquired during daily outdoor activities such as playing. Usually, the dirty dots are seen over the scalp but in this case, they are seen above the eyebrow probably due to the style of outdoor activities and also may be attributed to inadequate washing of this area.

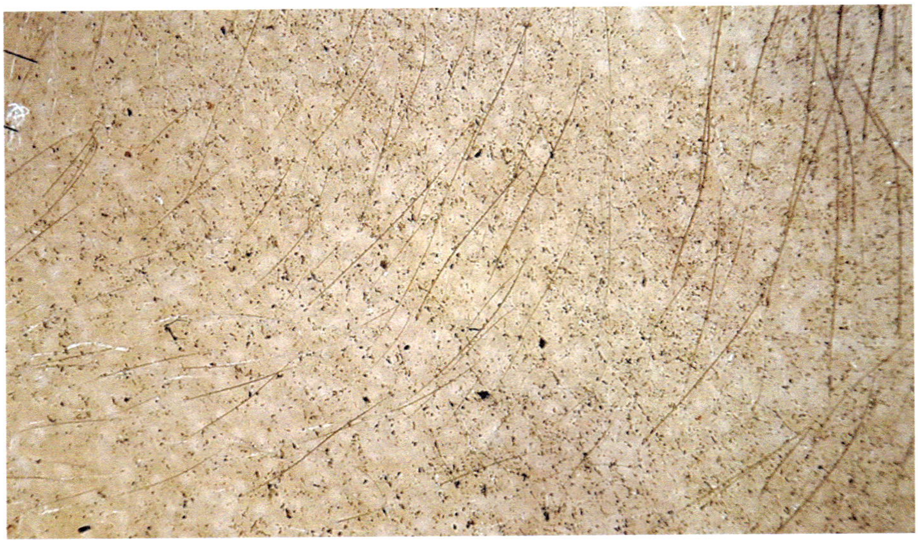

Below is a picture showing dirty dots[1,2] present over the scalp of a child.

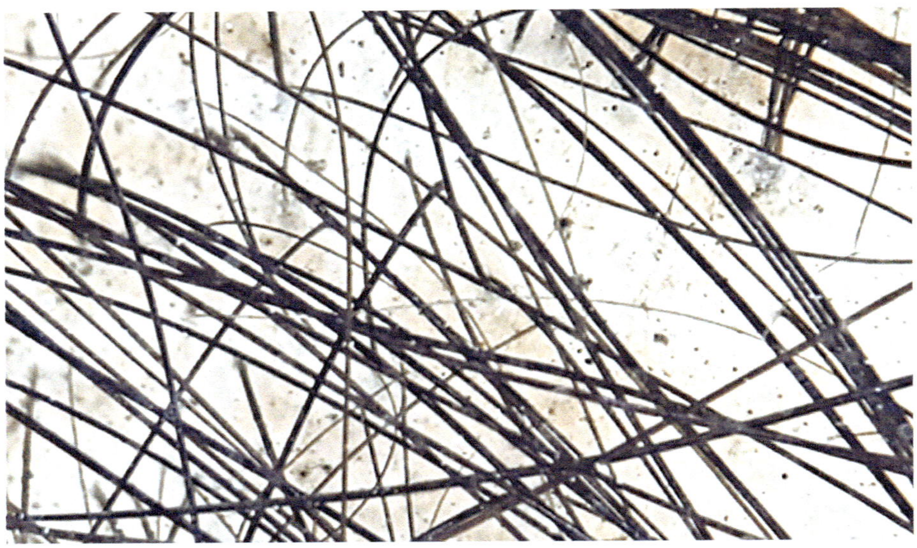

REFERENCES

1. Malakar S. Trichoscopy terminologies. In: Malakar S (Ed). Trichoscopy: A Text and Atlas. New Delhi: Jaypee Brothers Medical Publishers (P) Ltd.; 2017. pp. 27-8.
2. Tosti A. Normal scalp. In: Tosti A (Ed). Dermoscopy of the hair and nails. United States: CRC Press; 2016. p. 22.

CASE 2

Both the above cases of pediatric age group presented with erythematous, scaly papules of a few months duration. For the above two similar-looking clinical presentations, what are your differentials for A and B?

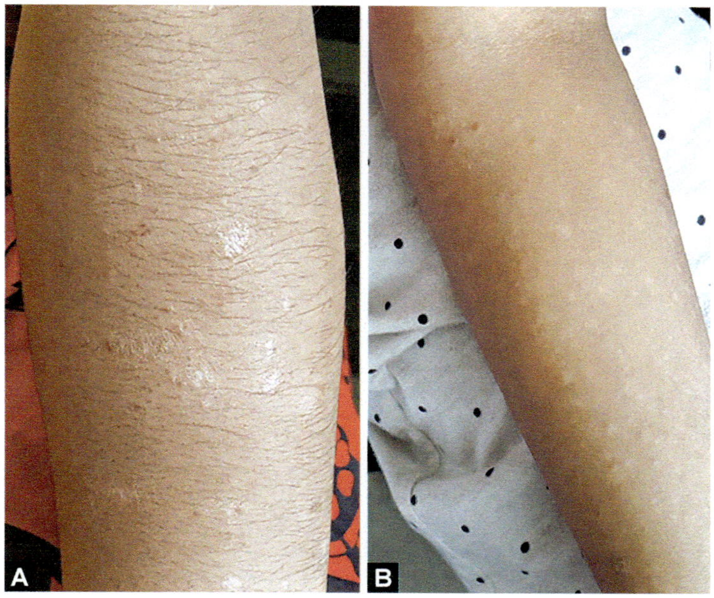

What are your differentials for A and B?

Differentials for A:

a. Guttate psoriasis
b. Pityriasis lichenoides chronica
c. Polymorphic light eruption
d. Atopic dermatitis
e. None of the above

Differentials for B:

a. Papular urticaria
b. Pityriasis lichenoides chronica
c. Polymorphic light eruption
d. Guttate psoriasis
e. None of the above

By corroborating the dermoscopic findings with the clinical pictures, what is your final diagnosis?

Answer for A:

a. Guttate psoriasis

Answer for B:

b. Pityriasis lichenoides chronica

Explanation for A:

Dermoscopic finding shows regular red dots on an erythematous background, leading to the diagnosis of *guttate psoriasis*. Please note the presence of dermoscopic Auspitz sign.

Explanation for B:

On dermoscopy, *pityriasis lichenoides chronica* shows an orange-yellow background and both dotted as well as nondotted vessels.[1]

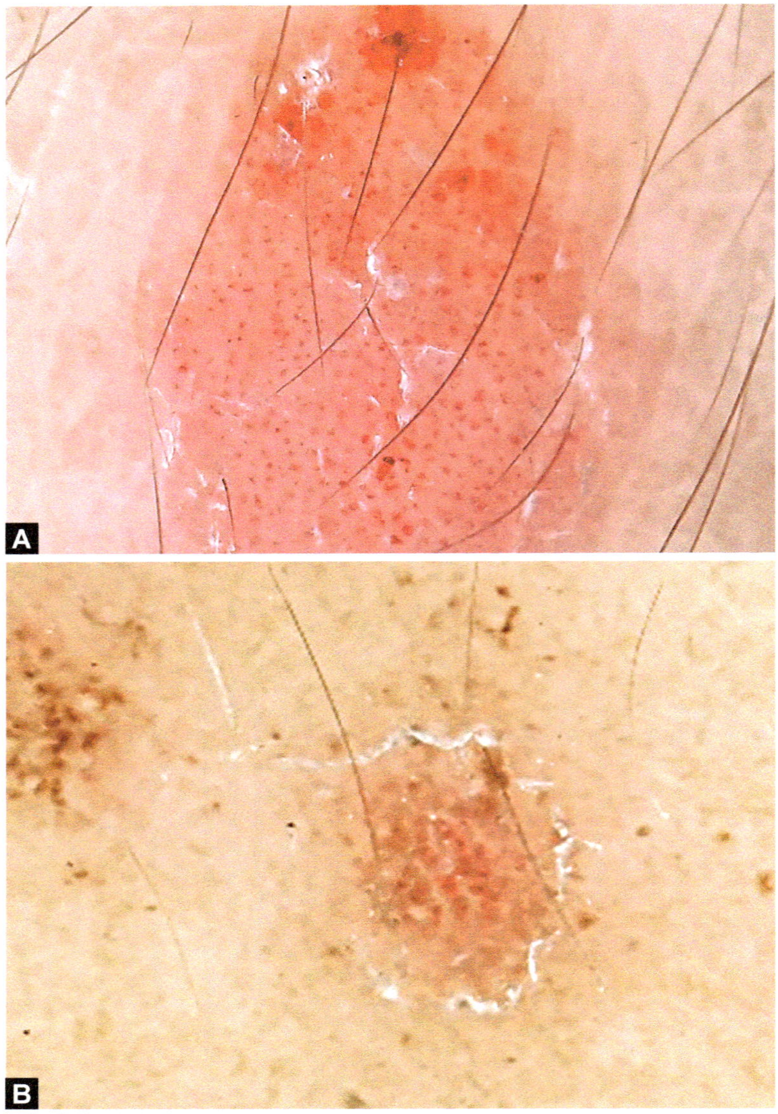

REFERENCE

1. Errichetti E, Lacarrubba F, Micali G, et al. Differentiation of pityriasis lichenoides chronica from guttate psoriasis by dermoscopy. Clin Exp Dermatol. 2015;40(7):804-6.

CASE 3

Cases A and B presented with nail changes. Splinter hemorrhages were noted in both and were highlighted by dermoscopy. But some other features differentiating the two conditions were also present. What are those features? Based on these, what will be your diagnosis for the two cases?

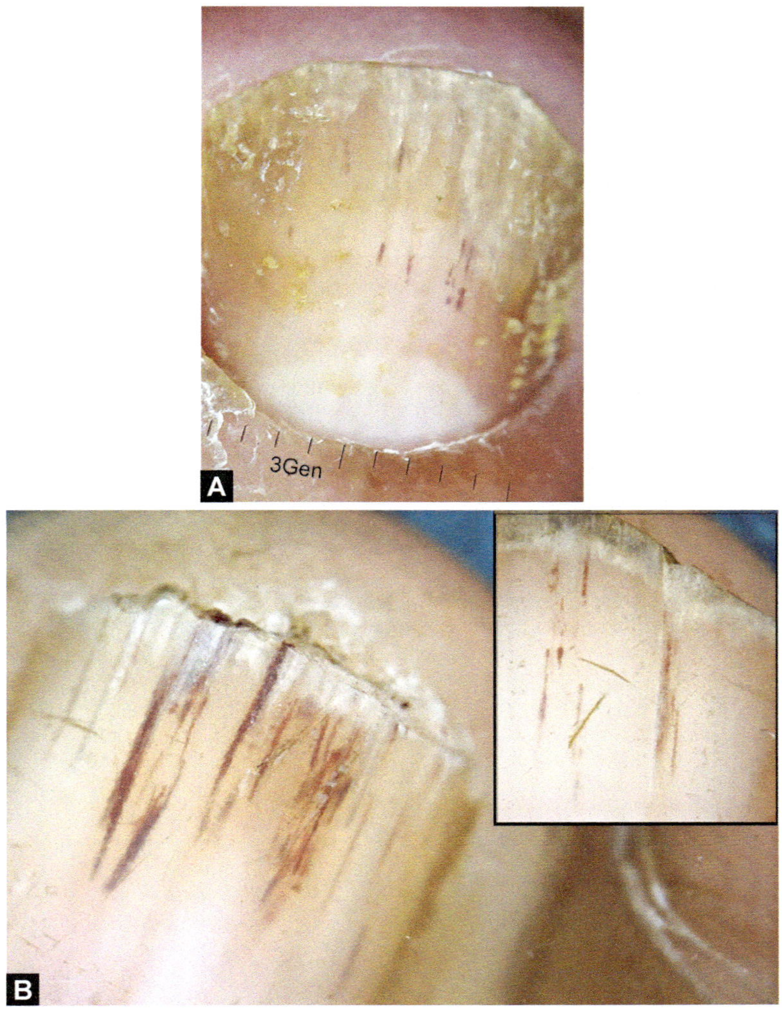

What are your differentials for A and B?

Differentials for A:

a. Trauma
b. Antiphospholipid syndrome
c. Psoriasis
d. Darier's disease
e. None of the above

Differentials for B:

a. Rheumatoid arthritis
b. Systemic lupus erythematosus (SLE)
c. Systemic scleroderma
d. Darier's disease
e. Subacute infective endocarditis

Answer for A:

c. Psoriasis

Answer for B:

d. Darier's disease

In case A, in addition to splinter hemorrhages,[1] other features present are coarse pits, salmon patch, and onycholysis, which hints toward the diagnosis of *psoriasis.*

In case B, apart from splinter hemorrhages, there are the following findings—V-shaped nicking at the distal edge of the nail (inset), subungual hyperkeratosis and on dermoscopic examination, alternating longitudinal red and white bands can be highlighted, confirming the diagnosis of *Darier's disease.*

REFERENCE

1. Errichetti E, Stinco G. Dermoscopy in general dermatology: a practical overview. Dermatol Ther (Heidelb). 2016;6(4):471-507.

CASE 4

A young girl presented with a mildly erythematous rash and burning sensation over the face for 1 year which was not responding to topical steroid or calcineurin inhibitors.

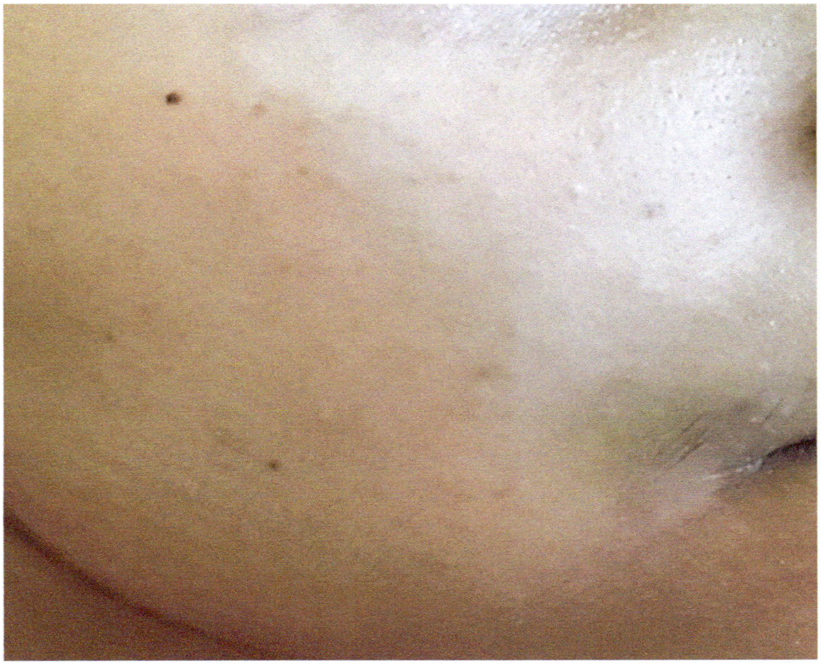

What is your differential diagnosis?

Differentials:

a. Sensitive skin
b. Long contd topical steroid
c. Polymorphous light eruption
d. Demodicosis
e. Rosacea
f. Perioral dermatitis

Here's a look at the dermoscopic findings in the above case. What is your final diagnosis on correlation of the two?

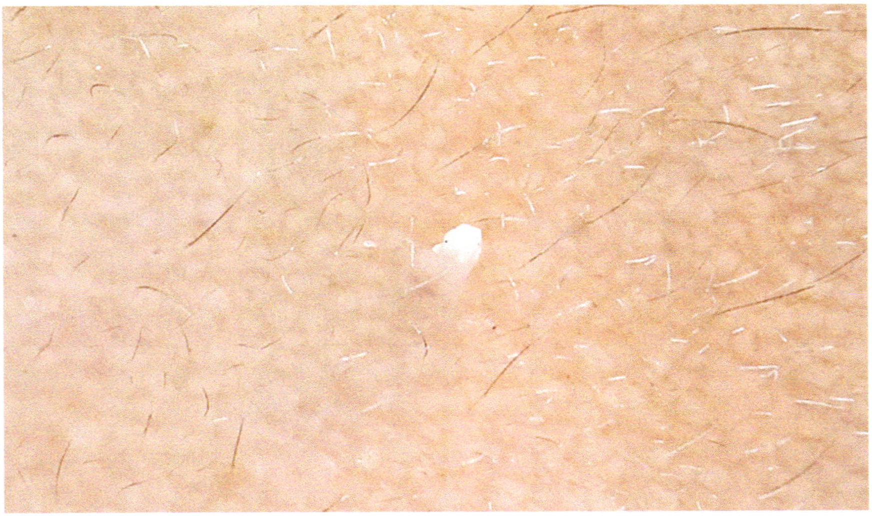

On trichoscopy of facial hairs, a white spicule is seen protruding from the follicular opening.

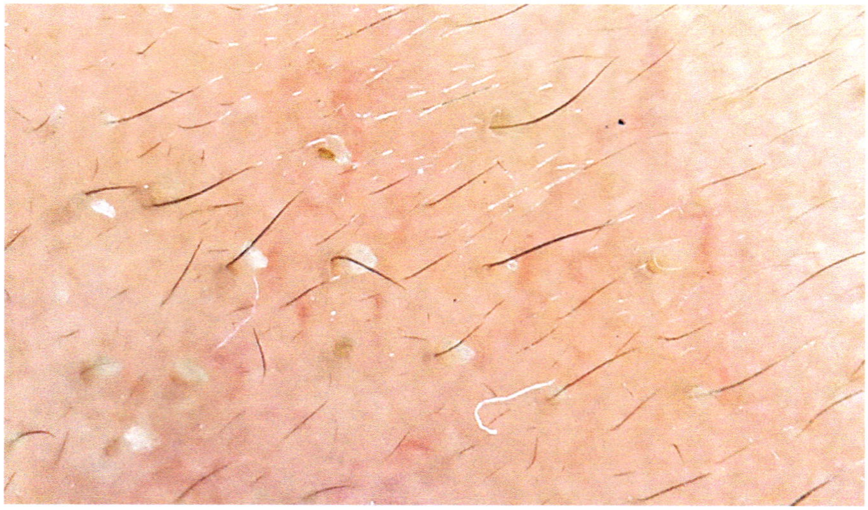

More white spicules and subtle reticular dilated vessels forming a pink network were also seen in another field.

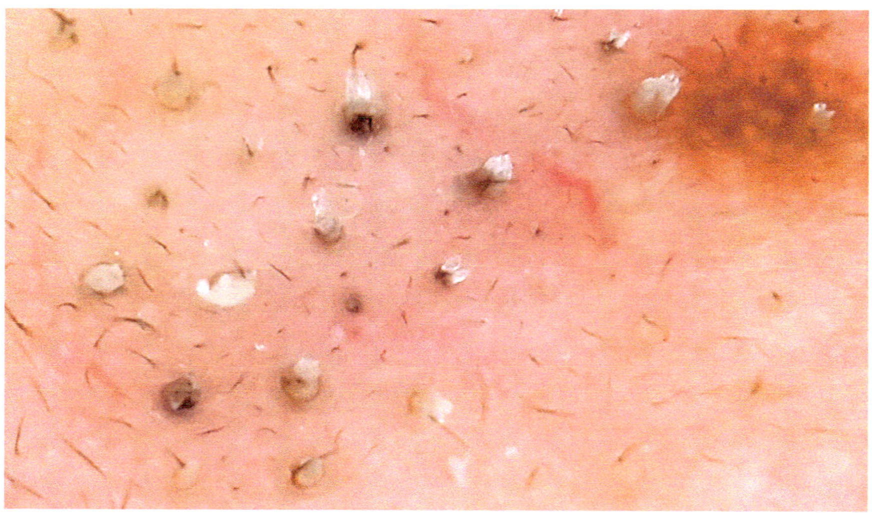

Dilated pores containing amorphous brown/gray plugs are also be associated with this disorder.

Answer:

d. Demodicosis

When a patient presents with sensitive skin, the differentials include long-term topical corticosteroid abuse, polymorphic light eruption, rosacea, perioral dermatitis, and *demodicosis*.

On dermoscopy, demodicosis is diagnosed when we find a high density (>5/mm^2) of white spicules at the follicular openings. These white spicules[1] represent the tails of the demodex mite.

REFERENCE

1. Malakar S. Infectious Dermatoses: In: Malakar S (Ed). Dermoscopy: Text and Atlas. New Delhi: Jaypee Brothers Medical Publishers (P) Ltd.; 2017. pp. 172-5.

CASE 5

A 4-year-old boy presented with lesions over the thigh and lower abdomen, which were of a few months duration. There was no associated itching.

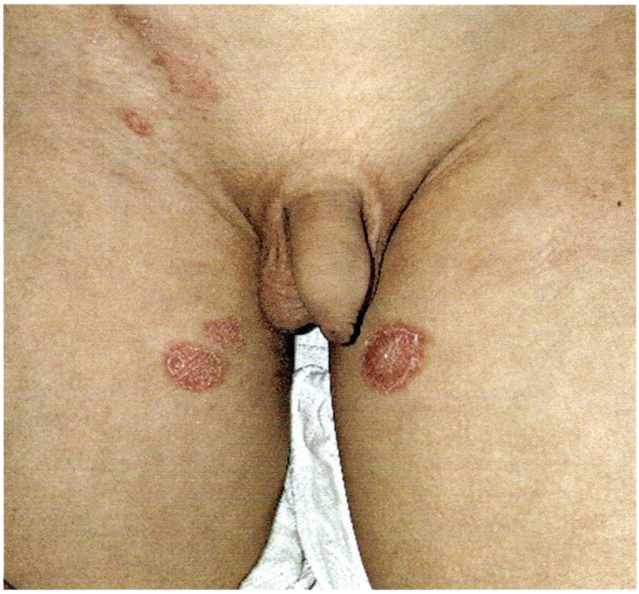

What are your clinical differentials for the above case?

Differentials:

a. Nummular eczema
b. Pityriasis rosea
c. Psoriasis
d. Tinea corporis

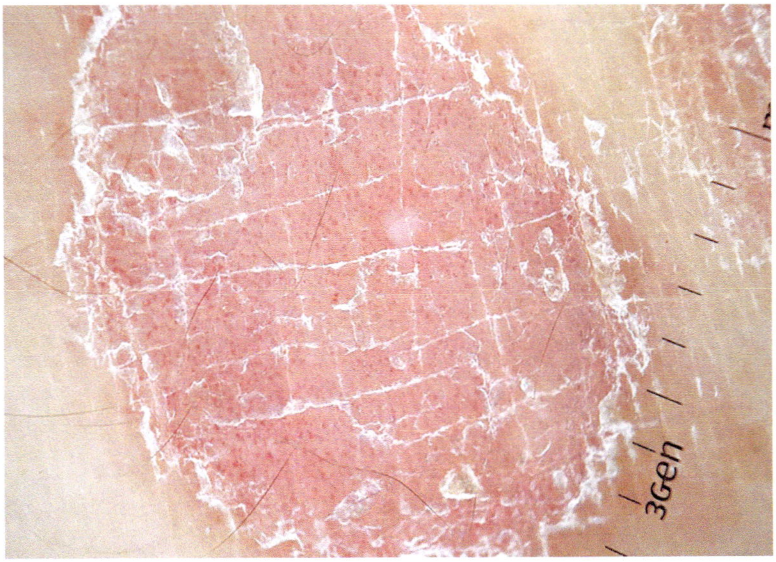

What is your final diagnosis on clinicodermoscopic correlation?

Answer:

c. Psoriasis

The presence of regular, red dots arranged on a dull red background point toward the diagnosis of *psoriasis*.[1] Thus, dermoscopy is a particularly useful tool in the diagnosis of psoriasis in pediatric patients, where it may be confused with dermatophytosis, candidiasis, and eczema.

REFERENCE

1. Malakar S. Papulosquamous disorders. In: Malakar S (Ed). Dermoscopy: Text and Atlas. New Delhi: Jaypee Brothers Medical Publishers (P) Ltd.; 2017. pp. 132-47.

CASE 6

Here are two similar-looking clinical cases. Both of them presented with hypopigmented lesions of about 3 months duration. What are your clinical differentials for each of these cases?

Differentials for A:

a. Lichen nitidus
b. Polymorphic light eruption
c. Lichen planus
d. Lichen sclerosus et atrophicus

Differentials for B:

a. Lichen nitidus
b. Polymorphic light eruption
c. Lichen planus
d. Lichen sclerosus et atrophicus

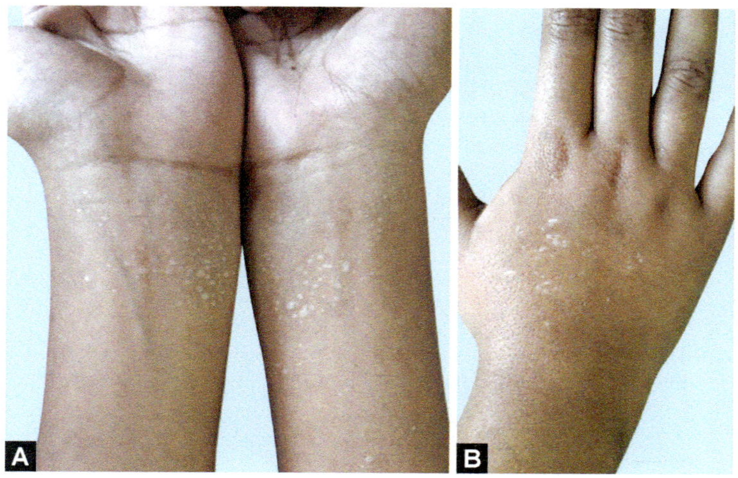

On dermoscopy, the picture was as follows:

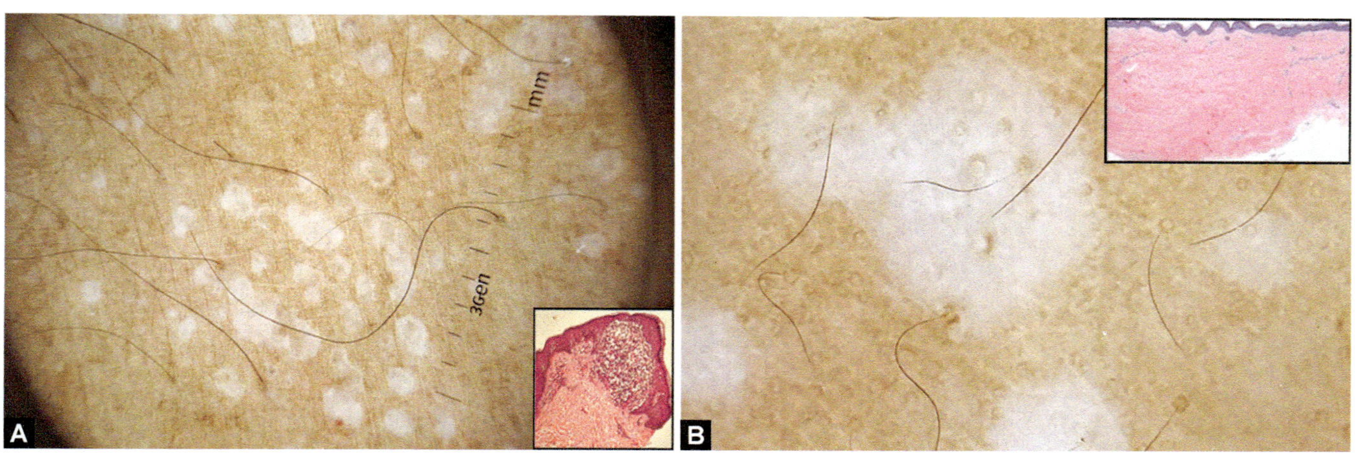

Now what is your diagnosis for each of the cases?

Answer for A:

a. Lichen nitidus

Answer for B:

d. Lichen sclerosus et atrophicus

Case A: The presence of brown shadow in the center, surrounded by a well-circumscribed, whitish area confirms the diagnosis of *lichen nitidus*.[1] This brown shadow corresponds to the subepidermal lymphohistiocytic infiltrate on histopathology.

Case B: Presence of comedo-like openings (which signify keratotic plugs) and presence of white structureless areas aids the diagnosis of *lichen sclerosus et atrophicus*.[2]

Thus, dermoscopy proves to be of great advantage in distinguishing between these two cases, with identical clinical presentation.

REFERENCES

1. Malakar S, Save S, Mehta P. Brown shadow in lichen nitidus: a dermoscopic marker!. Indian Dermatol Online J. 2018;9: 479-80.
2. Ankad BS, Beergouder SL. Dermoscopic patterns in lichen sclerosus: a report of three cases. Indian Dermatol Online J. 2015;6:237-40.

CASE 7

A 2-year-old child was brought to the outpatient department (OPD) by her parents, who had noticed a single, hypopigmented lesion on her left cheek 1 year back. The lesion was stable and asymptomatic.

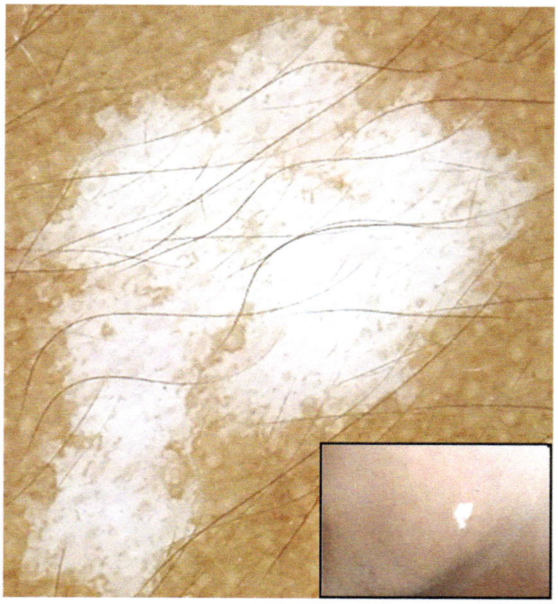

What would be your clinical differentials?

Differentials:

a. Nevus depigmentosus
b. Postinflammatory hypopigmentation
c. Vitiligo
d. Ash-leaf macule
e. None of the above

Now, what is your final diagnosis?

Answer:

e. None of the above

What would be your dermoscopic findings?

a. Uniform faint reticulate pigmentation
b. Zone of hypopigmentation and zone of normal pigmentation
c. Complete depigmentation
d. None of the above

Answer:

d. None of the above

This is a typical dermoscopic picture of *piebaldism*, characterized by *areas of distorted pigment* network on a background of complete depigmentation. Interspersed are a few areas of normal pigmentation.[1]

REFERENCE

1. Malakar S, Mukherjee SS, Malakar S. Looking through the dermoscope in a case of piebaldism. Our Dermatol Online. 2019;10(3):312-3.

CASE 8

A 4-year-old male child presented with lesions located symmetrically over both sides of the neck since birth, slowly improving with age. The mother gave a history of the lesion being like a whitish membrane at birth which is slowly improving to gain back the normal skin color. There was no history suggestive of any other systemic involvement. The lesion was treated as a post-traumatic ulcer at birth and managed conservatively. The child was off treatment for the past 2 years. Clinical examination revealed a discolored patch with a smooth surface and visible erythema symmetrically located on the lateral aspect of the neck. Palpation of the affected area revealed thinned out skin. The patch was characterized by areas of healing proceeding from the lower end of the lesion to the upper end demonstrated by hyperpigmentation of the lesion, decrease in erythema, and dilated vasculature.

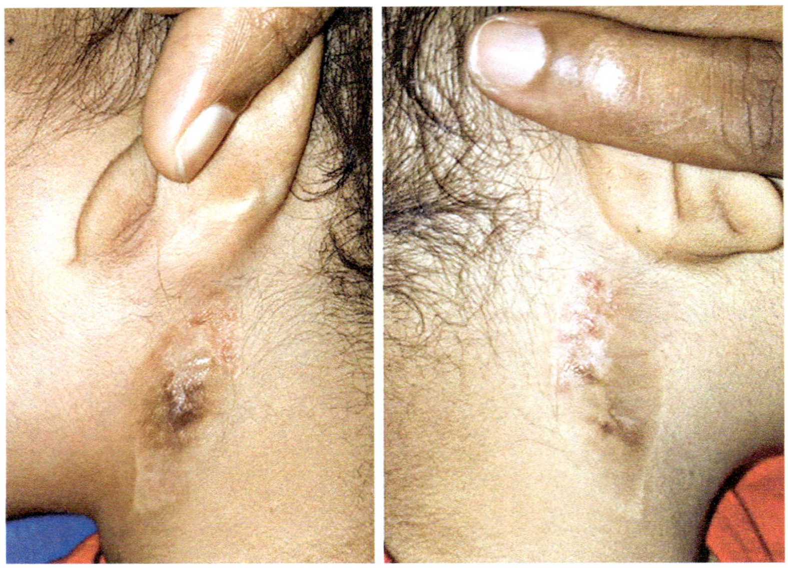

What are your clinical differentials?

Differentials:

a. Morphea
b. Atrophoderma
c. Post-trauma during delivery
d. None of the above

Following are the dermoscopic pictures with findings:

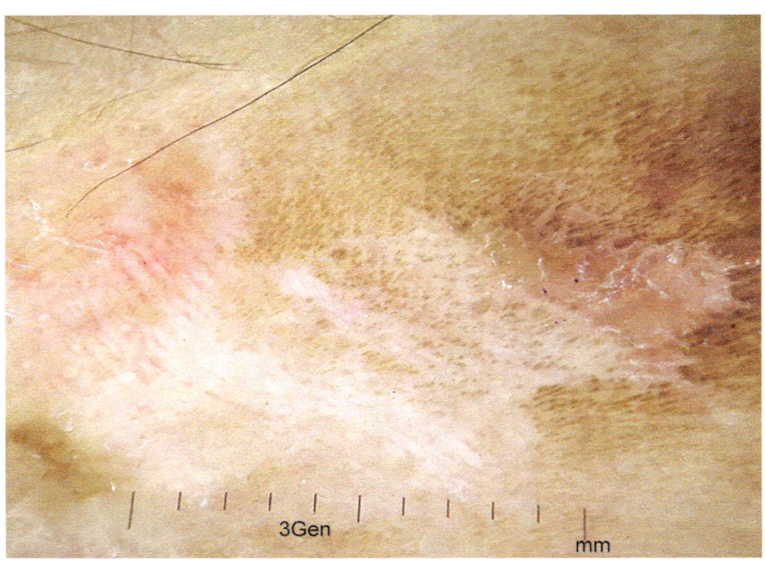

Dermoscopy of the left-sided lesion: Whitish membrane with linear vessels of increased caliber in association with erythema is present in the healing areas. The healed areas show marked melanin pigment network encroaching the center of the lesion from the periphery, suggestive of postinflammatory hyperpigmentation.

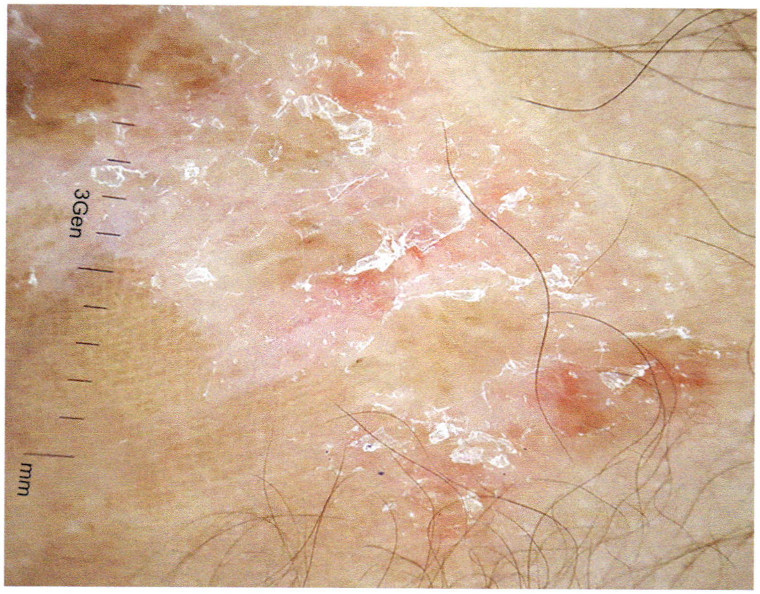

Dermoscopy of the right-sided lesion: Presence of a whitish membrane along with a few linear vessels and erythema in the healing part of the lesion. Note the lack of hair in the aplastic patch, whereas the surrounding skin shows presence of hair. Peripherally, increased melanin pigment can be seen.

What is your final diagnosis?

Answer:

d. None of the above

The presence of a thinned out whitish membrane with visible linear vessels of increased caliber and the perceptible erythema along with the history of the lesion being present since birth clinch the diagnosis of *aplasia cutis congenita (ACC)*.[1] ACC, though commonly seen on the scalp, may also present on the limbs and trunk.

For detailed description of ACC on scalp and nonscalp areas (*see* Chapter 6).

REFERENCE

1. Malakar S, Mukherje SS. Defining the dermoscopic characteristics of aplasia cutis congenita on the body. Indian J Paediatr Dermatol. 2019;20:347-9.

CASE 9

A 15-year-old girl presented with itchy lesions on both forearms, of 3 months duration.

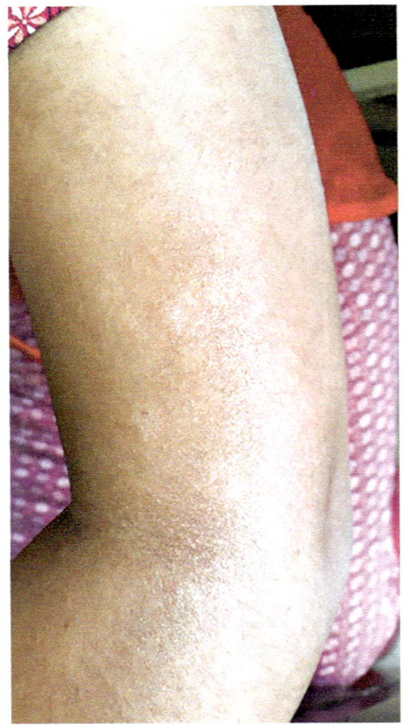

What is your clinical diagnosis?

Clinical differentials:

a. Atopic dermatitis
b. Polymorphic light eruption
c. Pityriasis versicolor
d. None of the above

See the dermoscopic picture for the clue of the diagnosis.

Dermoscopic examination revealed ring scales.

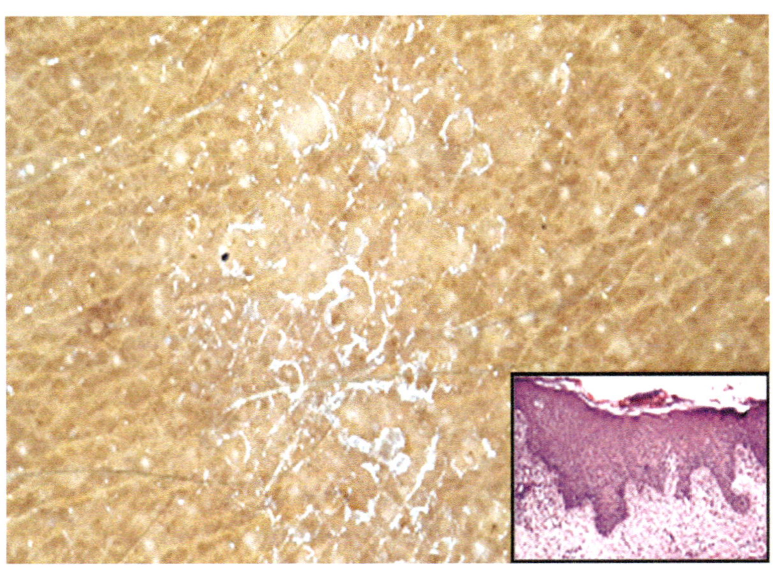

Based on the above informations, what is your final diagnosis?

Answer:

b. Polymorphic light eruption

This fits with the diagnosis of *polymorphic light eruption*. Ring scales are white, circular, and arranged continuously in a ring-shaped manner with central clearing against an ochre to light brown background.[1] Histologically, they signify the scale crust situated atop the stratum corneum.

Note that the ring scales of pityriasis rosea are yellow in color and seen against a yellowish background.

REFERENCE

1. Malakar S, Mehta P. Ring scales: a new dermoscopic sign in polymorphous light eruption. Int J Dermoscop. 2017;1(2):62-4.

CASE 10

An 8-year-old child presented with the following lesions.

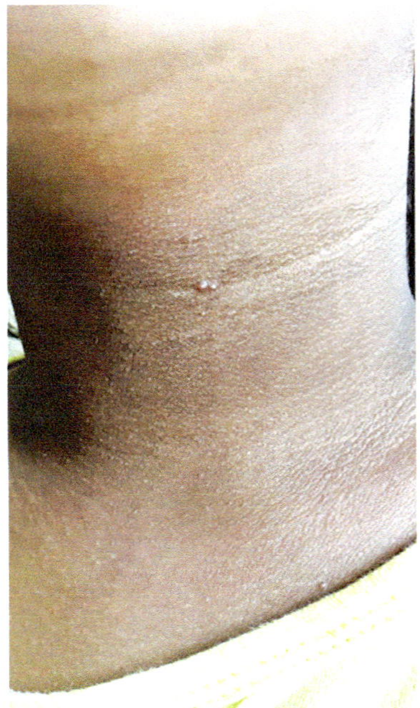

What are your clinical differentials?

Differentials:

a. Milia
b. Verruca plana
c. Miliaria
d. Molluscum contagiosum

Dermoscopic picture of the above condition shows:

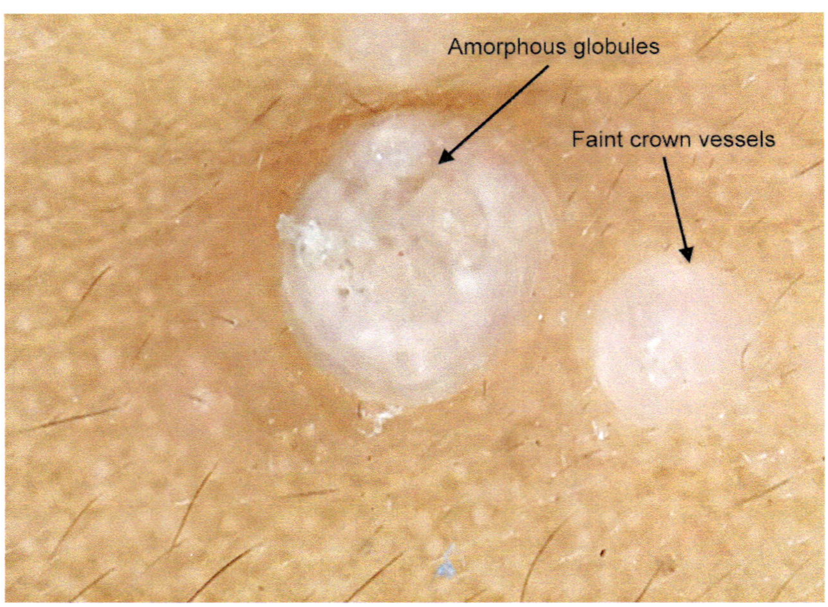

On clinicodermoscopic correlation, what is your final diagnosis?

Answer:

d. Molluscum contagiosum.

The typical findings in molluscum contagiosum of dermoscopy are central amorphous globular structures and peripheral crown vessels which may be faint or prominent.[1] Thus the diagnosis of the two tiny papules of the neck of the girl is *molluscum contagiosum*.

When the typical features are absent still the presence of rosettes are an important diagnostic criteria of molluscum contagiosum. Rosettes are dermoscopic structures characterized by 4 white points arranged as a 4-leaf clover, mainly localized over the follicular openings exclusively seen on polarized dermoscopy. Thus, in doubtful cases, even in the absence of crown vessels and central umbilication, a diagnosis of molluscum contagiosum can be confidently made.

REFERENCE

1. Malakar S. Infectious Dermatoses. In: Malakar S (Ed). Dermoscopy: Text and Atlas. New Delhi: Jaypee Brothers Medical Publishers (P) Ltd.; 2017. pp. 161-4.

CASE 11

An adolescent boy presented with the following lesion on her scalp, along with a 10-month long history of burning, itching, and pain over the scalp.

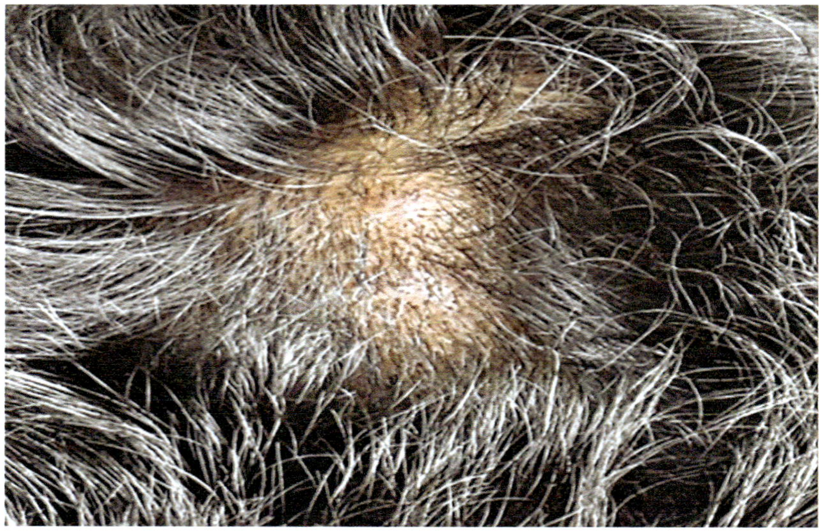

What are your clinical differentials?

Differentials:

a. Alopecia areata
b. Trichotillomania
c. Combined alopecia areata and trichotillomania
d. None of the above

Dermoscopy of the scalp shows the following features:

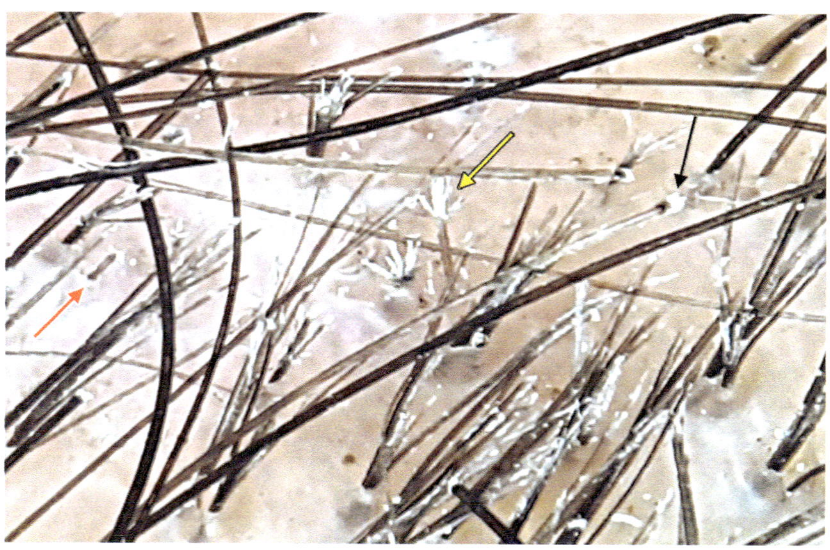

Dermoscopy shows extensive broom hairs (yellow arrow), block hair (red arrow), and trichorrhexis nodosa (black arrow).

What could be your final diagnosis?

Answer:

d. None of the above

The presence of several broom hair in the dermoscopic field, in keeping with the history, points to the diagnosis of *scalp dysesthesia*. Broom hair result from chronic rubbing, which damages the hair shafts.

Note: Scalp dysesthesia is defined as a single patch of alopecia with pruritus, burning sensation, and pain. On trichoscopy, there are broom hairs, block hairs, and trichorrhexis nodosa.[1]

REFERENCE

1. Rakowska A, Olszewska M, Rudnicka L. Trichoscopy of scalp dysesthesia. Postepy Dermatol Alergol. 2017;34(3):245-7.

CASE 12

An 11-year-old presented with patchy hair loss over the scalp, which was first noticed by her barber 4 months back.

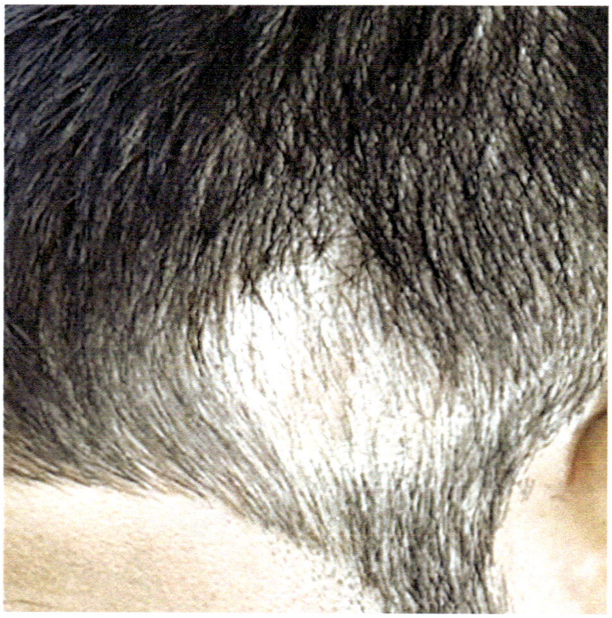

What is your clinical diagnosis?

Differentials:

a. Alopecia areata
b. Congenital triangular alopecia
c. Trichotillomania
d. None of the above

Dermoscopic area reveals the following:

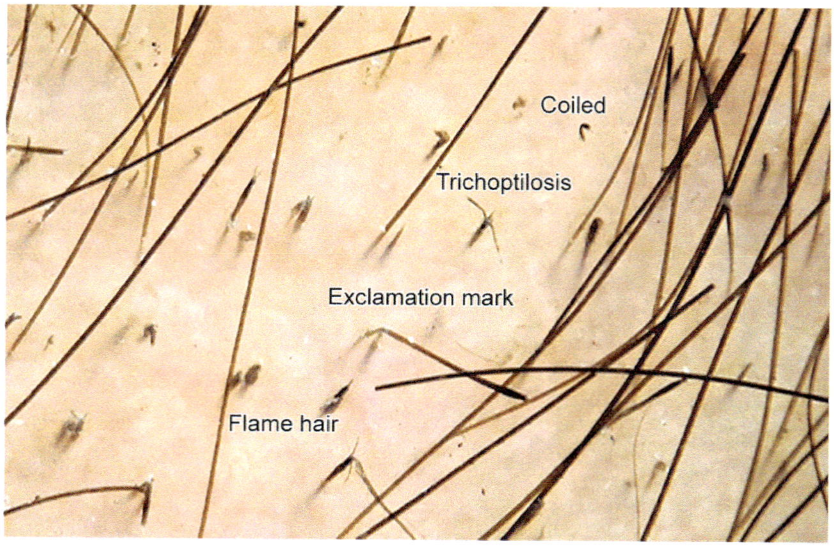

Dermoscopy shows both the features of alopecia areata (exclamation mark) and trichotillomania (flame hair, coiled hair, and trichoptilosis).

What is your final diagnosis?

Answer:

d. None of the above

The final diagnosis is *trichotillomania superimposed on alopecia areata.* Changes of both trichotillomania such as broken hair and of alopecia areata such as yellow dots, black dots, and exclamation hair can be seen here in this field.[1]

As soon as patients realize that there is an alopecic patch, they tend to manipulate the area by rubbing/scratching/pulling the hair, leading to secondary features of trichotillomania. Its importance lies in identifying and addresses this latter issue, as it may hamper response to treatment of alopecia areata.

REFERENCE

1. Sah DE, Koo J, Price VH. Trichotillomania. Dermatol Ther. 2008;21(1):13-21.

CASE 13

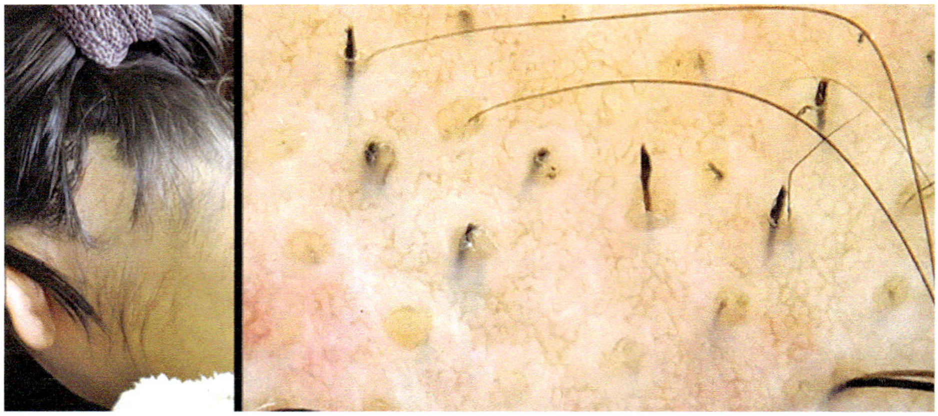

What are the trichoscopic features of this patchy alopecia?

a. Flame hairs
b. Yellow dots
c. Mace hair
d. Coiled hair
e. All of the above

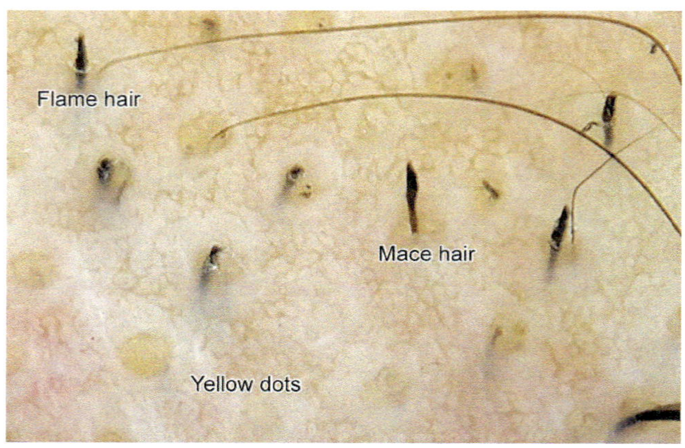

What are the trichoscopic features of the patchy alopecia?

a. Flame hairs
b. Yellow dots
c. Mace hair

What condition is it found in?

Trichotillomania.

Answer:

Mace hair is a trichoscopic sign characteristically seen in *trichotillomania*. The distal end of the hair shaft is bulbous, causing the hair to resemble a "mace". The hair shaft in mace sign is hyperpigmented throughout its length, and the upper half is rough in texture due to pulling of the hair shaft in trichotillomania.[1]

REFERENCE

1. Malakar S, Mukherjee SS. "Mace sign"—A definitive sign of trichotillomania? Our Dermatol Online. 2017;8(4):491-2.

CASE 14

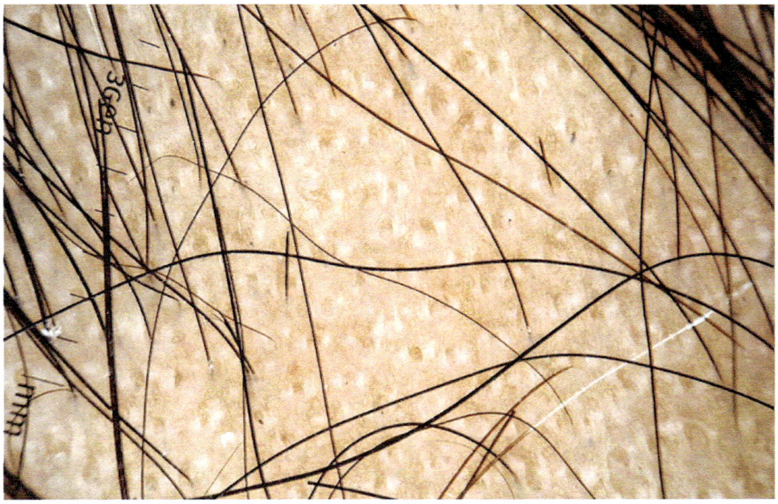

What is the trichoscopic finding?

A. *The findings*:
   a. Extensive yellow dots
   b. Exclamation mark
   c. a + b
   d. Extensive black dots

B. *Based on this, what is the most likely diagnosis?*
   a. Remission phase of alopecia areata
   b. Active phase of alopecia areata
   c. Not a case of alopecia areata
   d. Should be reviewed by biopsy

Answer for A:

c. a + b

Answer for B:

b. Active phase of alopecia areata

The major trichoscopic features here are yellow dots. Thus, the diagnosis is *alopecia areata*.

The presence of abundant yellow dots in alopecia areata signifies the active stage of the disease,[1] which needs to be treated in a timely fashion. This can also be used as a marker for disease course, progression, and response to treatment.

REFERENCE

1. Malakar S. Follicular and Perifollicular Patterns. In: Malakar S (Ed). Trichoscopy: A Text and Atlas. New Delhi: Jaypee Brothers Medical Publishers (P) Ltd.; 2017. pp. 58-60.

CASE 15

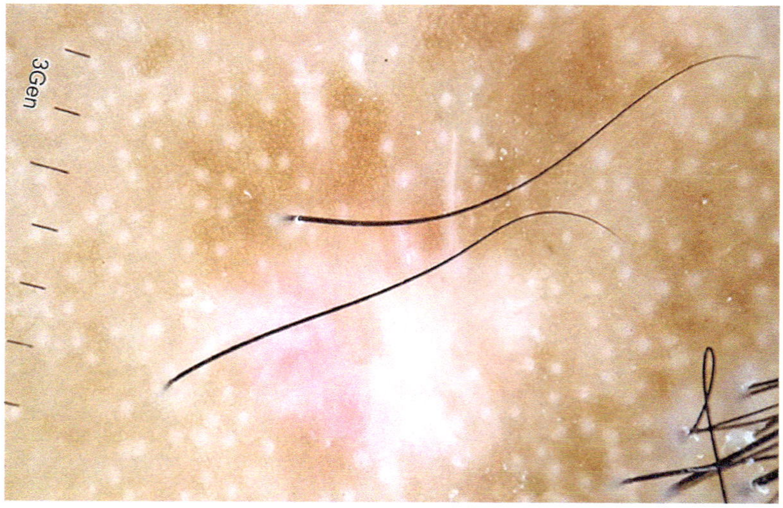

In the above trichoscopic image of a single large patch of alopecia, what are the findings?

The findings:

a. Extensive fibrotic white dots
b. Lone hairs
c. Milky white area and white fibrotic patch
d. All of the above
e. None of the above

Answer:

d. All of the above

This patch of cicatricial alopecia shows both milky white and white areas. The white areas denote established fibrosis whereas the milky white areas are a sign of evolving fibrosis.[1] If treatment is initiated at this early stage of milky white areas, irreversible damage can be prevented and some hair regrowth may be achieved. Hence, trichoscopic evaluation of any case of scarring alopecia is an essential tool.

The final diagnosis in this case is *lichen planopilaris*.[2]

REFERENCES

1. Olszewska M, Rakowska A, Slowinska M, et al. Classic lichen planopilaris and Graham-Little syndrome. Atlas of Trichoscopy: Verlag London: Springer; 2012. pp. 279-94.
2. Malakar S. Lichen Planopilaris. In: Malakar S (Ed). Trichoscopy: A Text and Atlas. New Delhi: Jaypee Brothers Medical Publishers (P) Ltd.; 2017. pp. 211-8.

Index

Page numbers followed by f refer to figure and t refer to table.